TANDEM MASS SPECTROMETRY - MOLECULAR CHARACTERIZATION

Edited by **Ana Varela Coelho**
and **Catarina de Matos Ferraz Franco**

Tandem Mass Spectrometry - Molecular Characterization
http://dx.doi.org/10.5772/56703
Edited by Ana Varela Coelho and Catarina de Matos Ferraz Franco

Contributors
Alan J Fischman, Xiao-Ming Lu, Ronald Tompkins, Diogo Ribeiro Demartini, Guilherme Sassaki, Lauro Souza, Maria Bronze, Ana Sitoe, Francisca Lopes, Rui Moreira, Ana Varela Coelho, Luigi Silvestro

Published by InTech
Janeza Trdine 9, 51000 Rijeka, Croatia

Publishing Process Manager Iva Simcic
Technical Editor InTech DTP team
Cover InTech Design team

Additional hard copies can be obtained from orders@intechopen.com

Tandem Mass Spectrometry - Molecular Characterization , Edited by Ana Varela Coelho and Catarina de Matos Ferraz Franco
p. cm.
ISBN 978-953-51-1136-8

Meet the editors

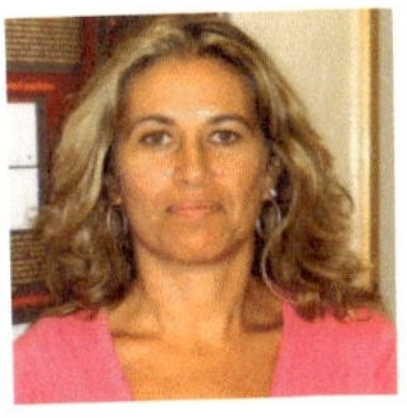

Ana Varela Coelho received her Ph.D. in 1998 from the University of Évora, Portugal, where she has taught several biochemistry curricular units for thirteen years. She was an Invited Professor at the Instituto de Tecnologia Química e Biológica – Universidade Nova de Lisboa, Oeiras, Portugal and then joined this Institute as an assistant researcher where she coordinates the Mass Spectrometry Laboratory since 2002. She has published more than eighty research articles in peer reviewed journal and participated in more than forty scientific projects. Her research interests include the use of tandem mass spectrometry in proteomic, peptidomic and metabolomic applications, in particular in the study of biological processes with biomedical applications, namely in tissue and organ regeneration.

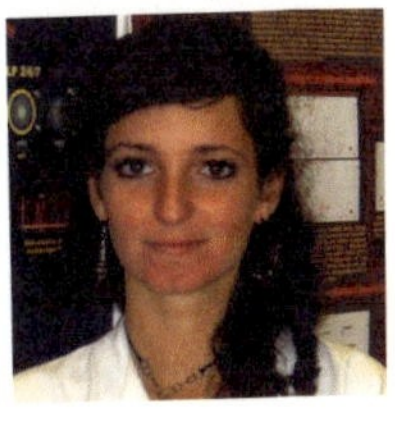

Catarina F. Franco concluded her Ph.D. in Biochemistry at New University of Lisbon in 2011. During this period Catarina studied the differential protein expression during arm tip regeneration events of starfish specie using proteomic and mass spectrometry based approaches. In 2012, Catarina started a post-doctoral fellow at Instituto de Tecnologia Química e Biológica. Currently she is interested in using tandem mass spectrometry tools for the characterization of protein post-translational modifications occurring during specific stages of regeneration of the starfish radial nerve cords.

Contents

Preface IX

Section 1 General Aspects 1

Chapter 1 **Matrix Effects in Mass Spectrometry Combined with Separation Methods — Comparison HPLC, GC and Discussion on Methods to Control these Effects 3**
Luigi Silvestro, Isabela Tarcomnicu and Simona Rizea Savu

Chapter 2 **A Short Overview of the Components in Mass Spectrometry Instrumentation for Proteomics Analyses 39**
Diogo Ribeiro Demartini

Section 2 Molecular Characterization by Mass Spectrometry 59

Chapter 3 **Contribution of Mass Spectrometry to the Study of Antimalarial Agents 61**
Ana Raquel Sitoe, Francisca Lopes, Rui Moreira, Ana Coelho and Maria Rosário Bronze

Chapter 4 **Mass Spectrometry Strategies for Structural Analysis of Carbohydrates and Glycoconjugates 81**
Guilherme L. Sassaki and Lauro Mera de Souza

Chapter 5 **Tandem MS and NMR: An Efficient Couple for the Characterization of Saponins 117**
Rita Laires, Kamila Koci, Elisabete Pires, Catarina Franco, Pedro Lamosa and Ana V. Coelho

Chapter 6 **Post-Translational Modification Profiling of Burn-Induced — Insulin Resistance and Muscle Wasting 137**
Xiao-Ming Lu, Ronald G. Tompkins and Alan J. Fischman

Preface

Tandem mass spectrometry started as a tool for the structural characterization of simple molecular components, presently, this analytical approach is being extensively used for the characterization and quantification of small molecules, and also of complex biomolecules.

The expeditious evolution at the instrumentation level and the increasing number of new applications in a variety of fields indicates that a lot should still be expected from this methodology.

This book comprises six chapters divided in two sections, which provides a current review of some general aspects in mass spectrometry and various applications of tandem mass spectrometry in the structural characterization of a diversity of compounds, complementing the previous books in this Tandem Mass Spectrometry series. In the first chapter are described several methods to overcome the matrix effects associated with mass spectrometry and its hyphenated chromatographic methods. The second chapter provides a description of the instrumental components relevant for proteomic applications. The second section includes four chapters on the characterization of antimalarial agents, carbohydrates, glycoconjugates, saponines and on the profiling of post-translational modifications.

Thanks are expressed to the contributing authors who provided their competence and leadership in the specific field attempting to provide comprehensive reviews. Finally, I would like to thank Ms. Iva Simcic, Publishing Process Manager, and other InTech publication staffs for their patience and professional support.

Ana Varela Coelho and Catarina de Matos Ferraz Franco
Institute of Technology, Chemistry and Biology (ITQB)
Mass Spectrometry Lab
Portugal

Section 1

General Aspects

Chapter 1

Matrix Effects in Mass Spectrometry Combined with Separation Methods — Comparison HPLC, GC and Discussion on Methods to Control these Effects

Luigi Silvestro, Isabela Tarcomnicu and
Simona Rizea Savu

Additional information is available at the end of the chapter

http://dx.doi.org/10.5772/55982

1. Introduction

1.1. The evolution of the concept of matrix

Even in the early times of chromatography with conventional detectors (i.e. UV/VIS, FID) it became evident that different sample matrices present peculiar interfering compounds, and the importance of using appropriate spiked matrix calibrators in order to get reliable quantitative results was recognized. In these conditions, however, the main concern was the presence of coeluting compounds giving similar detector responses, while the risk to alter the detector response of the analyte was not yet an issue.

Coupling liquid chromatography with mass spectrometry (LC-MS) was an important step forward because polar and thermally unstable compounds could be effectively analyzed and the poor specificity of previous detectors was overcome. The main steps to the hyphenation of the two separation techniques were made by Doles and Fenn with the development of the atmospheric pressure ionization (API) interfaces (Doles et al, 1968; Whitehouse et al, 1985; Fenn et al, 1989; Mallet et al, 2004). In short time LC-MS/MS has become an important tool for the analysis of drugs and metabolites from biological fluids, or for trace analysis from complex mixtures with many applications, e.g. pharmacokinetic studies of pharmaceuticals or the study of proteomics. John Fenn received in 2002 the Nobel Prize in Chemistry for his contribution to the development of the electrospray ionization (ESI) technique.

This huge improvement in selectivity brought quickly to a simplification of separation methods and/or sample preparation but on the other hand unexpected quantitative or even qualitative results were observed. Significant differences in peak intensities were observed comparing chromatograms recorded on neat solutions and biological extracts with equivalent concentrations. In most of the cases the signal intensity is reduced, although sometimes signal enhancement could also be detected. A new concept, that of matrix effect, was emerging, and coeluting components were recognized as very important in influencing analytes ionization and detector response. A much more complex vision of the matrix effect is now widely accepted and even matrix differences between samples of the same kind are in the center of attention.

As a matter of fact, a lot of emphasis is currently put on adequate validation procedures for analytical methods in order to be sure that correct quantitative or even qualitative data are obtained.

Matrix components of a sample can affect, most times negatively, the analytical measurement of the main compound. The phenomenon was called "matrix effect" and was defined at the Workshop on "Bioanalytical Method Validation-A Revisit with a Decade of Progress" (Workshop held in Arlington VA, January 12-14, 2000) as "The direct or indirect alteration or interference in response due to the presence of unintended analytes (for analysis) or other interfering substances in the sample" (Shah et al, 2000).

Mass spectrometry is a powerful analytical technique based on ions separation; therefore ionization is of key importance for high sensitivity and selectivity. The ionization efficiency depends on the physico-chemical properties of a molecule, and also on the conditions established in the ionization interface. In ESI the eluent from the chromatographic column, already containing ionic species, is pumped through a capillary; a high voltage is applied to the capillary producing charge separation at the surface of the liquid. The so-called "Taylor cone" is produced at the end of the capillary and liquid is nebulized into charged droplets. When the charge becomes sufficient to overcome the surface tension that holds the droplet together, gas-phase ions are released (Kebarle and Tang; 1993, Chech and Enke, 2001). Iribarne and Thomson published one of the first theories on gas-phase ions emission from charged droplets. The rate of ion emission from a droplet is proportional to the number of charges and will be higher for the more surface-active ion (Iribarne and Thompson, 1976 and 1979). It is very likely that here is where matrix components are interfering, competing in these processes; the mechanisms are not fully elucidated.

The ion suppression effect in ESI was first described by Kebarle and coworkers in the 1990s. They have shown that the ESI response is linear with the analyte concentration in the range from 10^{-8}M to 10^{-5}M, and in a mixture of organic basic compounds, the signal of an organic base ion measured as MH^+ could decrease with increasing concentration of another basic compound depending upon surface activity and Iribarne constants of the respective compounds. The decrease in ion intensities of the MH+ ions were attributed to gas-phase proton transfer reactions between the electrosprayed gas-phase ions and evaporated molecules of the stronger gas-phase base (Ikonomou et al 1990; Kebarle and Tang, 1993).

Buhrman and coworkers published in 1996 a study on ion suppression in plasma samples (Buhrman et al, 1996). The authors have validated a method for the quantitation of SR 27417 (a platelet-activating factor receptor antagonist) in human plasma. During method development, noticing a loss of signal in extracted samples compared to the neat solutions they studied the extraction efficiency of three sample clean-up procedures and their effect on analyte ionization. The matrix effect was evaluated by injecting: A) a neat solution of a concentration present in the sample considering an extraction efficiency of 100%; B) a spiked plasma sample extracted and C) a blank plasma extracted and spiked post-extraction with the solution from experiment A). Subsequently, the loss of intensity between A) and B) represents the efficiency of the total process, whilst the loss of intensity between A) and C) is the ion suppression (Buhrman et al, 1996).

Later, Matuszewski and coworkers compared the HPLC-MS/MS interface with a "chemical reactor" in which primary ions react with analyte molecules in a complex series of charge-transfer and ion-transfer reactions, depending of the ionization energies and proton activities of the present molecules (Matuszewski et al, 2003).

In such conditions, as the solvent evaporates, inside the droplet a competition starts between the proton affinity of the analyte and co-analyte, for the proton transfer to take place. If the co-analyte has a higher gas-phase proton affinity than the analyte this one will be protonated first, instead of the analyte, therefore the ion intensity of the last one will be reduced. In the same time, the presence of any nonvolatile matrix components will prevent the droplets to reach their critical radius and surface field by increasing their viscosity and surface tension and decreasing the solvent evaporating rate (Matuszewski et al, 2003). As observed also by King et al, the ionization suppression in biological extracts was the result of the high concentration of nonvolatile compounds present in the droplet solution and was not affected by the reactions occurring in the gas-phase (King et al, 2000).

Matrix effects are not attributed only to ESI interface, although some studies show that atmospheric pressure chemical ionization interfaces (APCI) are less susceptible to ion suppression, mainly due to the APCI mechanism, which occurs by charge transfer from the ionized solvent/additives when the analytes are already in gas-phase (King et al, 2000; Henion et al, 1998; Hsieh et al, 2001, Souverain et al, 2004). Nevertheless APCI and other types of ionization (e.g. atmospheric pressure photoioization – APPI) are not matrix effects-free but the ionization processes being different, the behavior is of course different from that of ESI. Ion suppression is not always directly related to the saturation of the charge available in ESI, but it may be related to changes either in the liquid-to-gas transfer efficiency or in the charge transfer efficiency (Sangster et al, 2004); experimental data obtained also by our group with these three ionization interface will be presented in the next sections.

Using the same sample preparation and chromatographic conditions, some studies compared the results obtained with a triple quadrupole MS interfaced with APCI or ESI, in order to evaluate the selectivity and reproducibility of an existing HPLC-MS/MS assay method (Fu et al, 1998, Matuszewski, et al, 2003).

Matuszewski and coworkers have introduced the concepts of quantitative assessment of the "absolute" and "relative" matrix effect. The absolute matrix effect was considered as the difference between response of the same concentration of standards spiked before and after extraction of the matrix. The variation of the absolute matrix effect between several lots of the same endogenous matrix was defined as relative matrix effect. Matrix effect (ME), recovery of the extraction (RE) and process efficiency (PE) were evaluated according with the equations:

ME(%)=B/Ax100

RE(%)=C/Bx100

PE(%)=C/Ax100=(MExRE)/100

Where A is the chromatographic peak area of the standard in neat solution, B is the peak area of the standard spiked into plasma after extraction and C is the peak area of standards spiked before extraction.

It is the same approach used by Buhrman group, but it also takes in consideration the potential for ion enhancement. In this study, Matuszewski and coworkers observed significant ionization enhancement with APCI interface (≈130%) and slight enhancement (analyte) or suppression (internal standards) with ESI interface (≈110% and ≈90%, respectively) (Matuszewski et al, 2003).

To conclude, the effect on the analytical signal of all compounds excepting the main analyte is therefore defined as "matrix effect" and is expressed as a matrix factor by the equation:

Matrix Factor (MF) = Peak response in presence of matrix ions/Peak response in the neat solution

MF=1 indicates no matrix effect

MF<1 indicates ion suppression

MF>1 indicates ion enhancement.

In bioanalysis, matrix effects are very specific and complex at the same time, because each biological matrix is unique and can affect differently any analytical technique used for the identification and quantitation of an analyte from the matrix. The extent of the matrix effect depends upon: 1) the sample matrix; 2) sample preparation procedure used for clean-up, 3) chromatographic separation (column, mobile phase,…) and, 4) ionization interface.

Phospholipids are a major source of matrix effects in bioanalysis. Most of them are ionized under positive mode due to the presence of quaternary nitrogen atoms. Glycerophosphocholines are the major phospholipids in plasma and are known to cause significant LC-MS/MS matrix ionization effects in the positive mode (Little et al, 2006, Bennet et al, 2006, Jemal et al, 2010).

The quantitative evaluation of the matrix effect is performed based on the approach described above (Buhrman et al, 1996, Matuszewski et al, 2003). For a qualitative evaluation, a classical experiment consists of injecting the extracts of blank (non-spiked) biological samples on the column, in the analysis conditions, while the target analyte is infused post-column at a concentration giving a high and flat signal. The influence of the co-extracted compounds will produce gaps (ion suppression) or peaks (ion enhancement) on the analyte signal. A lot of examples were presented in literature (Bonfiglio et al, 1999; Dams et al, 2003; Souverain et al, 2004 etc); in the second section of this chapter experimental data obtained for pramipexole in different analytical conditions will be presented.

The matrix effect became a critical parameter in bioanalytical method development and validation. For pharmacokinetic studies, FDA guidance documents (FDA 2001) require that this effect to be evaluated as a part of development and validation of a quantitative LC-MS/MS method, and more recent EMA guidelines as well (EMA 2011).

For an accurate quantitation of the requested analytes, the use of an isotope-labeled internal standard is required. This will reasonably compensate the eventual matrix effects, being chemically identical and hence it will be suppressed or enhanced in the same manner as the analyte (Viswanathan et al, 2007). When isotope-labeled standards are not easily available, structural analogues of the compound of interest or related molecules that match its extraction and chromatographic properties can be used, but in this case the matrix effects compensation can be different and the impact on results reliability should be evaluated.

2. Relevance of matrix effect in HPLC-MS/MS

Due to its high selectivity and sensitivity, mass spectrometry in tandem with liquid chromatography became quickly a powerful analytical tool and even took the supremacy over the coupling with gas-chromatography in various fields, like genomics and proteomics, metabolite identification and metabolomics, or regulated bioanalysis. Along with the development of HPLC-MS/MS instrumentation and its applications, the matrix interferences were observed and studied from the beginning. The importance of matrix effects was recognized especially in quantitative analysis, because they can heavily influence the reproducibility, linearity and accuracy of the method, leading to altered results (Trufelli et al, 2011). Although not so much considered, qualitative analysis can be also affected because some trace compounds will not be identified in a sample if their signal is excessively suppressed by matrix, thus giving erroneous assessment of the composition of the sample.

Matrix effects are different depending on the sample nature, and moreover variations are observed between different lots of the same type of sample. The phenomenon was defined by Matuszewski et al as "relative matrix effect". As discussed above, electrospray ionization is more influenced than other ionization techniques. Coming to chromatography, the matrix effect is usually higher on the early-eluting peaks, because all hydrophilic compounds from the biological sample are not well retained in reversed-phase columns and usually elute in the first minutes. This is not a 100% rule though, because some phospholipids, flavonoids or other classes of organic compounds can be strongly retained and in some cases, depending on the chromatographic conditions, they even accumulate in the column and elute periodically after a series of injections, thus a strong matrix effect being noticed only on the respective sample and not overall (Little et al, 2006; Jemal et al, 2010).

Some examples registered during routine work in our laboratory will be presented next. In the first case, we have developed and validated a method for quantitative determination of salicylic and acetylsalicylic acids in plasma by LC-MS/MS on an API4000 QTrap (AB Sciex) quadrupole-linear ion trap instrument, using an ESI interface, in negative mode. The chromatographic separation involved an Ascentis Express RP-Amide (10cmx2.1mm, 2.7μm) column, eluted in isocratic conditions, at 0.25 mL/min, with a mobile phase consisting of 0.1% formic acid in water/acetonitrile 45/55 (v/v). The concentration range to be measured in the biological samples being quite high (low limits of quantification/LLOQs of 5 and 50 ng/mL for acetylsalicylic and salicylic acid, respectively), a simple protein precipitation with acetonitrile was chosen for sample clean-up and further optimized. D4-salicylic and D4-acetylsalicylic acids were used as internal standards and matrix effects were evaluated during method validation.

Analysing a large set of plasma samples from a group of patients treated with acetylsalicylic acid, different matrix effects were observed in some volunteers compared to those registered on calibration curves and control samples (prepared by spiking a pooled plasma lot). Fig. 1 and 2 show the metric plots of D4-acetylsalicylic acid and D4-salicylic acid chromatographic peak areas, respectively, in one of the batches (including calibrator and OC samples); as expected stronger ion suppression can be seen on the transition of D4-acetylsalicylic acid, eluting first (retention time 1.15 min), compared to D4-salicylic acid (retention time 1.6 min).

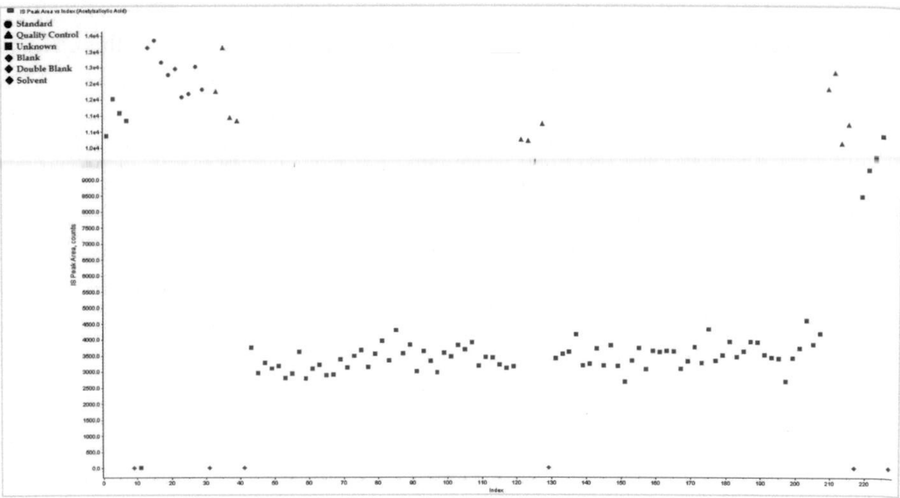

Figure 1. D4-acetylsalicylic acid (internal standard) chromatographic peak area plotted against the sample index in the results table, after the analysis of a batch containing unknown samples, calibration (CC) and control (QC) points. ESI ionization. Data legend on the left. High ion suppression can be observed between different plasma sources (unknown samples versus CC and QC samples).

Another situation often encountered in quantitative determinations is when the analyte signal is progressively suppressed after the injection of biological extracts, until a plateau is reached. For this reason, column equilibration by injecting an appropriate number of extracted samples is recommended before starting the analytical run.

Figure 3 shows the influence of the accumulated matrix on the signal of medroxyprogesretone17-acetate observed in our laboratory during method development. In this case the analysis was performed on an API 5000 triple quadruople mass spectrometer (AB Sciex), in positive ions mode, using an APCI interface. Medroxyprogesterone-17-acetate was used as internal standard for the quantitative analysis of chlormadinone acetate. The sample extracts

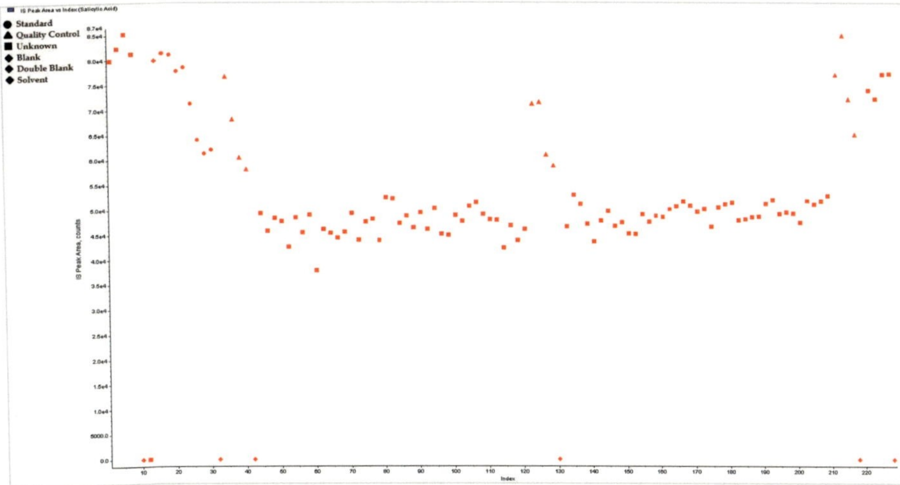

Figure 2. D4-salicylic acid (internal standard) chromatographic peak area plotted against the sample index in the results table, after the analysis of a batch (the same as in Fig. 1) containing unknown samples, calibration (CC) and control (QC) points. ESI ionization. Data legend on the left. High ion suppression can be observed between different plasma sources (unknown samples versus CC and QC samples). However, later-eluting D4-salicylic acid was less affected than D4-acetylsalicylic acid by matrix effects.

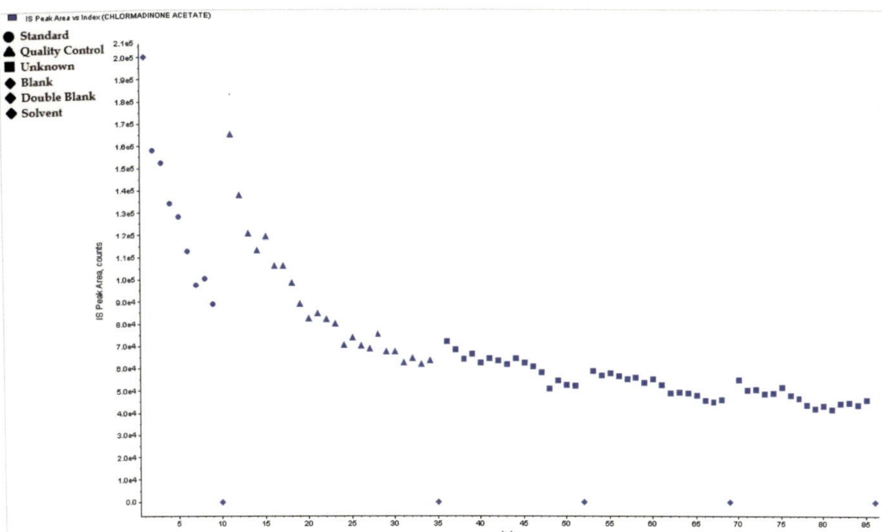

Figure 3. Medroxyprogesterone 17-acetate (internal standard) chromatographic peak area plotted against the sample index in the results table, after the analysis of a batch containing unknown samples, calibration (CC) and control (QC) points.APCI ionization. Data legend on the left. Progressive ion suppression is noticed after the injection of plasma extracts, until an equilibration of the system with the matrix components. The injection of a solvent sample is partially alleviating the matrix effects.

were separated on a LiChrospherRP-Select B (12.5 cmx3 mm, 5μm) column, eluted at 1.2 mL/min with a mobile phase composed of acetonitrile and water, in gradient conditions (starting from 70 to 97% acetonitrile). The low limit of quantification being in the low pg/mL range, a liquid-liquid extraction procedure was selected for sample clean-up. As it can be seen on the internal standard peak area metric plot, the sensitivity is quite high in the first samples of the run, then the signal goes down until stabilizing at a certain level. After the injection of a wash sample (mobile phase) the sensitivity increases again. The decreasing intensities could be produced by an instrument charging also caused by matrix components accumulated on some parts of the ion-path. This is an example of ion suppression in APCI and underlines the fact that co-extracted matrix can have an impact not only on the current but also on the next injections.

More recently we have conducted in our laboratory a series of experiments on pramipexole, a dopamine agonist in the non-ergoline class prescribed for the treatment of Parkinson's disease and restless leg syndrome. Because of its structure and its quite low molecular mass (211.324 g/mol), pramipexole quantification has proven to be a difficult problem to solve. Very good sensitivity and chromatographic separation were achieved with neat standards, but going further to plasma samples, issues of ion suppression and high chromatographic background have led to a long method development that covered almost all possible tests. For the final method, a separation on a pentafluorophenylpropyl stationary phase (Discovery HSF5, 10cmx2.1 mm, 5 μm, Supelco) was preferred, and elution was performed with a mixture of acetonitrile/ammonium formate 10mM, pH 6 (75/25, v/v) delivered at 0.7 mL/min. Mass spectrometer, API 3000 (AB Sciex) with HSID modified interface (Ionics) was operated in ESI positive ions mode. Measured concentrations being again in the low pg/mL range, a large number of experiments were conducted for a better clean-up and pre-concentration of the analyte from plasma. The matrix effects were explored with the classical test of post-column infusion of the target analyte. The results obtained after injecting blank plasma processed by solid-phase extraction (SPE, on cation-exchange Isolute SCX-3 100 mg cartridges, eluted with ammonia 5% in methanol), direct protein precipitation with solvent (acetonitrile) and supported liquid-liquid extraction (Isolute SLE 400mg cartridges, eluted with methyl-tert-butyl ether) are presented in Figure 4. As expected, direct protein precipitation produced the highest ion suppression, all over the recorded chromatogram and as well in the region of the target analyte peak (retention time 2 min).

In order to evaluate the contribution of phospholipids to these matrix effects, a second experiment, precursor ion scan of *m/z* 184, in positive mode, over a range from 200 to 1000 Da, was performed (Figure 5). This is used to detect all phosphatidylcholines (PC), lyso-phosphatidylcholines(lyso-PC) and sphingomyelins (SM) (Jemal et al, 2010).

The precursor ion experiment on the sample processed by direct precipitation with acetonitrile shows a correlation between ion suppression on the pramipexole main transition 212.2/153.1 and the presence of PC, lyso-PC and SM (Figure 5, A and B). The extracted masses (Figure 5 C and D) confirm the presence of lyso-PC in the beginning of the chromatogram (m/z 406.5, retention time 0.6) and SM in the same elution region with the analyte (m/z 703.8, retention time 2 min). The main suppression effect between 0.2-0.4 and 1.4-1.6 minutes seems in this case

http://dx.doi.org/10.5772/55982

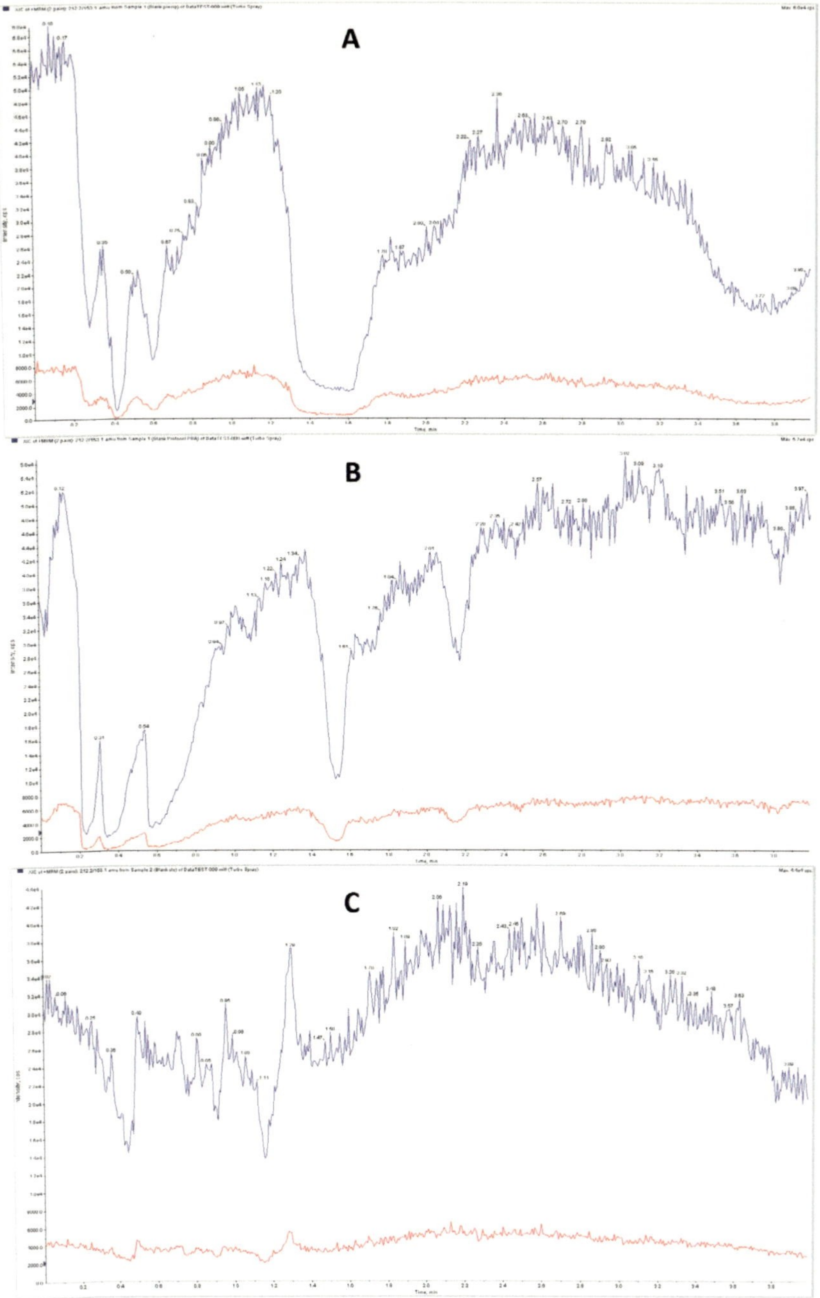

Figure 4. Ion-suppression monitored on the chromatographic traces of pramipexole (blue: 212.2/153.1, red: 212.2/111.1) in the conditions of the method described in the text, after the injection of A) blank plasma processed by direct precipitation of plasma proteins with acetonitrile, centrifugation, dilution 1:1 with mobile phase and injection in the LC-MS/MS system; B) blank plasma extracted on a cation-exchange cartridge Isolute SCX-3 100 mg, eluted with ammonia 5% in methanol and C) blank plasma extracted on an Isolute SLE400 mg cartridge eluted with 0.6 mL methyl-tert-butyl ether

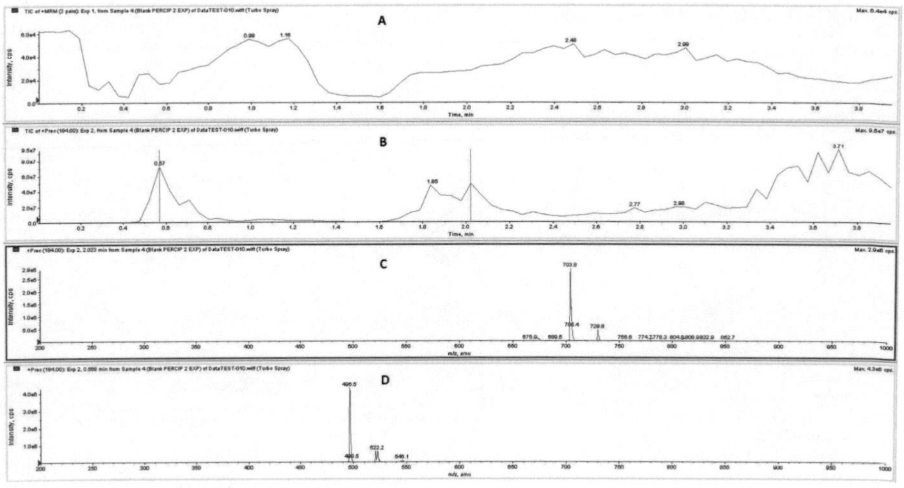

Figure 5. Ion-suppression monitored on the chromatographic traces of pramipexole (A) in the conditions of the method described in the text, after the injection of blank plasma processed by direct precipitation of plasma proteins with acetonitrile, centrifugation, dilution 1:1 with mobile phase and injection in the LC-MS/MS system. For correlation the precursor ion of *m/z* 184 scan (B) and extracted masses of two phospholipids (C and D) are presented below.

not produced by phospholipids; obviously salts and highly polar compounds are influencing the first region and some other lipids, amines, sterols etc could affect the second region.

Elemental sodium, potassium, iron, phosphorus and sulfur were measured in the same samples by ICP-MS (ELAN 6100 Perkin Elmer equipped with Apex-Q inlet system and PFA-ST nebulizer). Very high sodium and potassium concentrations were obviously measured in the plasma sample precipitated with acetonitrile, while in SLE the salts are not expected to be present, fact confirmed by ICP-MS (Figure 6). SPE also has high sodium levels (metal ions retained on the SCX-phase).

Similar experiments were presented in literature back in 1999, employing as model compounds caffeine and phenacetin (Bonfiglio et al). The authors have used a post-column infusion set-up and injected in the column plasma samples processed by protein precipitation with acetonitrile, liquid-liquid extraction with methyl-tert-butyl ether and SPE on Empore C2, C8, C18 and Oasis HLB. The highest ion suppression in ESI was observed for the protein precipitation, followed by Oasis SPE.

In conclusion, the sample nature, the ionization interface, mobile phase additives, stationary phases and last but most important, the sample clean-up technique, are all determining the extent of matrix effects in bioanalysis. Very interesting – and this makes the LC-MS/MS challenging but also beautiful – is that although some general rules can be established, these mechanisms are compound-dependent; in some cases there are no relevant matrix effects whilst in some others each parameter need to be optimized one by one for the best result. For our example analyte, pramipexole, positive electrospray ionization offered the best sensitivity. Different chromatographic conditions from reversed-phase at acidic or basic pH to HILIC and all three classical sample preparation methods were tested; in the end pentafluorophenylpropyl stationary phase was preferred, elution was performed with a mixture of acetonitrile/ammonium formate 10mM, pH 6 (75/25, v/v) and biological sample preparation by solid-phase extraction on cation-exchange Isolute SCX-3 96-well plates has given the best recovery and less interferences.

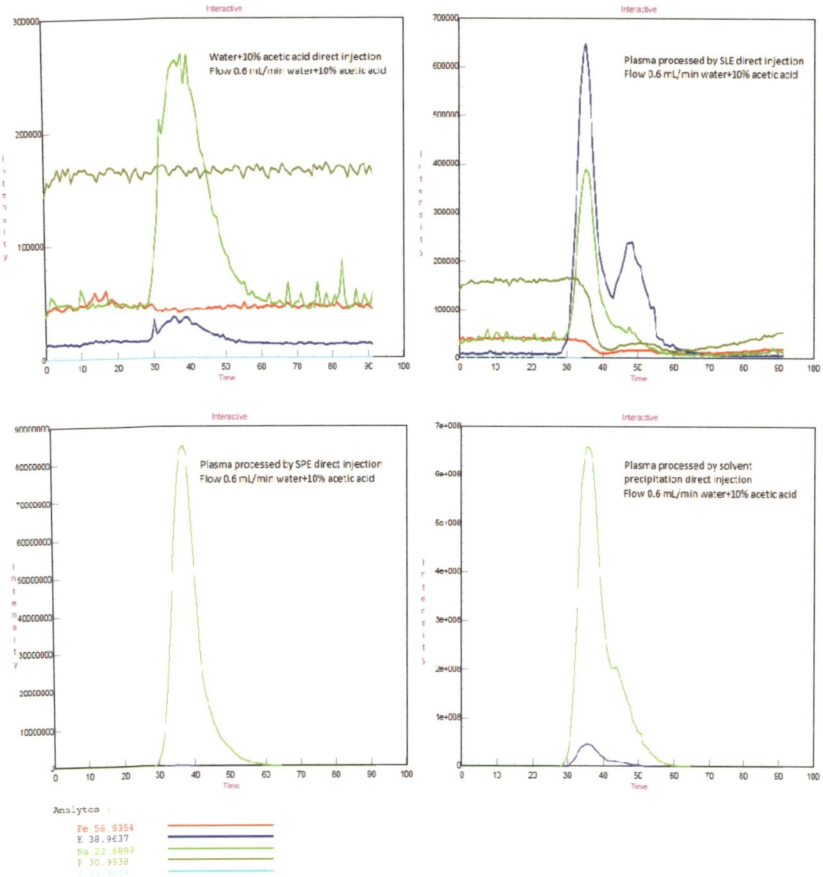

Figure 6. Elemental content (very interesting to notice the metal ion content) determined by ICP-MS in three plasma samples processed by SLE, SPE and solvent precipitation, as described in *Section 2*.

3. Relevance of matrix effect in GC-MS

In gas chromatography-mass spectrometry (GC-MS) the matrix effects were generally neglected, most probably due to the sophisticated sample preparation techniques employed for GC-MS, but they are not always negligible.

Gas chromatography involves chromatographic separation of volatile and thermally stable small molecules (in certain cases derivatization is needed to induce these properties), using a gaseous mobile phase. In GC-MS the analytes eluted from the chromatographic column enter directly into the mass spectrometer source where they are ionized by bombardment with free electrons (electron impact ionization), causing the fragmentation of molecules in a reproducible way, or they are ionized interacting with a reagent gas like ammonia or methane (chemical ionization).

The application of GC-MS to biochemical analysis and especially in metabolomics is based on the pioneering a work of Horning and coworkers who have demonstrated in 1971 that this technique could be used to measure different compounds present in urine and extracts. It was for the first time when the metabolic profile terminology was used (Horning et al, 1971). The next step was the diagnose of metabolic disorders by a urine test, introduced by Tanaka and coworkers (1982).

Due to the different mechanisms involved in the ionization process, there is a big difference between the matrix effects produced in LC-MS and GC-MS. While in LC-MS the co-eluted compounds affect the soft ionization mechanism in the interface, in GC-MS the ionization energy is high enough to overcome competing ionization processes, therefore mostly the GC inlet and the chromatographic column are affected by the matrix compounds, this being reflected in a high background in cases of very dirty samples or improper separation. Even though, several groups of researchers have noticed peculiar results.

In gas-chromatography the ion enhancement effect was described for the first time as "matrix induced chromatographic response" by Erney and coworkers while they were analyzing organophosphorous pesticides in extracts from milk and butterfat (Erney et al, 1993). According to their theory, during injection of standards in neat solvents, analytes could be adsorbed and thermo-degraded on the active sites of the injector or column, represented by the free silanol groups. When a real sample extract is analysed, matrix compounds block the active sites and less analyte molecules will be adsorbed, consequently enhancing their signal. In such conditions an overestimation of the calculated concentration of analytes will occur if a matrix-matched calibration curve is not used.

In the same time, the increase of the number of new active sites by gradual accumulation of non-volatile matrix compounds in the GC inlet and front part of the chromatographic column, could decrease the analyte response as "matrix – induced diminishment effect" (Hajslova et al, 2007).

Compared to LC-MS, the two phenomena of the matrix effect occur simultaneously and practically is impossible to control the formation of new actives sites from deposited non volatiles matrixes. To compensate the matrix effect phenomena, the thorough clean-up of the sample to be injected (with or without derivatization) by different extraction techniques, the use of alternative calibration methods like addition of isotopically labeled internal standards or the standard addition method, as well as masking the actives sites of the system by different reagents, have been adopted.

http://dx.doi.org/10.5772/55982

To compensate the matrix effect analyte protectants are used in GC-MS. These compounds are added both to the sample and standard solution to interact strongly with the active sites of the GCsystem, mainly with the silanol groups, and minimizing the matrix effect (Mastovka et al, 2005).

The evaluation of the matrix effect was used as a validation parameter for the GC-MS assay in plasma, urine, saliva and sweat of Salvinorin A, the main active ingredient of the hallucinogenic mint Salvia divinorum. The peak areas of extracted blank samples spiked with standards after extraction procedure were compared with the peak areas of pure diluted substances. The recovery was very good and results showed analytical signal suppression less than 10% due to co-eluting endogeneous substances (Pichini et al, 2005).

4. Different approaches to minimize the matrix effect during sample preparation both in HPLC-MS and GC-MS

The techniques used for sample preparation in order to decrease the matrix effects can be grouped in five classes:

1. Non selective methods to eliminate proteins (i.e. protein precipitation)
2. Non selective methods to separate hydrophobic compounds, generally but not always containing the analyte, from the hydrophilic fraction (i.e. liquid/liquid extraction)
3. Selective chromatographic methods to separate off-line the analyte from the matrix (i.e. SPE)
4. On-line chromatographic methods to separate the analyte from the matrix (i.e. column switch two-dimensions HPLC methods with different stationary phases)
5. Analyte pre/post column derivatization to enhance analyte separation from matrix components, and ionization; this approach can be combined with any one of the previous.

1. Non selective method to eliminate proteins

It is first of all clear that these methods are useful in samples containing important amount of proteins. Protein precipitation is of modest use in normal urine samples almost free of proteins while in case of pathologic urine with high protein content it makes sense; in case of plasma there are no doubts that the protein precipitation is quite effective.

A few basic observations are important to understand the fundamentals of protein precipitation methods:

- The precipitation method used must avoid introducing a new matrix factor that we cannot separate from the analyte of interest, like heavy salt contamination;
- The precipitated samples must have a final composition adequate to guarantee the solubility of the analyte; usually, poor water soluble compounds are better precipitated in solvent then in mineral acid;

- Many precipitation methods, like those with solvents, will introduce a relevant dilution that may limit the application if the instrumental analytical sensitivity was not good enough;
- Not any precipitation conditions will bring to samples compatible with any HPLC method, like aqueous samples in case of a HILIC separation. In such cases solvent evaporation and sample reconstitution with an appropriate mobile phase is needed;
- The precipitating agent may alter, for example by chemical degradation or chemical reaction, the analyte of interest; this factor must be adequately verified;
- The precipitation process will transform relatively homogenous samples, like those of plasma, in a non-homogenous mass; adequate mixing procedures and precipitation times must be used to guarantee a complete precipitation within the all sample.

Keeping in mind the above aspects the main precipitation methods are:

a. Solvent precipitation – Methanol, ethanol, acetonitrile and acetone, are probably the most widely employed solvents; this is also the most suitable procedure for LC/MS analysis;

b. Acid precipitation – Another widely used approach of precipitation based most often on halogenated organic acids like trichloroacetic acid but also on inorganic acids like perchloric acid, tungstic acid.

c. Salt precipitation – A less used approach in combination with LC-MS/MS exactly because of the risk of high ion suppression, but with certain established applications, e.g. zinc sulfate in immunosuppressant analysis (Koster et al, 2009)

d. Thermal precipitation – This is for sure the oldest method of protein precipitation but it is seldom used nowadays for analytical purposes (Fan et al, 2001). The technique remains important for protein purification.

e. Support assisted precipitation – similar with the solvent precipitation but using a solid phase bed (e.g. 96-well format PPT plate) that filters/retains the precipitate after centrifugation (Biotage).

2. Non selective methods to separate hydrophobic compounds from the hydrophilic fraction

In case of hydrophobic compounds, mixing the biological sample, generally aqueous, with a suitable non miscible organic solvent, will bring to a partition of the analyte in the solvent, leaving the proteins and salts in the aqueous phase. This process of liquid-liquid extraction is giving the cleanest extracts from biological matrices and it is the main sample preparation procedure for CG-MS and also widely used in HPLC-MS/MS.

The following basic procedures are used for this type of extraction:

a. Classical liquid/liquid extraction (LLE) – In this system the aqueous based samples are mixed with an adequate solvent, shaken for a fixed period of time, allowed separating (usually by centrifugation) and the solvent is recovered and further used for analyses, after evaporation and reconstitution with an appropriate mobile phase, but some studies even optimized conditions for direct injection of hydrophobic extracts in reversed-phase conditions (Medvedovici et al, 2011)

b. On-line liquid/liquid extraction – In this case the extraction procedure is performed by flowing the two non-miscible phases (the aqueous samples and the organic extraction solvent), generally countercurrent, in a chamber of adequate design. The organic eluent, enriched by the analyte of interest is directly analyzed without further processing, or it is evaporated and reconstituted with an appropriate mobile phase, depending on the chromatographic method.

c. Supported liquid extraction – In this particular technique the biological samples (necessarily fluids) are absorbed over a solid support capable to retain a thin layer of liquid on its hydrophilic surface. A non-miscible solvent is then passed through the solid support containing the samples and the analyte is partitioned in the solvent; this will be recovered and further used for analysis.

The liquid-liquid extraction is also used, although currently to lesser extent, for the washing/removal of the impurities from the sample. In some cases, a series of extraction and back-extraction steps are carried out, in order to obtain a better clean-up of very dirty samples, or when the analyte suffer from high background interferences.

3. Selective chromatographic methods to separate off-line the analyte from the matrix (i.e. SPE)

Solid phase extraction techniques are widespread and very valuable sample preparation techniques. Based on the retention of the analyte on a stationary phase by different mechanisms (adsorption, ion-exchange, size-exclusion) and elution with an appropriate organic solvent at the right pH, solid-phase extraction has some advantages over liquid-liquid extraction. First of all the broad range of stationary phase beds can cover all classes of compounds, including highly polar ones; second, larger volumes of sample, even 1 L, can be loaded on the SPE cartridges, while in LLE such volumes are more difficult to handle. Of course here one must take into account that increasing pre-concentration will apply not only to the target analyte but also to the co-extracted compounds, therefore stronger matrix effects could be expected; careful optimization of SPE conditions is needed for best results.

Off-line SPE can be performed in tubular cartridges, 96-well format beds, flat disks, thin film (SPME) etc., under vacuum or applying a positive pressure from above. Solid phase micro extraction (SPME) is already routinely used in GC/MS and literature data were reviewed by Vas and Vekey (2004). SPME helps to minimize effects due to interfering organic compounds in complex matrices (Sigma Aldrich). Applications were developed for forensic, environmental or food analysis. Brown and coworkers developed and applied a SPME-GC-MS method for measuring four club drugs, gamma-hydroxybutyrate, ketamine, methamphetamine, and methylenedioxymethamphetamine, in human urine using deuterium labeled internal standards. The drugs were spiked into human urine and derivatized using pyridine and hexylchloroformate to make them suitable for GC-MS analysis. The SPME conditions of extraction time/temperature and desorption time/temperature were optimized to yield the highest peak area for each of the four drugs (Brown et al, 2007). Headspace solid-phase micro-extraction (HS-SPME) integrates sampling, extraction, concentration and sample introduction into a single step for GC analysis of biological fluids and materials. Compared to liquid-liquid extraction and solid phase extraction, extracts are very clean and despite the absolute recoveries of the analytes from whole blood are rather low, generally <10% (Mills and Walker, 2000), due to the possibility of a good pre-concentration, interesting LLOQs are achievable. The same technique was used for the determination of volatile organic compounds released by packaging expanded polystyrene by GC/MS (Kusch and Knupp, 2004).

With respect to ion suppression, for any LC-MSMS analysis is good to know whether the loss of the sensitivity is due to poor recovery or to matrix effects on the analyte ionization. A combination between an anionic – exchange SPE for sample preparation and a pre-column – analytical column switching approach was used to minimize the matrix effect and to achieve the LLOQ to 2.5 pg/ml for salmeterol in plasma (Capka and Carter, 2007).

4. On-line chromatographic methods to separate the analyte from the matrix (i.e. column switch two-dimensions HPLC methods with different stationary phases)

The isolation of the target analyte from matrix can be performed also on-line, typically with the help of a dual HPLC-system and a column-switching valve (of course more complex multiplexing systems are commercially available). On-line methods have several advantages: direct injection of the biological material (if fluid), easier for automation, therefore reducing health risks correlated with handling of hazardous material, not generating waste as used cartridges, and not the least, in a long run less expensive. As a drawback, the amount of sample loaded is limited, but the coupling with a very sensitive mass spectrometer will overcome the limited sample enrichment.

For on-line sample preparation, different stationary phases embedded as classical SPE columns, or as restricted access media (RAM) and perfusion chromatography (POROS) columns are available; another technique of interest is turbulent flow chromatography.

5. Analyte pre/post column derivatization to enhance analyte separation from matrix components, and ionization; this approach can be combined with any one of the previous.

Derivatization is commonly applied in GC/MS analysis in order to increase volatility and thermal stability of various compounds. In LC-MS/MS derivatization reactions are less used; they become important when the ionization of the target analyte is poor or matrix interferences are high. A classical example is the quantitative determination of estradiol and estrone via dansylated derivatives, in positive ionization (Nelson et al, 2004) or the determination of bisphosphonates after methylation (Tarcomnicu et al, 2007 and 2009). Because the retention time is shifted and peaks of interest elute in a region with less interferences and matrix effects, both in GC and LC-MS, derivatization is useful to improve the separation. Ionization is generally enhanced, too.

The derivatization process is carried out mostly during sample extraction or on the dried extract, but sometimes even in the injector, in case of GC-MS, or post-column in LC-MS/MS. It is done by sylilation, acylation, alkylation (methylation), Schiff base formation etc.

The analyte features and sample nature (solid, fluid), amount, additives used (e.g. anticoagulant or stabilizer in case of plasma or urine) are first considerations to give an orientation in order to choose a sample preparation method. Fortunately in general it is not necessary to test all the aforementioned techniques, but sometimes a concurrence of factors with negative impact on the results will require a step-by step approach.

A strategy to minimize the matrix effect produced by endogeneous phospholipids from plasma was developed by evaluating sample preparation and chromatographic techniques with respect to extract cleanliness, matrix effect and analyte recovery (Chambers et al, 2007). Comparisons were made between protein precipitation, liquid-liquid extraction, pure cation exchange solid-phase extraction, reverse-phase SPE and mixed mode – SPE. Two chromatographic techniques, UPLC and HPLC were used to compare resolution and matrix sensitivity. A combination of mixed-mode SPE and UPLC was proved to be the most sensitive and robust method for removing phospholipids (up to 99% relative to protein precipitation) and for determination of trace levels of drugs in plasma.

Figures 4 shows the ion suppression induced by matrix on the analyte signal; protein precipitation with solvent, SLE and SPE have been tested for the model compound, pramipexole. This example and other presented in literature (Bonfiglio, et al, 1999; Dams et al, 2003; Matuzsewski et al; 2003, Souverain et al, 2004; Mastovka et al, 2005; Pichini et al, 2005, Annesley, et al, 2007, Capiello et al, 2008) illustrate the effect of co-extracted matrix compounds on the target analyte separation and ionization. For sophisticated research, with demands of very high sensitivity and specificity, sample preparation may become very complex and need laborious optimization but the results will be rewarding.

5. How to minimize matrix effect by chromatography (HPLC and GC)

Beside sample matrix components, other potential sources of matrix effects are mobile phase impurities or additives used in HPLC (Annesley et al, 2007). For mass spectrometry pure solvents like acetonitrile or methanol are the most suitable and flow rate, applied voltage, conductivity, liquid surface tension must be properly balanced for the formation of a stable ESI spray (Chech and Enke, 2001). Higher percentage of organic solvent in the mobile phase with decreased surface tension and low boiling point will result in a more efficient desolvation of the analyte. The conductivity of the solution is also important in ESI, therefore the presence of ionic species in the solution is necessary. In positive ESI the protonated solvent clusters of methanol/water or acetonitrile/water, formic or acetic acid are ideal for facilitating the protonation. Diluted salt solutions like ammonium acetate or formate facilitate adduct formation, especially in APCI, and also improve the chromatographic peak shape. For negative ionization, diluted ammonium hydroxide is added to the aqueous solution to facilitate deprotonation (Loo et al, 1992) although formic acid, halogenated solvents (e.g. trifluoroethanol) and diluted volatile buffers (ammonium acetate or formate) are suitable as well (Chech and Enke, 2001). However protonated analytes can be observed with high pH mobile phases and deprotonated analytes under low pH conditions, as already reported (Zhou and Cook, 2000).

Ion-pairing reagents like trifluoroacetic, pentafluoropropionic, or heptafluorobutiric acids, widely used in HPLC with conventional detectors due to good retention and peak shape in the analysis of polar compounds, have known ion-suppressing effect in negative ESI; the same for tetraalkyl ammonium hydroxide and salts in ESI positive. These additives should be carefully used in LC/MS. When the use of strong acidic ion-pair reagent is unavoidable for chromatography reasons, post-column addition of a weak acid like propionic acid could overcome the ion suppression (the so-called "TFA fix") (Apffel et al, 1995, Kuhlman et al, 1995, Annesley et al, 2007). Inorganic non-volatile buffers like phosphate and sulfate are not recommended in mass-spectrometry; they can cause salt deposits on the metal surfaces disturbing conductivity and being detrimental for ion formation and transmission (Chech and Enke, 2001).

TFA presents also matrix effects in positive ionization and an experiment confirming the well-known suppression of the ionization was described by Mallet et al. They compared the intensities of m/z 472 ion of terfenadine $[M+H]^+$, acquired in a solution containing 50/50 methanol/water, by mixing to an equivalent flow rate of 0.5% TFA and 0.5% ammonium hydroxide. In the presence of ammonium hydroxide the ion m/z 472 has shown an increase of 41% in the signal intensity compared to a decrease of 75% in the presence of TFA. With this experiment Mallet studied the influence of pH, to the ionization effects in positive and negative mode of 16 basic drugs and acidic compounds with a diversity of mass range, polarity and structure; compared to TFA formic acid and acetic acid shown less suppression effect (Mallet et al, 2004).

Benijts and coworkers have used the basic SPE procedure to study the influence of acetic acid and formic acid at two concentration levels, 0.01 and 0.1%, and of ammonium acetate and ammonium formate at the concentration 1mM and 5mM in positive and negative ionization modes, for 35 endocrine disrupting chemicals. In negative ionization mode a significant suppression of the signal was recorded at the concentration of 0.01% for both acids. The addition of buffers like ammonium formate in the mobile phase produced a slight enhancement of the ionization for all compounds excepting estradiol with a ME% of 172% (Benijts et al, 2004).

Steroids are among the compounds prone to suffer from matrix interferences both in terms of ion suppression and background interferences. We have selected here, as an example, the analysis of desogestrel from human plasma; in this case the type of ionization method was first carefully studied (as it will be presented in the next section of this chapter) and APPI (photo-spray) has given the best results in terms of sensitivity and background cleanliness (Figures 7-9). The sample clean-up was performed by SLE with a mixture of diethyl ether/tert-butyl methyl ether, which offered a good recovery and pre-concentration (obviously solvent precipitation is not suitable the molecule being highly non-polar, while SPE method needed evaporation of methanol, very time-consuming compared to the ether mixture).

Various stationary phases from different producers were tested during method development (octadecyl, octyl, pentafluorophenylpropyl, phenyl). Figure 8 presents the chromatograms recorded on the transitions selected for desogestrel after the injection of blank plasma spiked with analyte at 1 ng/mL, clean-up by SLE. Separation from the interfering matrix peak in the vicinity on the octadecyl column (Eternity C18 10 cmx2.1 mm, 2.7μm) was not satisfactory at first; playing on the gradient a cleaner delimitation of desogestrel peak was achieved.

http://dx.doi.org/10.5772/55982

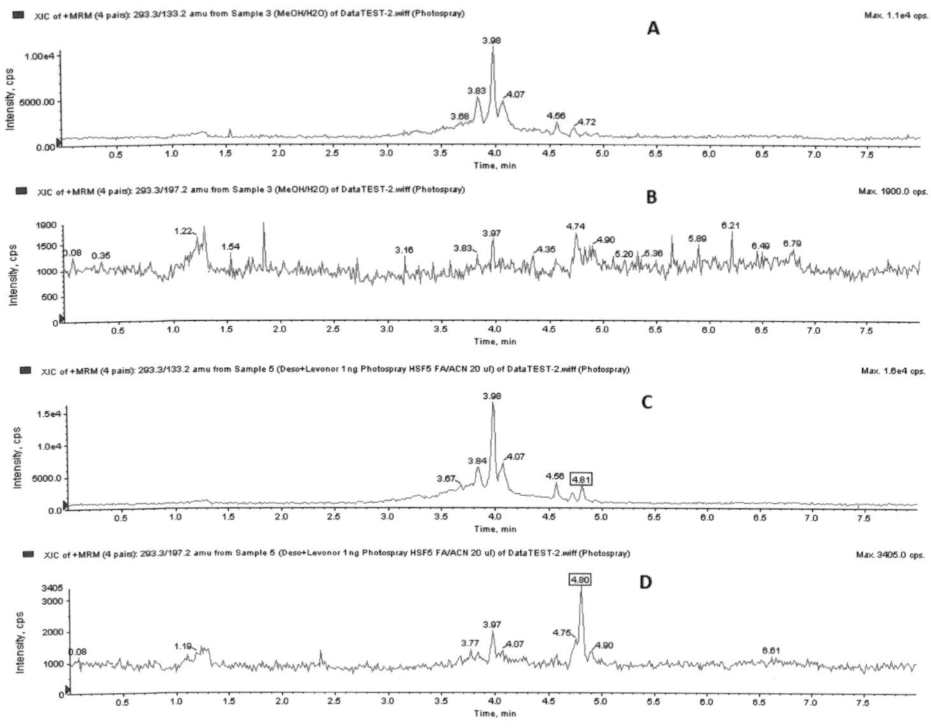

Figure 7. Chromatograms recorded on two transitions selected for desogestrel (A, C: 293.3/133.2 and B, D: 293.3/197.2) in APPI ionization after the injection of pure methanol (A, B) or Desogestrel solution at 1ng/ml in water/methanol (1:1, v/v). Desogestrel elutes at 4.8 min. As it can be observed each transition is differently affected by matrix components. Column: HSF5 10 cmx2.1 mm, 5µm (Supelco); Mobile phase: aqueous formic acid 0.1% and acetonitrile; Flow: 0.3 mL/min; gradient elution; injection volume: 30µL In the next step, chromatography was optimized further for minimizing matrix effects.

Figure 9 shows an overlay plot of two extracted plasma samples, a blank and a spiked concentration (1ng/mL), in the new chromatographic conditions. Desogestrel peak is clearly visible, as indicated by the arrow. Good results were obtained with the phenyl stationary phase as well.

A huge selection of stationary phases and mobile phases is available at the moment and their right combination can make significant improvements in the chromatographic separation, thus in diminishing matrix effects. As already mentioned before, sample preparation must be also seen in view of the chromatographic technique selected.

As it can be observed in Figure 7, on the chromatographic traces selected for desogestrel several quite intense peaks were recorded even after injecting pure methanol.

No miraculous HPLC or GC separation method permit to escape of matrix effects but a few general considerations are reported next and they may serve as a guideline to improve the analytical work minimizing matrix effect:

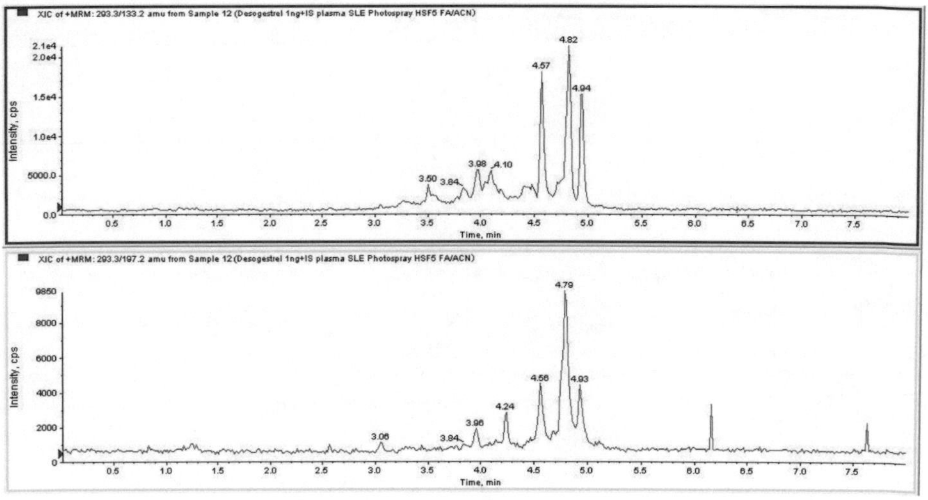

Figure 8. Chromatograms recorded on two transitions selected for desogestrel (293.3/133.2 and 293.3/197.2) in APPI ionization. Desogestrel spiked at 1 ng/mL in plasma, extracted by SLE. Column: Eternity C18 10 cmx2.1 mm, 2.7μm (Akzo Nobel); Mobile phase: aqueous formic acid 0.1% and acetonitrile; Flow: 0.2 mL/min; gradient elution; injection volume: 30μL. Desogestrel eluted at 4.94 min.

1. Void peak and source contamination – As aforementioned, salts, peptides and other polar compounds generally not retained in the chromatographic column are important matrix factors. These compounds tend also to deposit on the ionization sources extending the matrix effects far beyond the elution times, often accumulating from one injection to the following. It is nonetheless very useful and simple introducing in the chromatographic system, both in case of HPLC and GC, of a diverter valve (controlled by the computer system or the HPLC pump) to send to waste the initial chromatographic peak. This approach will avoid heavy source contamination improving the system stability. In case of GC separations, conventional valves can be used but other interesting alternative are fluidic switches without moving parts and no risks of introducing cold spots in the chromatographic system and/or deteriorate the peak shape;

2. Fast separations are good but if the resolution is maintained – It is always convenient to get faster methods but it is important to avoid inadequate separation in order to be quick; the matrix peaks must be adequately isolated from the peaks of interest.

3. LC x LC or GC x GC methods – It is clear that two dimension separations permit to get the maximum in term of isolation of the compound to be analyzed from matrix peaks. In case of difficult analyses it is always difficult to evaluate if a complex sample preparation is convenient and more effective than a better HPLC/GC separation, in principle both approaches must be each time evaluated. Experiments carried out by Pascoe and coworkers are a good example; the authors tested a series of stationary phases with a column-switching set-up and reported a reduction in matrix effects (Pascoe et al, 2001).

As a general rule, the use of stationary phases with different retention mechanisms (i.e. ion exchange and reversed phase or hydrophobic with polar GC columns) is the most effective

http://dx.doi.org/10.5772/55982

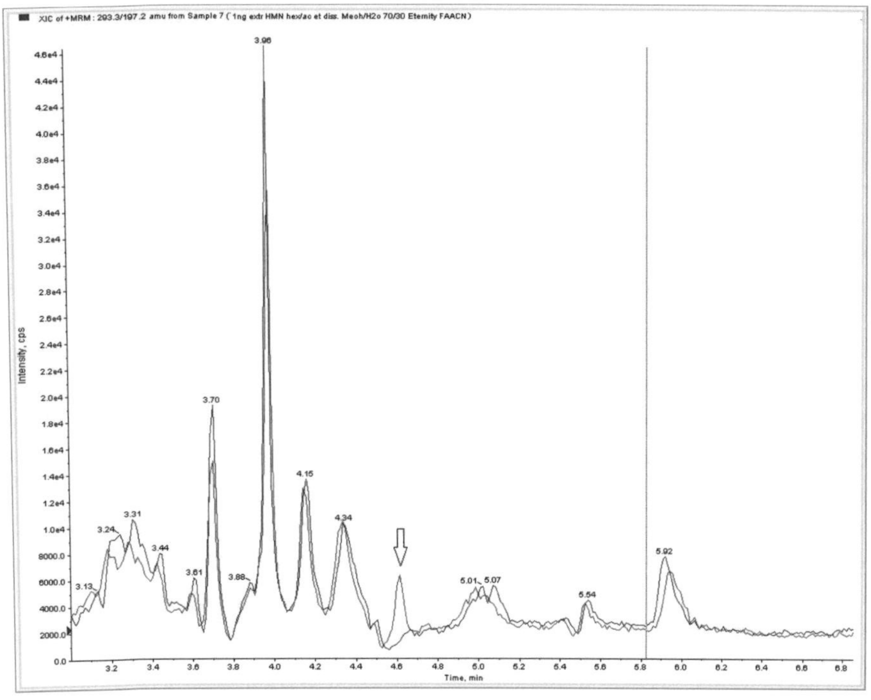

Figure 9. APPI ionization. Desogestrel - An overlay of blank plasma extract and plasma spiked with desogestrel at 1 ng/mL. Chromatograms recorded on the transition 293.3/197.2, in APPI ionization. Column: Eternity C18 10 cmx2.1 mm, 2.7μm (Akzo Nobel); Mobile phase: aqueous formic acid 0.1% and acetonitrile; Flow: 0.2 mL/min; gradient elution; injection volume: 30μL. Desogestrel peak is indicated by the arrow.

combination to maximize the separation of analytes from matrix and, at the same time, to increase the selectivity.

4. Column overload and source overload – A common trend is to increase the loop size when the sensitivity is inadequate considering that more analyte in the source is increasing the chromatographic peak; this fact is often wrong for two important reasons. First, increasing the injection volume may bring to a column overload with modification of peak shape and a peak normally not affected by matrix can become disturbed by it due to a broadening of the matrix peak. A deterioration of peak shape is often observed with large injection volumes making no advantage in terms of S/N ratio improvement. As a paradox, in complex matrices, in case of inadequate sensitivity it is often interesting to test the injection of a more diluted sample to understand if the low sensitivity is really due to inadequate amount of sample or an excessive matrix effect.

5. Mobile phase composition – As discussed above, in HPLC it is always important to remember that different mobile phases may present quite different matrix results; the same also for the type of MS ionization (see next section). It is therefore important to test several mobile phases and ionization conditions in order to minimize the matrix effects.

6. Flow rate – Using lower flow rate is a big advantage in order to minimize matrix effects. The ionization efficiency improves significantly with lower flow rate, less contaminants are introduced in the source contributing to keep the ion optics cleaner, higher content of water (this means often better separation) in the mobile phase can be handled without too much loss in sensitivity and less heating is needed in the source often resulting in a less important chemical background, partially responsible of matrix effects.

7. Stationary phases – Evidently, it is not possible to review all existing columns and to suggest special kinds because each analyte has its own properties and such detailed presentation is outside the scope of this chapter. It is however interesting to summarize a few key points in order to minimize matrix effects and get the maximum of results. First, when developing a new analytical method it is important to consider the polarity of the analyte and, in comparison, the expected type of matrix present in the sample. As an example in urine one will not have problems with proteins while a high salt content (e.g. biliary salts) and other polar compounds will dominate the matrix. In such conditions, for the analysis of highly polar compounds, it can be interesting to consider ion exchange columns or HILIC chromatography, instead of classical reversed phase columns. In case of non-polar compounds in plasma, matrix effects from phospholipids are critical and these endogenous products are also quite apolar creating peculiar matrix problems. In such cases a careful choice of a column able to retain differentially the analyte is important; columns like phenyl or pentafluorophenylpropyl can be quite selective in retaining the analyte if it has an aromatic group normally absent in phospholipids. The possibilities are endless but the problem must be evaluated before screening blindly a large number of stationary phases.

8. Analyte derivatization – Derivatization methods, despite not being strictly chromatographic methods can often bring to results otherwise impossible, especially when the derivatization changes the analyte polarity. Several examples are available where highly polar compounds, like aminoacids, biphosphonate, catecholamines, aminoglycosides, can be transformed by derivatization in less polar compounds easily separated by GC or HPLC.

9. High resolution mass spectrometry can be very useful for the analysis of dirty biological extracts, through a better separation of the analyte from background interferences. Ultra-high pressure liquid chromatography (UHPLC), micro, capillary and nano-LC provide high resolution separations (increased number of theoretical plates) with very narrow peaks thus easing the possibility of changing the analyte retention time towards regions in the chromatogram less affected by matrix. Many labs are transferring their methods now towards ultra-high-pressure chromatography (UHPLC); matrix effects have been evaluated and improvement reported (Van de Steene and Lambert, 2008).

10. HPLC column, solvents, plastic and polymer residues, reagents as source of matrix – Never forget that column bleeding both in GC and HPLC can be an important cause of matrix effect. In case of poor chromatographic sensitivity with compounds otherwise ionizing properly it is useful to check different columns, also within the same type of bonding, for matrix effects. Unfortunately similar problems may come also from solvents, water and

http://dx.doi.org/10.5772/55982

salts employed in HPLC, as well as from plastic and polymer residues from tubes, 96-well plates, caps and lids, filters, SPE beds, etc. (Mei et al, 2003; Capiello et al, 2008).

6. Optimization of MS interfaces and ionization conditions to minimize matrix effect

The first point to consider is the choice of interface type. In this respect it is important to observe that matrix effects are more evident in conditions of poor ionization, therefore generally the source with the best ion efficiency is the first choice. A second point to consider is that matrix effects also derive from a competition between matrix ions and analyte ions at the level of ion sampling in the orifice area. Clearly, a source giving minimum ionization efficiency for the matrix is also effective in minimize matrix effects over the analyte ionization; this fact can be well appreciated with sources having specific ionization mechanisms, like the atmospheric pressure photoionization source (APPI), that may give interesting advantages in terms of matrix effects. However, only experimental tests will confirm and help to define the most appropriate ionization interface.

Once defined the source to be used an important step is the definition of the ionization polarity. In this respect the chemical structure of the analyte may impose a choice but it is also important to consider the restriction coming from the mobile phase composition: one will never get a reasonable negative ionization in presence of trifluoroacetic acid, while formic or acetic acids are fine; no chance to work in positive mode with a strong base like tetrapropylammonium in the mobile phase but diluted ammonium hydroxide is good.

The aspects of mobile phase composition and ionization mode being clarified, an important stage in the source optimization is not only to play on the best signal for the analyte but also to look for the lowest background ionization. It is in fact important to find the situation where the ratio between background ions and analyte is the most convenient. Ion transfer voltage (ESI, APPI) or needle current (in case of APCI), declustering (orifice) voltage, nebulization conditions (temperature, gas flow rates) and source position optimization (depending upon the kind of source) are some of the key elements of optimization aiming to improve this ionization ratio.

In our example, we have optimized the ionization interface for the analysis of desogestrel. Due to the high background in ESI on the most intense multiple reaction monitoring (MRM) transitions corresponding to the analyte, several other less intense transitions were explored under selected chromatographic conditions (column HSF5 10 cmx2.1 mm, 5μm, mobile phase: aqueous formic acid 0.1% and acetonitrile in gradient elution at 0.3 mL/min, mass spectrometer: API 5000 triple quadrupole). The result is presented in Figure 10. Further development included testing of APCI (Figure 10) and APPI (Figures 7-9) ionization interfaces.

Photoionization can give excellent results in terms of ionization efficiency for aromatic compounds or structures with multiple conjugated double bonds (Yang and Henion, 2002, Tiedong 2004, Yamamoto 2006) and proved to be the best also for our target compound,

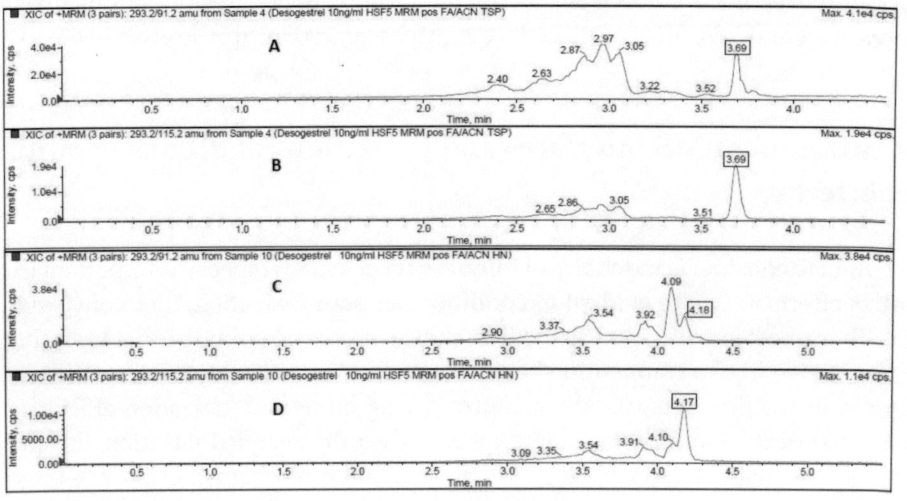

Figure 10. Chromatograms recorded on two transitions selected for desogestrel (293.2/91.2 and 293.2/115.2) in ESI ionization (A, B) and APCI ionization (C, D). Desogestrel – 10ng/mL standard in water/methanol (1:1, v/v). Column: HSF5 10 cmx2.1 mm, 5μm (Supelco); Mobile phase: aqueous formic acid 0.1% and acetonitrile; Flow: 0.3 mL/min; injection volume: 30μL. The same gradient was used in both ionization modes; the difference in retention time (3.69 vs. 4.17 min) resulted because the acquisition was 0.5 min later triggered in chromatograms A and B.

although matrix issues were not completely solved. APPI was selected for the final method; chromatography experiments were presented in *Section 5*.

As demonstrated by Mei and coworkers, matrix effects are also not only ionization mode dependent but also source-design dependent (Mei et al, 2003). They have injected plasma processed by solvent precipitation, using identical LC set-up, into three instruments from different manufacturers, equipped with ESI as well as with APCI interfaces. The measurements were performed in positive ions mode, monitoring 8 MRM transitions, chromatographic separation employing a Metachem Basic 4.6x50 mm, 5 μm column eluted in gradient with ammonium acetate 10mM containing 0.005% acetic acid and methanol. For the Micromass Quattro tandem mass spectrometer, Mei et al found that APCI source is more sensitive to matrix effects in the studied conditions. Overall, 22 examples of matrix effects were identified across various regions of the chromatographic gradient; most of these involved early-eluting polar compounds. One of the monitored molecules showed ionization enhancement in presence of Li-heparin as anticoagulant.

Capiello and coworkers have studied as an alternative to ESI an efficient LC-MS interface based on direct electron ionization (Direct-EI) for the analysis of small and medium molecular mass compounds (Capiello et al, 2008). They have quantitatively evaluated the impact of matrix effects on this type of ionization, using for experiments plasma or river water samples. Phenacetin and ibuprofen were used as model compounds. Plasma samples were extracted by LLE or SPE; water samples by SPE. The majority of matrix effects observed in LC-ESI-MS were surmounted using the LC-Direct EI-MS interface. There is to mention though that in this

http://dx.doi.org/10.5772/55982

case also the LC set-up was different, respectively a nano-LC system was used in combination with Direct-EI; nano-LC itself brings improvement in overcoming matrix effects also when ESI is employed. (More on this topic in *Section 8*)

7. Accepting matrix effects as unavoidable in analyses of real samples; approaches to obtain reliable quantitative results

As a conclusion of the discussion so far, there is no doubt that both in quantitative and qualitative bioanalysis, matrix effects are present. These effects are unseen in the chromatogram but can have deleterious impact on methods accuracy and sensitivity; it is important that they are identified and addressed in method development, validation, and routine use of HPLC–ESI–MS/MS (Taylor, 2009, Hall et al, 2012).

Adequate measures must be taken to guarantee that results are reliable; these actions can be divided in two groups:

1. Identification of the relevance of matrix effect in the analytical conditions used
2. Introduction of corrective factors to compensate the unavoidable matrix effects inherent to the analytical method employed.

First kind of actions groups the procedures used to detect and/or quantify the matrix effects present in an analytical procedure. The first method was proposed by Bonfiglio et al (1999) and it is based on the continuous infusion of the compound to be analyzed in the mass spectrometer equipped with the selected ionization sources. Just before entering in the source, this is mixed with the mobile phase from the HPLC pump to be used for the analytical procedure. Blank matrix samples extracted using certain procedure are injected in this system, with or without chromatographic column. A few examples of this method were presented in Figure 4 (*Section* 2). As it can be seen this approach allows very well to test different HPLC procedures, especially in order to improve separation conditions, trying to avoid the co-elution of the analytes of interest with peaks having an important matrix effect. Weak points of this approach are its complexity, the difficulty to quantitatively define the impact of the matrix effect and the risk to contaminate the interface with high amount of analyte through infusion.

In order to overcome this fact, the alternative approach was proposed by Buhrman et al (1996) then by Matuszewski et al (2003). In such method extracted blank samples (representative of matrix and analytical procedures to be tested) are spiked with a known amount of the analyte and the results are compared to the-ones obtained analyzing the same compound at the same concentration dissolved in mobile phase. Ratios between these data are now employed and recommended from several regulatory authorities as a quantitative "matrix factor", with well-defined limits of acceptance (Viswanathan et al, 2007).

Considering the corrective actions, in order to compensate the matrix factor, the use of internal standards (in particular analogue of the analyte labeled with stable isotopes) is definitively the main approach to solve the problem (Tranfo et al, 2007). In case of other chemically related analogues, normally used in HPLC with UV or fluorescence detectors to correct for extraction and/or injection variation, their matrix factor in LC-MS can be quite different from that of the analyte; in such cases a verification of the matrix factor for analyte and as well for the internal standard is useful even if they eluted in the same retention time with the analytes. When the internal standard is not co-eluting with the analyte, the influence of interfering compounds on the ionization can be different thus the quantitative results could be biased. It is noteworthy that also in case of stable isotope labeled internal standards significant differences of retention time, versus the non labeled compound, can be observed sometimes (especially when the mass difference is high, e.g. d7- or d9-labeled molecules, or in case of HILIC separations), making critical the matrix effect correction if a sharply eluting peak of an interfering compound is present. Due to this fact different labeling, like ^{13}C, could be used instead of the more commonly employed deuterium to minimize the chromatographic shift.

In case an internal standard cannot be used or it is not available blank samples spiked with the analyte of interest must be always analyzed in parallel to be sure that the analyte is not influenced by matrix avoiding unreliable results. A spiking of a known analyte concentration on the same sample to be analyzed is also an interesting approach (if the sample amount is enough) to guarantee the appropriateness of the measurement performed.

8. Future perspectives

After so many evidences of the relevance of matrix effects in bioanalytics what can we expect next? Do we have possibilities to further improve this situation?

In the next we will consider the main three areas explored in this paper and the chances of development for the future:

1. *Sample preparation* – This area knows continuous improvements; more and more selective extraction methods provide cleaner sample extracts, with reduced matrix content. In this context the development of better immunopurification media (more chemically stable, easier on-line applications) for an always larger palette of antigens, the appearance of newer molecular imprinted polymer (MIP) columns for specific chemical groups and the possibility to do automated solid-phase micro-extraction (SPME) processing large number of samples at the same time are between the most attractive opportunities. SPME seems to be potentially very interesting, its simplicity minimizing liquid handling, the possibility for reusing the sorbent by adequate washing (much simpler than in SPE), the possibility to introduce immunopurification media or MIP, and finally the potential for down scaling to the micro level are between the most intriguing aspects.
2. *HPLC methods* – The choice of stationary phases, with enhanced separation properties, is constantly growing, and one of the directions with a lot of potential is currently hydrophilic interaction liquid chromatography (HILIC), with increasing number of applications in bioanalysis fields (Hsieh, 2008, Van Nuijs et al, 2011).

http://dx.doi.org/10.5772/55982

However the improvement in equipment seems to be the most interesting part. Years are passed from the time when LC/MS producers were struggling to get higher flow rate sources pushed by customers acquainted to large HPLC columns and unsatisfied by the technical performance of micro-column on micro-HPLC system. UHPLC is nowadays widespread and better results in terms of matrix effects compared with classical HPLC were already reported (Novakova et al, 2006, Van de Steene et al, 2008).

Micro, capillary, nano-HPLC columns are now easily available, robust, reliable and performing very well in terms of separation. All this also thanks to better HPLC systems, permitting to exploit adequately these columns. It is well recognized that matrix effects are reduced at lower flow rates, with a concomitant increase in term of sensitivity; it has to be seen if a revolution will take place in LC/MS as it happened in GC-MS years ago when going from packed to capillary GC columns. A lot of improvement will come for sure passing to packed columns in the sub millimeter diameter range and below, eluted with very low flow rate. Experiments performed recently in our laboratory with a 0.3 mm inner diameter column were very promising. An example is presented in Figure 11.

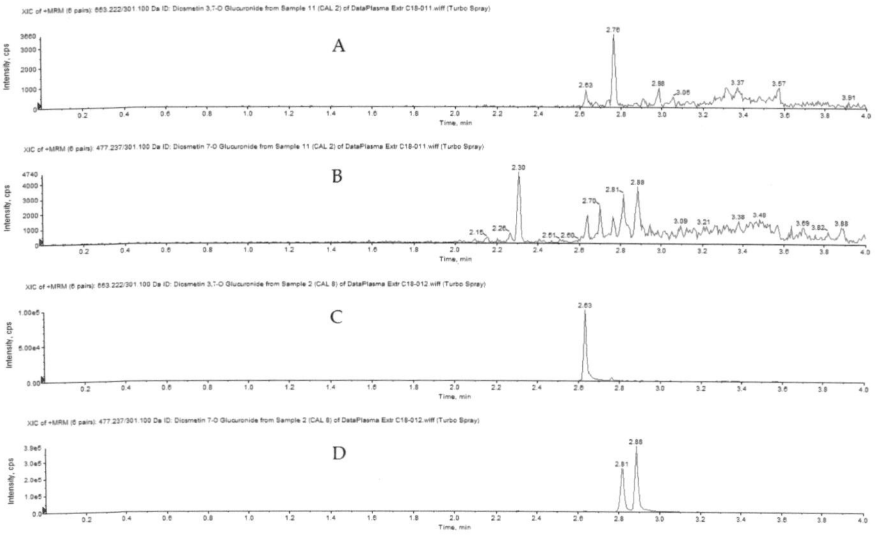

Figure 11. Chromatograms recorded on the MRM transitions of Diosmetin-3,7-O-Glucuronide (A, C - 653.222/301.1) and Diosmetin-7-O-Glucuronide/ Diosmetin-3-O-Glucuronide (B, D – 477.237/301.1) after the injection of extracted plasma samples spiked at 0.1 ng/mL (A, B) or 15 ng/mL (C, D); elution at 50 µL/min on Halo C18 (0.3x50 mm, 2.7 µm, 90A packing – Eksigent) column. Diosmetin-7-O-Glucuronide – retention time 2.88 min; Diosmetin-3-O-Glucuronide – retention time 2.81 min

Diosmetin is a metabolite of diosmin, a natural flavonoid found in most fruits and vegetables; moreover these contain a series of compounds with the same mass and related structure giving numerous interferences, therefore on conventional LC columns the separation was not possible below certain concentrations. Figure 11 presents the chromatograms recorded using a sub-millimeter column, Halo C18 (0.3x50 mm, 2.7 μm, 90A packing – Eksigent) eluted at 50 μL/min in gradient with a mobile phase containing water+0.5% formic acid and acetonitrile with 0.5% formic acid. Plasma spiked at 0.1 ng/mL or 15 ng/mL was injected. As it can be noticed, five peaks were distinctly separated in the biological extract within an interval of 0.25 min; in these conditions it was possible to obtain a blank sample from patients with special diet. This powerful separation helps in reducing matrix effects and benefits also from the advantage of very low flow-rate.

The hyphenation of separation techniques like isothacophoresys/capillary electrophoresis and HPLC is another area not yet well exploited but offering a lot of potential to get cleaner samples with minimal matrix effects.

3. *MS Ionization interfaces* – An exhaustive presentation is not possible in this area; however a few examples of potential new ways to reduce matrix can be introduced.

In the last years ion mobility become more and more present in the MS analytic instrumentation range. In particular ion mobility (IM) techniques have created a possibility to play on the gas phase in front of the sampling orifice of the mass spectrometers, selecting the relevant ions to be analyzed. These applications are quite at the beginning and the real impact on the matrix effects has not been fully explored, until now the focus being more on the enhancement of the analytical selectivity. The difference in cleaning the matrix interferences can be impressive, as it can be seen in the example of clenbuterol analysis from human urine (Figure 12) without further processing; the sample is just diluted 1:1 and injected in the LC-MS system (AB Sciex).

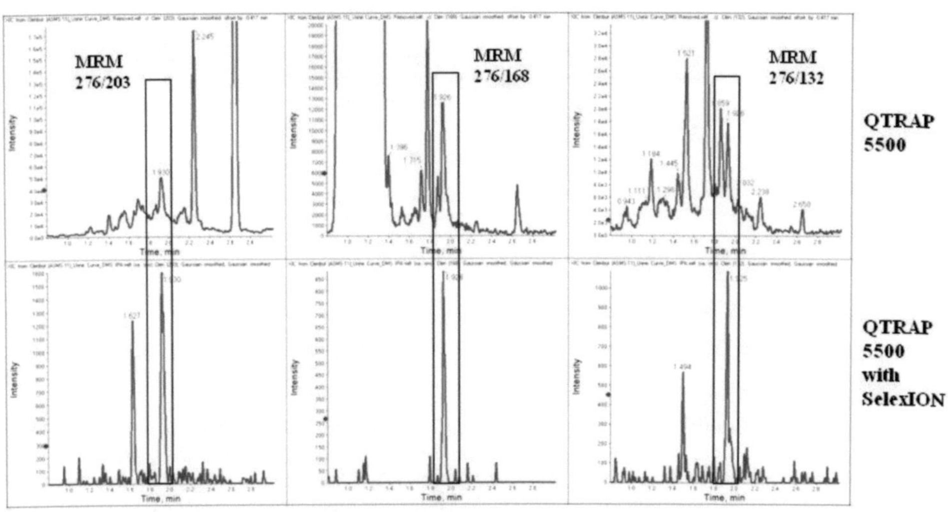

Figure 12. Clenbuterol Spiked in Human Urine (diluted 1:1 prior to analysis). QTRAP® 5500 vs 5500 with SelexION™ Technology. (Reproduced with the permission of AB Sciex).

Other groups are also focusing on very low molecular mass ions analysis, that most often are considered background ions, hence optimizing instruments for liquid or gaseous matrices. An

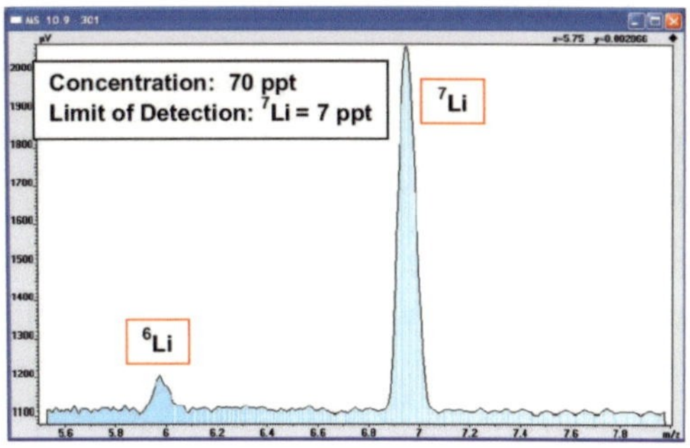

Figure 13. Analysis of the Lithium isotopes at a concentration of 10^{-8} mol/L using an instrument specially designed for low molecular mass compounds. (Reproduced with the permission of AMD Intectra).

API Interface with ESI/APCI Glow Discharge on a double beam magnetic sector was developed by AMD; the interface can switch between LC, GC or CE inlet without needs of any system modification. The high-resolution results (Figure 13) obtained in the low mass range (like alkali metals from m/z 6 to 39), generally affected by huge interferences of artifacts, are very interesting (AMD Intectra GmbH).

Most probably exciting results will come next from this kind of sources in combination with newer techniques of ion sampling from the atmospheric pressure side to the high vacuum chamber. We are going from orifice – skimmer sources always more to ion guide systems (with small quadrupoles or lens cascade) permitting to obtain a higher transmission and improving the separation from neutral molecules, solvent clusters and allowing a cut-off based on ion characteristics.

This brief example of future progress in ion sources wants to be just a message on how much the hardware development remains open for important improvement in the matrix effects control.

To conclude let's hope that new developments will be so impressive to make matrix effects something of the past and all problems presented in this chapter just scientific curiosity. Who knows?

Author details

Luigi Silvestro[1], Isabela Tarcomnicu[2] and Simona Rizea Savu[1]

1 3S-Pharmacological Consultation & Research GmbH, Harpstedt, Germany

2 Pharma Serv International SRL, Bucharest, Romania

References

[1] Annesley, T. M. (2007). Methanol-associated matrix effects in electrospray ionization tandem mass spectrometry. Clin Chem , 53, 1827-1834.

[2] Apffel, A, Fisher, S, Goldberg, G, Goodley, P. C, & Kuhlmann, F. E. (1995). Enhanced sensitivity for peptide-mapping with electrospray liquid-chromatography mass-spectrometry in the presence of signal suppression due to trifluoroacetic acid-containing mobile phases. J Chrom A , 712, 177-190.

[3] Benijts, T, Dams, R, Lambert, W, & De Leenheer, A. (2004). Countering Matrix effects in Environmental Liquid Chromatography-Electrospray Ionization Tandem MassSpectrometry Water Analysis for Endocrine Disrupting Chemicals", J.Chrom.A, , 1029, 153-159.

[4] Bennett, P. K, Meng, M, & Capka, V. Managing Phospholipids-Based Matrix Effects in Bioanalysis". (2006). www.tandemlabs.com/documents/IMSC-web.pdf

[5] Bonfiglio, R, King, R. C, Olah, T. V, & Merkle, K. (1999). The Effects of Sample Preparation Methods on the Variability of the Electrospray Ionization Response for Model Drug Compounds. Rapid Commun. Mass Spectrom. , 13, 1175-1185

[6] Brown, S. D, Rhodes, D. J, & Pritchard, B. J. (2007). A validated SPME-GC-MS method for simultaneous quantification of club drugs in human urine. Forensic Sci Int., 171(2-3):142-50

[7] Buhrman, D. L, Price, P. I, & Rudewicz, P. J. (1996). Quantitation of SR 27417 in Human Plasma Using Electrospray Liquid Chromatography-Tandem Mass Spectrometry: A Study of Ion Suppression", J. Am. Soc. Mass Spectrom. 7, 1099

[8] Capka, V, & Carter, S. J. (2007). Minimizing matrix effects in the development of a method for the determination of salmeterol in human plasma by LC/MS/MS at low pg/mL concentration levels", J. Chromatogr. B, , 856, 285-293.

[9] Cappiello, A, Famiglini, G, Palma, P, Pierini, E, Termopoli, V, & Trufelli, H. (2008). Overcoming matrix effects in liquid chromatography-mass spectrometry. Anal Chem , 80, 9343-9348.

[10] Cech, N. M, & Enke, C. G. (2001). Practical implications of some recent studies in electrospray ionization fundamentals. Mass Spectrometry Reviews, , 20, 362-387.

[11] Chambers, E, & Wagrowski-diehl, D. M. Ziling Lu, Z, Mazzeo, JR. (2007). Systematic and comprehensivre strategy for reducing matrix effects in LC-MS/MS analyses" J.Chromatogr. B, , 852, 22-34.

[12] Dams, R, Huestis, M. A, Lambert, W. E, & Murphy, C. M. (2003). Matrix Effect in Bio-Analysis of Illicit Drugs with LC-MS/MS: Influence of Ionization Type, Sample Preparation, and Biofluid" J.Am.Soc.Mass Spectrom , 14, 1290-1294.

[13] (Doles M, Hines RL, Mack RC, Mobbley RC, Ferguson LD, Alice MB, Molecular beams of macroions, J.Chem.Phys. 1968; 49:2240).

[14] EMAGuideline on validation of bioanalytical methods. Nov (2009). Doc. Ref: EMEA/CHMP/EWP/192217/2009

[15] Erney, D. R, Gillespie, A. M, & Gilvydis, D. M. (1993). Explanation of the matrix-induced chromatographic response enhancement of organophosphorus pesticides during open tubular column gas chromatography with splitless or hot on-column injection and flame photometric detection" Journal of Chromatography A, , 638(1), 57-63.

[16] Fan, J, Huang, B, Wang, X, & Zhang, X. C. (2011). Thermal precipitation fluorescence assay for protein stability screening. J Struct. Biol. 175 (3), 465-468

[17] Fenn, J. B, Mann, M, Meng, C. K, Wong, S. F, & Whitehouse, C. M. (1989). Electrospray ionization for mass spectrometry of large biomolecules. Science , 246(4926), 64-71.

[18] Food and Drug Administration (May 2001) Guidance for Industry / Bioanalytical method validation

[19] Fu, I, Woolf, E. J, & Matuszewski, B. K. (1998). Effect on of the Sample Matrix on the Determination of Indinavir in Human Urine by HPLC with Turbo Ion Spray Tandem Mass Spectrometric Detection", J.Pharm.Biomed.Anal. 18, 347

[20] Guo, T, Chan, M, & Soldin, S. J. (2004). Steroid Profiles Using Liquid Chromatography--Tandem Mass Spectrometry With Atmospheric Pressure Photoionization Source. Archives of Pathology & Laboratory Medicine,128 (4), 469

[21] Hajslova, J, & Cajka, T. (2007). Gas chromatography- mass spectrometry (GC-MS) in Food Toxicants Analysis, Y.Pico (Editor), Chapter 12.

[22] Hall, T. G, Smukste, I, Bresciano, K. R, Wang, Y, Mckearn, D, & Savage, R. E. (2012). Identifying and Overcoming Matrix Effects in Drug Discovery and Development, Tandem Mass Spectrometry- Applications and Principles, Dr Jeevan Prasain (Ed.), 978-9-53510-141-3InTech, Available from: http://www.intechopen.com/books/tandem-mass-spectrometry-applications-andprinciples/identifying-and-overcoming-matrix-effects-in-drug-discovery-and-development

[23] Henion, J, Brewer, E, & Rule, E. G. (1998). Sample preparation for LC/MS analysis of biological and environmental samples, Anal. Chem. 70(19), 650A-656A.

[24] Horning, E. C, & Horning, M. G. (1971). Human metabolic profiles obtained by GC and GC/MS" J. Chromatogr. Sci., , 9, 129-140.

[25] Hsieh, Y, Wang, G, Wang, Y, Chackalamannil, S, Brisson, J. M, Ng, K, & Korfmacher, W. A. (2002). Simultaneous determination of a drug candidate and its metabolite in rat plasma samples using ultrafast monolithic column high-performance liquid chro-

matography/tandem mass spectrometry. Rapid Commun Mass Spectrom. , 16(10), 944-50.

[26] Hsieh, Y. (2008). Potential HILIC-MS in quantitative bioanalysis of drugs and drug metabolites. J. Sep.Sci., , 31, 1481-1491.

[27] http://wwwabsciex.com/Documents/Downloads/Literature/SelexION-Technology-New-Solution-Selectivity-Challenges-TN%20pdf, 2960211-2960201.

[28] http://wwwamd-intectra.de/

[29] http://wwwbiotage.com/DynPage.aspx?id=22317

[30] http://wwwsigmaaldrich.com/analytical-chromatography/sample-preparation/spme/spme-resolves.html

[31] Ikonomou, M. G, Blades, A. T, & Kebarle, P. (1990). Electrospray-ion spray: a comparison of mechanisms and performance. Anal Chem. , 62, 957-967.

[32] Iribarne, J. V, & Thomson, B. A. (1976). On the evaporation of small ions from charged droplets. Chem. Phys. 64, 2287

[33] Jemal, M, Ouyang, Z, & Xia, Y. Q. MS Bioanalytical Method Development that Incorporates Plasma Phospholipids Risk Avoidance, Usage of Incurred Sample and Well Thought-Out Chromatography" Biomed.Chromatogr. , 24, 2-19.

[34] Kebarle, P, & Tang, L. (1993). From ions in solution to ions in the gas phase- the mechanism of electrospray mass spectrometry, Anal. Chem., 65 (22), , 972A-986A.

[35] King, R, Bonfiglio, R, Fernandez-metzler, C, Miller-stein, C, & Olah, T. (2000). Mechanistic Investigation of Ionization Suppression in Electrospray Ionization" J.Am.Soc.Mass Spectrom.11, 942

[36] Koster, R. A. Dijkers, ECF, Uges, DRA. (2009). Robust, High-Throughput LC-MS/MS Method for Therapeutic Drug Monitoring of Cyclosporine, Tacrolimus, Everolimus, and Sirolimus in Whole Blood. Ther Drug Monit _31 (1), 116-125

[37] Kuhlmann, F. E, Apffel, A, Fisher, S. M, Goldberg, G, & Goodley, P. C. (1995). Signal enhancement for gradient reverse-phase high-performance liquid-chromatography electrosprayionization mass spectrometry analysis with trifluoroacetic and other strong acid modifiers by postcolumn addition of propionic-acid and isopropanol. J Am Soc Mass Spectrom , 6, 1221-1225.

[38] Little, J. L, Wempe, M. F, & Buchanan, C. M. (2006). Liquid chromatography mass spectrometry/mass spectrometry method development for drug metabolism studies: examining lipid matrix ionization effects in plasma", J.Chromatogr. B., , 833, 291-230.

[39] Loo, J. A. Ogorzalek Loo RR, Light KJ, Edmonds CG, and Smith RD. (1992). Multiply Charged Negative Ions by Electrospray Ionization of Polypeptides and Proteins." Anal Chem , 64, 81-88.

[40] Mallet, C, Ziling, R, Lu, Z, & Mazeo, J. R. (2004). A Study of Ion Suppression Effects in Electrospray Ionization from Mobile Phase Additives and Solid-Phase Extracts", Rapid Commun.Mass Spectrom., , 18, 49-58.

[41] Mastovka, K, Lehotay, S. J, & Anastassiades, M. (2005). Combination of Analyte Protectants To Overcome Matrix Effects in Routine GC Analysis of Pesticide Residues in Food Matrixes", Anal.Chem. 77, 8129

[42] Matuszewski, B. K, Constanzer, M. L, & Chavez-eng, C. M. (2003). Strategies for the Assessment of Matrix Effect in Quantitative Bioanalytical Methods Based on HPLC-MS/MS, Anal. Chem. , 75, 3019-3030.

[43] Medvedovici, A, Udrescu, S, Albu, F, Tache, F, & David, V. (2001). Large-volume injection of sample diluents not miscible with the mobile phase as an alternative approach in sample preparation for bioanalysis: an application for fenspiride bioequivalence. Bioanalysis., , 3(17), 1935-47.

[44] Mei, H, Hsieh, Y, Nardo, C, Xu, X, Wang, S, Ng, K, & Korfmacher, W. A. (2003). Investigation of matrix effects in bioanalytical high-performance liquid chromatography/tandem mass spectrometric assays: application to drug discovery. Rapid Commun Mass Spectrom , 17, 97-103.

[45] Mills, G. A, & Walker, V. (2000). Headspace solid-phase microextraction procedures for gaschromatographic analysis of biological fluids and materials", J.Chromatogr. A, , 902, 267-287.

[46] Nelson, R. E, Grebe, S. K, Kane, O, & Singh, D. J. RJ. (2004). Liquid Chromatography-Tandem Mass Spectrometry Assay for Simultaneous Measurement of Estradiol and Estrone in Human Plasma. Clin. Chem. , 50, 2-373.

[47] Novakova, L, Solichova, D, & Solich, P. (2006). Advantages of ultra performance liquid chromatography over high-performance liquid chromatography: comparison of different analytical approaches during analysis of diclofenac gel. J Sep Sci , 29, 2433-2443.

[48] Pascoe, R, Foley, J. P, & Gusev, A. I. (2001). Reduction in matrix-related signal suppression effects in electrospray ionization mass spectrometry using on-line two-dimensional liquid chromatography. Anal Chem , 73, 6014-6023.

[49] Paul, J. Taylor ((2005). Matrix effects: the Achilles heel of quantitative high-performance liquid chromatography-electrospray-tandem mass spectrometry. Clinical Biochemistry 38, April 2005, (4), 328-334.

[50] Peter KuschGerd Knupp. (2004). Headspace-SPME-GC-MS Identification of Volatile Organic Compounds Released from Expanded Polystyrene. J. Polym. and the Environ. , 12(2), 83-87.

[51] Pichini, S, Abanades, S, Farre, M, Pellegrini, M, Marchei, E, & Pacifici, R. dela Torre, R, Zuccaro, Quantification of the plant-derived hallucinogen Salvinorin A in conven-

tional and non-conventional biological fluids by gas-chromatography/mass spectrometry after Salvia divinorum smoking", Rapid Commun.Mass Spectrom., 19, 1649-1656, 2005.

[52] Sangster, T, Spence, M, Sinclair, P, Payne, R, & Smith, C. (2004). Unexpected observation of ion suppression in a liquid chromatography/atmospheric pressure chemical ionization mass spectrometric bioanalytical method. Rapid Commun Mass Spectrom, , 18, 1361-1364.

[53] Souverain, S, & Rudaz, S. Veuthey, JL "Matrix effect in LC-ESI-MS and LC-APCI-MS with off-line and on-line extraction procedures". (2004). J. Chrom. A 1058 (1-2), 61-66

[54] Tanaka, K, & Hine, G. (1982). Compilation of gas chromatographic retention indices of 163 metabolically important organic acids, and their use in detection of patients with organic acidurias" J.Chroamtogr. A, 239, 301

[55] Tarcomnicu, I, Gheorghe, M. C, & Silvestro, L. Rizea Savu, S, Boaru, I, Tudoroniu, A. (2009). High-throughput HPLC-MS/MS method to determine ibandronate in human plasma for pharmacokinetic applications. J Chromatogr B Analyt Technol Biomed Life Sci. , 877(27), 3159-68.

[56] Tarcomnicu, I, & Silvestro, L. Rizea Savu, S, Gherase, A, Dulea, C. (2007). Development and application of a high-performance liquid chromatography-mass spectrometry method to determine alendronate in human urine. J Chromatogr A , 1160, 21-33.

[57] ThomsonIribarne, J. Field induced ion evaporation from liquid surfaces at atmospheric pressure. Chem. Phys. 71, 4451., 1979

[58] Tranfo, G, Ciadella, A. M, Paci, E, & Pigini, D. (2007). Matrix effect in the determination of occupational biomarkers in urine by HPLC-MS/MS. Prevention Today, , 3, 57-64.

[59] Trufelli, H, Palma, P, Famiglini, G, & Capiello, A. (2011). An overview of matrix effects in liquid chromatography-mass spectrometry. Mass Spec. Reviews, 30 (3), 491-509

[60] Van de SteeneJ, Lambert W. (2008). Comparison of matrix effects in HPLC-MS/MS and UPLC-MS/MS analysis of nine basic pharmaceuticals in surface waters. J Am Soc Mass Spectrom. , 19(5), 713-8.

[61] Van Nuijs, A, Tarcomnicu, I, & Covaci, A. (2011). Application of hydrophilic interaction chromatography for the analysis of polar contaminants in food and environmental samples. *Journal of Chromatography A, 1218*, 5964-5974.

[62] Vas, G, & Vekey, K. (2004). Solid-phase microextraction: a powerful sample preparation tool prior to mass spectrometric analysis. J. Mass Spectrom., , 39, 233-254.

[63] Vinod, P. Shah and all, Workshop/Conference Report "Bioanalytical Method Validation-A Revisit with a Decade of Progress", Pharmaceutical Research, 17, (2000). (12)

[64] Viswanathan, C. T, Bansal, S, Booth, B, Destefano, A. J, Rose, M. J, Sailstad, J, Pshah, V. P, Skelly, J. P, Swann, P. G, & Weiner, R. (2007). Workshop/conference report-Quantitative bioanalytical methods validation and implementation: Best practices for chromatographic and ligand binding assays. AAPS Journal, 9 (1):EE42, 30.

[65] Whitehouse, C. M, Dreyer, R. N, Yamashita, M, & Fenn, J. B. (1985). Electrospray interface for liquid chromatographs and mass spectrometers, Whitehouse CM, Dreyer RN, Yamashita M, Fenn JB, Anal.Chem. 57:675

[66] Yamamoto, A, Kakutani, N, Yamamoto, K, Kamiura, T, & Miyakoda, H. (2006). Steroid Hormone Profiles of Urban and Tidal Rivers Using LC/MS/MS Equipped with Electrospray Ionization and Atmospheric Pressure Photoionization Sources. Environ. Sci. Technol., 40 (13), , 4132-4137.

[67] Yang, C, & Henion, J. (2002). Atmospheric pressure photoionization liquid chromatographic-mass spectrometric determination of idoxifene and its metabolites in human plasma. J Chromatogr A. 970(1-2):155-65.

[68] Zhou, S, & Cook, K. D. (2000). Protonation in electrospray mass spectrometry: wrong way round or right-way-round? J Am Soc Mass Spectrom , 11, 961-966.

Chapter 2

A Short Overview of the Components in Mass Spectrometry Instrumentation for Proteomics Analyses

Diogo Ribeiro Demartini

Additional information is available at the end of the chapter

http://dx.doi.org/10.5772/54484

1. Introduction

Mass spectrometry has been widely used for analyses of biomolecules such as proteins. The soft ionization methods available nowadays, the faster and more accurate mass spectrometers, a diversity of protein databases resulting from large scale genome studies and the advances in the bioinformatics field for optimized data mining, altogether significantly contributed to high quality outputs in the proteomics area [1-3].

In order to achieve the higher number of identified proteins (and perhaps quantified), in proteomics studies, some steps are equally important and required: 1) sample preparation; 2) sample pre-fractionation; 3) peptidase digestion; 4) mass spectrometry analysis; 5) data mining. Each of these steps can be extremely challenging and the final conclusions will be based on their success [4-6].

Samples used for proteomics studies are always complex and the abundant proteins mask the low abundance proteins in several cases. Tryptic peptides originated from abundant proteins predominate, no matter what kind of analysis is performed in the mass spectrometer. Highly abundant proteins such as albumin in blood samples, cytoskeleton proteins in pelleted cells, among other examples, need to be removed to allow detection of less abundant ones, and require separate analyses [7]. The same situation happens in plant derived materials, in which the amount of RuBisCO in leaves and of storage proteins in seeds and seedlings mask the non abundant proteins in the samples. To deal with this situation, several approaches can be used. For example, these proteins can be depleted from the source sample by immunoprecipitation. Another strategy used is to create exclusion lists for the mass spectrometer during data analysis. In this case, the selected peptides will be ignored during data acquisition. Another approach widely used is the dynamic exclusion. In this case, according to user definitions, the mass spectrometer will ignore the most abundant peaks in the MS1 (for example, 5), and will analyze the next top 5. However, if the mass spectrometer used is not fast enough during each cycle, important information could be lost [8,9].

A nice example of a proteomic study is the quantification of 1,323 proteins from *Arabidopsis thaliana* chloroplasts, using label-free spectral counting. This was achieved by coupling organelle fractionation (thylakoids and stroma) and different extractions methods, applied to enrich the abundant proteins fraction (ammonium acetate precipitation and alkaline extraction), and analysis of all fraction separately. Protein pre-fractionation using sodium dodecyl sulfate one-dimension polyacrylamide gel electrophoresis and high-resolution mass spectrometry analysis performed with two different machines, also contributed to this high number of identified and quantified proteins [10].

The challenge grows even more when the samples to be analyzed consist of membrane proteins [11]. Membrane proteins usually are highly hydrophobic and in this case chaotropic agents combined with high amounts of detergents are employed to make them soluble. However, these additives can interfere in the trypsin digestion process. The concentration of these agents must be reduced in order to maintain the trypsin activity. In case of *in solution* digestion, besides chaotropes and detergents, reducing and alkylation agents (usually dithiothreitol and iodoacetimide, respectively) must also be removed. These steps, designated as desalting process, can be performed in several ways. Most commonly it involves reverse phase chromatography in which the pH of the digested sample (peptides) is reduced using trifluoroacetic acid, formic acid, or others. The peptides are bound to a C-18 matrix and eluted with increasing concentrations of acetonitrile. After drying the samples under vacuum, they are prepared for mass spectrometry analyses [3,4,12].

The mass spectrometer itself must be correctly chosen to obtain a satisfactory balance between accuracy and speed. Fast scan rates instruments can lose accuracy in their measurements, and *vice versa.*

Tandem mass spectrometry (MS/MS) is a method where the gaseous ions are subjected to two or more sequential stages of mass analysis, which can be separated spatially or temporally, according to their mass to charge ratio, *m/z* [13,14]. The mass analyzers characterize the ions according to their *m/z*. The ion selected in the first stage of analysis is subjected to different reactions and charged products from this reaction are analyzed in a second step (a second mass analyzer or other types of analyzers) [15]. The "reaction" step is critical for data quality and performance.

A brief overview of the most used components in a mass spectrometer applied in proteomics research is discussed, specially focused on the newest researchers on the field.

2. Most used components for mass spectrometers in proteomics analyses

In this section a brief overview of the components of a mass spectrometer used in proteomics will be given.

http://dx.doi.org/10.5772/54484

2.1. Ionization

In order to be analyzed in a mass spectrometer, the sample must be ionized and it is imperative that the ionized molecules (proteins or peptides) turn into a gas phase to allow analysis, fragmentation and detection [14]. The extensive advance of mass spectrometry in protein analyses happened after the advance of the ESI (electrospray ionization) [16], and MALDI (matrix-assisted laser desorption/ionization) ionization methods, which allowed analysis by mass spectrometry to be extended to non-volatile and thermolabile compounds. In both cases, the production of intact molecular ions is achieved under adequate experimental conditions, with minimal fragmentation. Due to this fact, these two ionization processes are referred as soft ionization methods [13,16-18].

2.1.1. Electrospray Ionization (ESI)

Shortly, in electrospray ionization the sample (proteins or peptides) is nebulized when high voltage is applied. As previously said, this ionization process allowed extensive studies on proteomics field because almost no energy is retained by the analyte and, in general, no fragmentation happens during the ionization process [17,18]. Another important aspect is that it generates multiple charges species (specially for ionized peptides), and the *m/z* values are detectable in most mass analyzers [13].

The ionization process is based on a liquid dispersion [14] and the process takes place following three main steps: production of charged droplets, the fission of the charged droplets and production of desolvated ions [13,14,19,20]. The production of charged droplets takes place when high-voltage is applied at the capillary tip where the analyte solution is being injected. At this stage, the electric field causes a separation of the positive and negative charges in the solution containing the analyte. In case of operation in positive ion mode (when the capillary is set at positive potential), the positive ions move towards the counter electrode. It causes an accumulation of positive ions at the surface of the liquid in the tip. The reverse polarity will produce negatively charges. There is a deformation of the meniscus of the liquid in the tip at a critical potential forming the Taylor cone [16,17] which is a static description and does not include spraying behavior [14]. The electric potential applied to the liquid at the tip pulls it into an elliptic shape. However, there is an equilibrium between the surface tension trying to pull the liquid back and the electrostatic attraction which pushes the liquid to the counter electrode [13,14].

The capillary tip is under a constant neutral gas flow, such as nitrogen. In this case, the collision of the gas with the droplet from the tip causes the solvent evaporation, a key step in the ESI method. The second step in the electrospray process is the Rayleigh fission of the droplets. The droplets fission happens when the Coulombic repulsion between the charges is stronger than the surface tension of the liquid, due to a constant decrease of the droplet radius. The limit in which this phenomenon happens is called the Rayleigh limit: the balance between the surface tension and electrostatic attraction is lost. At this stage, the droplets decrease considerably in size and charges states [13,14].

The next step is the solvent evaporation process from the charged droplet forming a gas-phase ion-analyte [13]. Two main mechanisms explain the production of desolvated ions in the gas phase: ion evaporation mechanism and charged residue mechanism. The assumption of the ion evaporation mechanism is that, at a specific time, the electric field on the surface of the droplet is sufficiently high, which causes the emission of the solvated ion from the charged droplet [17,21]. The charged residue mechanism assumes that a series of fission events leads to a final droplet, which contains a single analyte molecule completely free of solvating solvent [17,22].

An important advantage of ESI is that it can be easily coupled with liquid chromatography systems, specially those working at nanoflow range. In a *bottom up* approach, in which the proteins are digested with a peptidase and the resulting peptides are separated in a reverse phase column, the electrospray ionization is widely used. Typical columns used to the separate the complex sample mixture of peptides are made of reverse phase materials (C-18, 3–10 μm diameter) packed into fused silica capillaries (12–100 μm diameter) with sintered silica particles or silicate-polymerized ceramics as frits [5]. The dead volume between the at the end of the column and the ionization region must be as short as possible to avoid peak broadening and mixture of the peptides which were just separated in the reverse phase column. The ESI process is the same when the sample is continuously infused without previous separation in the LC system. In these cases, the flow must be adjusted to higher values to compensate the lack of the packed resin.

A capillary column coupled to a LC system and the ESI process is represented in figure 1A.

2.1.2. Matrix-Assisted Laser Desorption/Ionization (MALDI)

In MALDI analyses, the sample must be mixed with matrix and spotted in a stainless steel plate prior the analysis in the mass spectrometer. The sample is co-crystallized with the matrix, which has an essential function in MALDI. The co-crystallized sample is ionized by short laser pulses (Figure 1B). Subsequently, the ions are accelerated and the time that they spend to flight in a vacuum tube to reach the detector is measured in a TOF (time-of-flight) analyzer [23].

The matrix has to absorb the laser energy via electronic or vibrational excitation and it must also isolate the analyte molecules by diluting during preparation/crystallization preventing their aggregation. Finally, it must be able to perform the sample ionization [24]. The ionization method by MALDI can be divided, according to Zenobi and co-workers, into two main categories. In the "primary ionization", the first ions are generated from neutral molecules, mostly matrix-derived ions. In the "secondary" ionization the ions come mostly from the analyte samples, with few contamination from the matrix [24,25]. The disintegration of the condensed phase by the laser energy has to take place without excessive destructive heating of the embedded analyte molecules. The most straightforward explanation for ions formation in MALDI, assumes that ions from primary ionization result from a laser excitation of an absorbing organic material by molecule multiphoton ionization, which leads to a matrix radical cation [25,26]. The secondary ion formation mechanism take place in the MALDI plume, which is a solid-to-gas phase transition state formed, shortly after the laser pulse

[25-28]. In case of proteins or peptides, the proton transfer mechanism is probably the most important secondary reaction. In most proteomics approaches, samples are spotted in a MALDI plate with acidic matrixes, and data collected in positive mode. Some analytes do not have a high proton affinity, then negative ions could be collected or the sample could be prepared with a more basic matrix [26]. Other important types of secondary reaction mechanisms that take place in the MALDI plume are the cation transfer, electron transfer and electron capture [26].

Ionization by MALDI can be coupled to a liquid chromatography system similar to ESI, however, since the sample must be mixed with the matrix prior analysis, a spotter must be used. MALDI works with wide dynamic ranges [29], such as 2 kDa up to 7 kDa, or more [30]. The dominance of singly charged ions, specially for proteins or peptides with molecular weighs 20 kDa is a characteristic of MALDI, in contrast with ESI which produces much more species in higher charges states [31].

An important advantage of MALDI is that this ionization process is more tolerant to salts and high concentrations of buffer. However, determination of lower masses can be sometimes difficult. This happens because the matrix is also ionized in the process and "flies" in the same range of low molecular masses molecules [32,33]. Most of the matrices used nowadays are small organic molecules, which absorb UV in the range of 266– 355 nm. Nowadays, the number of choices for matrixes is quite small for proteomics analyses, derived from benzoic or cinnamic acid. It is important to point that not all matrixes are useful only for certain all types of analytes [25], causing different ways to prepare the sample.

Different MALDI matrices that can be used according to the type of analytes [24-26,34]. In case of biological samples, some matrixes can be selected [24,35,36]:

a. nicotinic acid: absorption at 266 nm and used for proteins and peptides;

b. 2,5-dihydroxybenzoic acid: absorption 337-353 nm, and can be used for proteins, peptides, carbohydrates and some synthetic polymers;

c. sinapinic acid: absorption 337-353 nm and widely used for proteins and peptides;

d. α-cyano-4-hydroxycinnamic acid: absorption 337-353 nm and mostly used for peptides analyses;

e. 3-hydroxy-picolinic acid: absorption 337-353 and it is suitable for nucleic acids;

When the sample solution is mixed with the matrix, placed/spotted in a MALDI plate, and dried without vacuum, the distribution of the sample is the plate can be quite distorted. However, if vacuum is used to help drying the sample, a better chemical distribution can be achieved in each sample spot [37]. In most cases, the sample preparation is done by the "dried droplet" method, which is quite simple. The sample and the matrix are separately dissolved in a common solvent system (such as 0.1 % trifluoroacetic acid), and then mixed either before or on the MALDI plate. After that, the solvent evaporation will take place, helped or not by a gas flow. By the end, the sample will be co-crystallized with the analyte and will be ready for analyses.

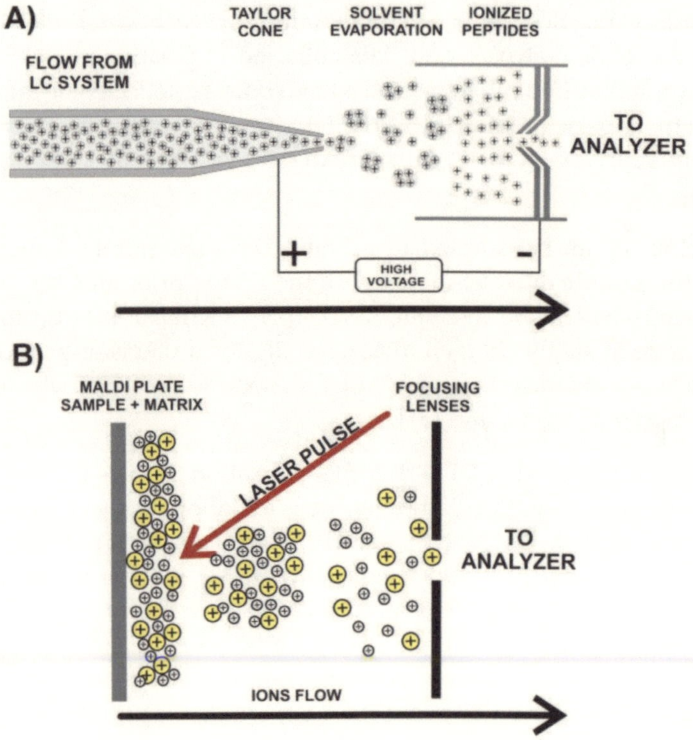

Figure 1. A simplified representation of electrospray ionization (ESI) is represented in **A**. The positively charged droplets and desolvated peptides are represented by the signal +. The superficial tension tends to pull back the charged droplets to the column, while the voltage applied pushes the drop away from the column. The solvent evaporates and the ionized peptides reach the skimmer and go to further analysis. In **B**, the ionization process by matrix-assisted laser desorption/ionization (MALDI) is represented. The laser pulse strikes the MALDI plate, in which the sample is (yellow circles) is co-crystallized with the matrix (grey circles). Either matrix or sample can reach the detector.

2.2. Analyzers

Once the sample is ionized, it enters the mass spectrometer itself. The mass analyzers explore different characteristics of the parent or fragmented ions. In case of tandem experiments, the parent ion must be selected for further fragmentation, and the generated fragment ions will be detected. The combination of two or more analyzers in the same mass spectrometer yielded the high performance and resolution of the nowadays equipments. These characteristics will be briefly detailed ahead.

The main function of a mass analyzer is to separate the ions according to their *m/z* ratio [38], basically by their behavior in electric or magnetic fields [39]. Nowadays, there are few types of analyzers widely used analyzers in tandem mass spectrometry experiments, for proteomics analyses: quadrupole, quadrupole ion trap, time of flight and orbitrap. These analyzers vary in terms of size, price, resolution, mass range, and the ability to perform tandem mass spectrometry experiments.

In case the ions are separated "in space" (time of flight, TOF; sector; quadrupoles), the techniques are called beam techniques, because the ions "travel" across the analyzer in a "pulsed beam" mode. In this case, the MS or MS/MS analyses are performed in separated events. The ion trap analyzers, such as quadruploe ion traps and orbitraps characterize ions based on the frequency of their motion in a defined space [15]. Thus MS and MS/MS events can be performed in the same analyzer, being separated by time and not by "space" [15,40]. The analyzers use magnetic or electric fields, or even combinations of both to select ions. To avoid undesired collisions with neutral gases during analyses, the operation is performed under high vacuum [41].

2.2.1. *Quadrupole mass filter*

A quadrupole analyzer can work as a linear ion trap, in which ions are confined radially by a two-dimensional (2D) radio frequency field, and axially by stopping potentials applied to end electrodes.

A quadrupole mass analyzer is widely used as a "filter" prior fragmentation of the desired ions. Basically it consists of four roods assembled in two pairs, as shown in figure 2A. The first two opposite roods have the same applied voltage, which is different from that of the second two opposite roods establishing a two dimensional quadrupole field in the x-y plane (Figure 2A) [38]. The mass analysis depends on the radio frequency, and direct current voltages which are applied to the four roods [1]. Due to that reason, ions travelling in the quadrupole during analysis will be, at the same time, attracted by one set of roods and repulsed by the second set of roods. Considering the ion population being injected in a quadrupole analyzer, a selection can be made according to their m/z ratio, making some ions to have a stable trajectory in the analyzer, while a considerable number of other ions will not go all the way through (Figure 2A, arrows). The ion path occurs in the z direction, while the attraction and repulsion are occurring simultaneously in the x and y direction (Figure 2A) [38,42]. If the oscillations of an ion are stable, the ion will continue to drift down the rod assembly and reach the detector. The stable ions which "travel" all the analyzer length will go to the next steps, which can be detection, fragmentation and a second round of analysis.

The above explanation is quite simple for a complex situation. In a quadrupole mass filter ions of a single m/z maintain stable trajectories from the ion source to the detector, whereas ions with different m/z values are unable to maintain stable trajectories and do not reach the detector or collision cell [1]. The quadrupole filter is frequently used as mass filter device prior fragmentation in the collision cell, in the case of MS/MS analysis.

2.2.2. *Quadrupole ion trap analyzers*

Another largely employed type of analyzers is the quadrupole ion trap. The quadrupole ion trap devices are found as two-dimension (2D) also known as linear traps, or three dimension (3D) assembly. In case of 2D traps, ions are confined radially by a two-dimensional radio frequency field, and axially by stopping potentials applied to end electrodes. It traps the ions in a two dimensional field. When compared to 3D traps [43], linear traps have higher injection efficiencies and higher ion storage capacities [38]. Besides storing ions, they can be combined with other mass analyzers in hybrid instruments and used to isolate ions of selected mass to charge ratios, to perform tandem mass spectrometry experiments [38,44].

In all cases, the ion trap is able to store either positively and negatively charged ions, or ions of one specific polarity [38]. In short words, the operation mode of an ion trap is quite similar to that of a quadrupole mass filter; the key difference is that a linear quadrupole is mainly used as a mass filter while the three-dimensional quadrupole used as an ion trap [38,39,44,45]. As the name says, these analyzers are able to trap ions for a specific period of time or to an "amount" of accumulated ions. The quadrupole ion traps analyzers are the best suitable to miniaturization among all kinds of mass analyzers, mainly because they tolerate higher pressures and can work at lower voltages. However, the extreme precision in manufacturing these devices and the lower trapping capacities, can be pointed as disadvantages [44].

When the voltage is applied to the electrodes in the trap, a "trapping potential" is formed, which keeps the ions inside the trap [38,42]. In a ion trap, the trajectories of trapped ions of consecutive specific *m/z* rations are affected and become unstable when the field within the trap is changed. The ions leave the trap according to their *m/z* ratio and reach the detector [45].

In case of 3D traps (also known as 3D Paul traps [43]), three shaped electrodes (two hyperbolic and practically identical) compose the quadrupole ion trap. A simple representation of a 3D ion-trap analyzer is shown in figure 2C. In the case of the regular 3D ion trap shown in figure 2C, the hyperbolic geometry is advantage of the ion traps is that they are used as storage chambers, mass analyzers or both [46]. Each of the end-cap electrodes has holes in the center for transmission of electrons and ions. The electrons and ions "entrance" is found in one of the endcaps, while the other one endap is the exit "electrode" through which ions will pass to a detector. The ring electrode has an internal hyperbolical surface and it is positioned symmetrically between the two end-cap electrodes [38,44,47]. These traps have mass selective detection, storage and ejection capabilities [38].

2.2.3. Time of flight analyzer

Another kind of widely used analyzer is the time-of-flight, TOF. Theoretically the mass range in a TOF analyzer is unlimited [48]. However, in practice, the range is limited by the loss of control over the kinetic energy and spatial distributions of the ions with increasing mass as they are injected into the acceleration region of the mass spectrometer. Consequently, the mass accuracy and resolution decrease as the ion mass increases [48,49]. Compared with quadrupole analyzers, the majority of the ions will reach the detector and the lost of ion will not be as expressive as in quadrupole analyzers [39,45].

In TOF analyzers, the desorbed and ionized molecules are accelerated by an electrostatic field and are then ejected through a flight tube under vacuum. In this tube, smaller ions fly faster than larger ions. The detector measures the time of flight for each particular ion. This time to reach the detector depends on the *m/z* of the molecule being analyzed; theoretically, all ions leave the accelerator chamber with the same kinetic energy, and the time to reach the detector will be dependent on the mass of that particular ion (Figure 2B). The ions sepa-

http://dx.doi.org/10.5772/54484

rated by their TOF reach the detector, and a spectrum is presented. Since MALDI produces mostly single charged species, the *m/z* values correspond to the mass of the ion [50].

The TOF analyzer can operate in the linear mode or reflectron mode (presented in Figure 2B). In case of the linear mode, the ions fly in the tube and reach the detector. In case of the reflectron mode, the ions fly towards the reflectron which focuses ions with the same *m/z* values, making these ions reach the detector at the same time. Also, there is an adjustment of the kinetic energy since the ions decelerate and accelerate again inside the reflectron. The results are considerable more accurate in the reflectron mode than in the linear mode [23,50,51].

2.2.4. *Orbitrap*

A couple of years ago, an orbital analyzer, named as the Orbitrap was introduced [40]. The mechanism of analysis is quite different. In an Orbitrap, quoting Michalski and co-workers [52], "the signal is recorded from the image current produced by ion packets which oscillate around and along the spindle-shaped inner electrode of the trap". An extremely simple representation of this principle is shown in figure 2D. This analyzer traps the ions radially around a central spindle electrode. The ion injection is performed perpendicularly to the longer axis of the trap (*z* axis) [40].

In an Orbitrap, the potential distribution of the field is a combination of quadrupole and logarithmic potentials. There are no magnetic or radio frequency fields, so ion stability is achieved exclusively due to ions which orbit around an axial electrode and also perform harmonic oscillations along the electrode [40,53].

The necessity of an external ion storage device prior Orbitrap analysis was pointed by Makarov when the analyzer was developed [53]. In recent years, the common feature of commercially available mass spectrometers which use an Orbitrap as analyzer is that the trap is preceded by the C-trap, which is an external injection device [54]. The process of capturing ions in the C-trap following by the injection into the Orbitrap is fast and can be easily interfaced and synchronized to any external device such as a linear ion trap mass spectrometer or directly to an ion source. The process of detection is considerably longer, since the sensitivity is proportional to the square root of number of detected oscillations [40,53,54]. Since the commercial release of the Orbitrap analyzer, there were several changes to the design of the C-trap and the higher-energy collision induced dissociation, which have improved the efficiency and speed of fragmentation [54].

The high resolution achieved by the Orbitrap helped the fast adoption of this kind of analyzer, which is considered easy to use, robust and shows excellent performance capabilities [55].

2.3. Fragmentation

2.3.1. *Importance of sample preparation for tandem mass spectrometry in proteomics*

There is no doubt that the fragmentation step of a precursor ion is a key point in proteomics analyses since it enables analyzes at the MS/MS or MSn levels. In tandem mass spectrometry analyses, the first analyzer selects the ion(s) which proceeds to a subsequent section, where the excitation and dissociation steps will happen. Tandem mass spectrometry analyses are the result of two or more sequential separations of ions usually coupling two or more mass analyzers [1,39].

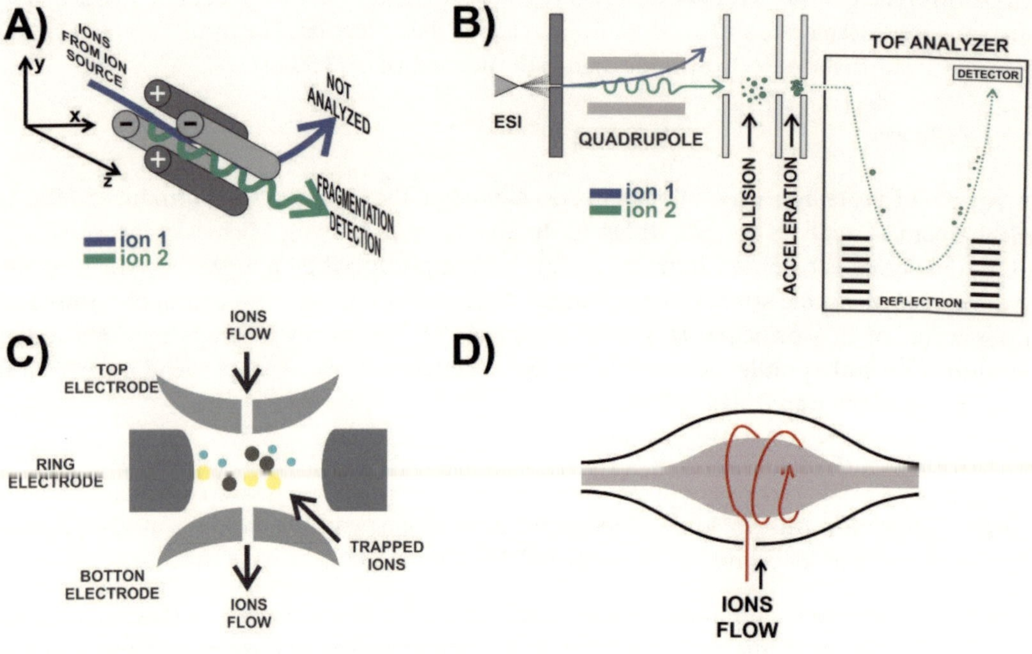

Figure 2. In **A**, there is a representation of a quadrupole mass filter. The ions generated in the ion source migrate through the quadrupole in the *z* direction and at the same time are exposed to simultaneous attraction and repulsion by opposite roods. Ions with stable trajectory are separated in the analyzer and travel all way across (ion 2, green). However, some ions with unstable trajectory are ejected before (ion 1, dark blue). In **B**, the ionization by electrospray and the quadrupole (two roods are shown) and time of flight analyzer is represented. Products from precursor ions previously analyzed and selected for fragmentation (ion 2, green) are accelerated and analyzed in the TOF analyzer. The analyzer might have the reflectron mode or not. The time that the ions spend to travel all way into the TOF is measured and spectrum is recorded. In **C**, the quadrupole ion trap is represented. Ions are trapped for a selected period of time or "amount of ions" before being released. A simple representation of the orbitrap analyzer is presented in **D** in which ions are separated based on their orbital movement around the trap.

A typical workflow for protein identification based on tandem mass spectrometry can be divided in three main steps: reduce sample complexity, perform the mass spectrometry analysis and search the data collected against a protein database. First, it is necessary to reduce complexity of a crude biological sample: several strategies can be used in this step [56]. At the protein level it may include organelle fractionation, protein enrichment by immunopercipitation, removal of abundant proteins and fractionation by sodium dodecyl sulfate polyacrylamide electrophoresis. Multidimensional chromatography is widely used at the peptide at level [57]. The digestion of the proteins present in the sample by a peptidase can be performed in solution or in gel after SDS-PAGE fractionation. In case of liquid chromatography tandem mass spectrometry approach, the peptides from the digested proteins are separated by reverse phase chromatography, ionized by ESI and analyzed by tandem mass spectrometry. Abundant proteins will produce abundant peptides, in most cases. These peptides will be selected for fragmentation regardless the approach, and will mask the low abundant proteins. Besides different strategies used to deal with this situation (exclusion lists, dynamic exclusion, affinity columns), it is still challenging and will not be focused in this chapter. For further reading, please refer to selected references cited ahead [7-10]. The last step is to combine the peptide identification results into a list of proteins that are most likely present in the sample [56,58].

The most used fragmentation methods used in proteomics analyses are briefly discussed ahead.

2.3.2. *Collision Induced Dissociation - CID*

In collision induced dissociation, also known by collision activated dissociation, the excitation of the precursor ion is achieved by energetic collisions with an inert gas, usually helium or argon [59]. In CID, the ions selected in the first analyzer are focused in a reaction or collision cell, which in several cases is a quadrupole [52,60], prior the reaction in gas phase. In case of peptides, precursor ions are dissociated into fragments along the backbone cleaving at the amide bonds [59,61]. Activation of peptides under low-energy collision conditions happens mainly by charge directed reactions [59].

Generally, collisions between the precursor ion and the target gas are accompanied by an increase in the internal energy, which induces decomposition with high probability of fragmentation [62]. The overall process supplies sufficient internal energy to induce covalent bond breakage, and the preferred sites of protonation are the amide bonds of the peptide backbone [62,63]. The protonated amide linkages are weakened and favored to create a series of homologous products ions upon collision-activation. Fragmentation of peptides by CID creates the complementary *b* (in case the charge is retained in the C-terminus) and *y* (in case the charge is retained in the *N*-terminus) ions [64].

The overall CID process can be divided in two steps: the excitation of the precursor ions and their fragmentation/dissociation. The fragmentation of a precursor ion can occur if the collision energy is sufficiently high that the ion is excited beyond its threshold for dissociation. The CID processes can be separated in low and high energy-collisions. Usually, low energy collisions (1-100 eV) is used for organic compounds of moderate masses (hundreds of daltons), while high energy collision (keV range) are produced in TOF/TOF instruments and the CID spectra resulted from low and high energy collisions are considerably different [62].

There are a number of proteins for which the digestion by trypsin will not be a good choice either because it produces too short or too long peptides. In both cases, CID fragmentation will not be effective for them. Collision-induced dissociation is very effective for short and low charged tryptic peptides, usually less than 20 residues and no more that 4 charges [65,66]. In case of posttranslational modification studies, CID helps mostly to identify the sites and types of the modification (such as phosphorylation, acetylation, etc) in a particular protein [66,67]. Even though the sequence of the protein is known, in complexes samples they are not pure. For this reason, individual digestion of the same by two different peptidases and analyses by different fragmentation methods in tandem mass spectrometry approaches is used.

2.3.3. *Electron Capture Dissociation - ECD*

Electron capture dissociation is based on the dissociative recombination of multiply protonated polypeptide molecules with low-energy electrons [68]. The mechanism of ECD is not completely understood, however, in general terms, can be explained as follow. Polypeptide polycations initially capture an electron in a high orbit, followed by a charge neutralization, which leads to an excited radical species that undergoes bond cleavage [64,68]. The radical species dissociates through N–Cα bond cleavages to produce *c*- and *z*-type product ions. The mechanism (s) by which the N–Cα bond cleavages occur is believed that following electron capture, a hydrogen atom is transferred to an amide carbonyl [68-70] or a proton is transferred to an amide anion radical [68,71], both resulting in the formation of an aminoketyl radical intermediate, which dissociates through N–Cα bond cleavages.

Fragmentation in ECD happens at a very high rate, however, the time required for electron capture by precursor ions exceeds the residence time in most mass spectrometers, such as those with TOF and quadrupole analyzers. Another important point is that ECD efficiency is highest for low energy electrons [69], which is difficult to provide in ion traps, for example. For that reason, ECD is mostly used in Fourier transform ion cyclotron resonance mass spectrometry [68].

Electron capture dissociation has been shown advantageous in sequence characterization, *de novo* sequencing, disulphide bond analysis [69,71], and posttranslational modification analyses [68]. The information obtained by ECD is complementary to those obtained by CID in traditional MS/MS methods [68-70]. One important advantage of ECD is to promote a lower energy pathway than CID; even though fragmentation happens, fragile posttranslational modifications are preserved [66].

2.3.4. *Electron Transfer Dissociation - ETD*

The electron-transfer dissociation (ETD) is based on ion/ion chemistry [66,72,73]. It involves transferring an electron from a radical anion to a protonated peptide [72,73], resulting in cleavages at the N-Cα bond of the peptide backbone and preserving most of the posttranslational modifications [66]. Differently from CID, but similar to ECD, ETD creates the complementary *c*- and *z*-type ions. The ETD is widely used for posttranslational modification studies, such as phosphorylation specially because the predominant loss of the phosphate moiety by neutral loss generally precludes further fragmentation.

Different from ECD, in which the primary source of excess energy is the recombination energy released when the electron is captured, in EDT this recombination energy is reduced by the electron binding energy to the anion donor; ETD involves transfer of an electron to the multiply protonated precursor ion from a singly charged radical [64,71]. However, similar to ECD, ETD also induces relatively non-selective cleavage of the N–Cα bond on a peptide's backbone and will produce the *c*- and *z*-product ions [64,66,68]. As ECD, ETD prevents fragile posttranslational modifications from fragmentation [64,66].

The ion/ion chemistry in EDT requires few milliseconds to be completed. Besides that, ETD can be performed with femtomole amount of sample and on a compatible timescale to liquid chromatography and MS analyses. Also, ETD is advantageous in the study of larger peptides, which carry three or more charges. These larger and highly charged peptides offer favorable cleavage conditions during ETD [66]. However, it is important to remember that when working with ETD, a different protease must be used, instead of trypsin, to produce larger peptides (25 aminoacids or more). Longer peptides tend to gain more charges (13 to 16) based on the increased number of basic residues [66]. Endopeptidases Lys-C and Asp-N usually yield longer peptides, and make a good choice with ETD fragmentation [66,73].

3. Concluding remarks

The main idea of this chapter was to provide an overview on the most used components/methods in proteomics analyses employing mass spectrometer. A brief overview on the ionization methods, analyzers and fragmentation was given and can be used as a support for new researches on the field.

Acknowledgements

The author´s research is supported in part by CNPq, CAPES and FAPERGS (Brazil). The author would like to express his gratitude to Dr. Celia Carlini, for critical reading of this chapter.

Author details

Diogo Ribeiro Demartini

Address all correspondence to: diogord@terra.com.br

Department of Biophysics and Center of Biotechnology – Universidade Federal do Rio Grande do Sul, Porto Alegre, RS, Brazil

References

[1] Glish GL, Vachet RW. The Basics of Mass Spectrometry in the Twenty-First Century. Nature Reviews Drug Discovery 2003;2(2) 140-150.

[2] Ong SE, Mann M. Mass Spectrometry-Based Proteomics Turns Quantitative. Nature Chemical Biology 2005;1(5) 252-262.

[3] Wong JW, Cagney G. An Overview of Label-Free Quantitation Methods in Proteomics by Mass Spectrometry. Methods in Molecular Biology (Clifton, N. J.) 2010;604273-283.

[4] Aebersold R, Mann M. Mass Spectrometry-Based Proteomics. Nature 2003;422(6928) 198-207.

[5] Ishihama Y. Proteomic LC-MS Systems Using Nanoscale Liquid Chromatography With Tandem Mass Spectrometry. Journal of Chromatography. A 2005;1067(1-2) 73-83.

[6] Granvogl B, Plöcher M, Eichacker LA. Sample Preparation by in-Gel Digestion for Mass Spectrometry-Based Proteomics. Analytical and Bioanalytical Chemistry 2007;389(4) 991-1002.

[7] Fong KP, Barry C, Tran AN, Traxler EA, Wannemacher KM, Tang HY, Speicher KD, Blair IA, Speicher DW, Grosser T, Brass LF. Deciphering the Human Platelet Sheddome. Blood 2011;117(1) e15-e26.

[8] Muntel J, Hecker M, Becher D. An Exclusion List Based Label-Free Proteome Quantification Approach Using an LTQ Orbitrap. Rapid Communications in Mass Spectrometry 2012;26(6) 701-709.

[9] Zhang Y, Wen Z, Washburn MP, Florens L. Effect of Dynamic Exclusion Duration on Spectral Count Based Quantitative Proteomics. Analytical Chemistry 2009;81(15) 6317-6326.

[10] Ferro M, Brugiere S, Salvi D, Seigneurin-Berny D, Court M, Moyet L, Ramus C, Miras S, Mellal M, Le GS, Kieffer-Jaquinod S, Bruley C, Garin J, Joyard J, Masselon C, Rolland N. AT_CHLORO: A Comprehensive Chloroplast Proteome Database With Subplastidiallocalization and Curated Information on Envelope Proteins. Molecular & Cellular Proteomics: MCP 2010;9(6) 1063-1084.

[11] Seigneurin-Berny D, Rolland N, Garin J, Joyard J. Differential Extraction of Hydrophobic Proteins From Chloroplast Envelope Membranes: A Subcellular-Specific Proteomic Approach to Identify Rare Intrinsic Membrane Proteins. Plant Journal 1999;19(2) 217-228.

[12] Bantscheff M, Schirle M, Sweetman G, Rick J, Kuster B. Quantitative Mass Spectrometry in Proteomics: a Critical Review. Analytical and Bioanalytical Chemistry 2007;389(4) 1017-1031.

[13] Banerjee S, Mazumdar S. Electrospray Ionization Mass Spectrometry: a Technique to Access the Information Beyond the Molecular Weight of the Analyte. International Journal of Analytical Chemistry 2012;20121-40.

[14] Wilm M. Principles of Electrospray Ionization. Molecular & Cellular Proteomics: MCP 2011;10(7) 1-8.

[15] Glish GL, Burinsky DJ. Hybrid Mass Spectrometers for Tandem Mass Spectrometry. Journal of the American Society for Mass Spectrometry 2008;19(2) 161-172.

[16] Fenn JB, Mann M, Meng CK, Wong SF, Whitehouse CM. Electrospray Ionization for Mass Spectrometry of Large Biomolecules. Science 1989;246(4926) 64-71.

[17] Gabelica V, De PE. Internal Energy and Fragmentation of Ions Produced in Electrospray Sources. Mass Spectrometry Reviews 2005;24(4) 566-587.

[18] Goodlett DR, Yi EC. Proteomics Without Polyacrylamide: Qualitative and Quantitative Uses of Tandem Mass Spectrometry in Proteome Analysis. Functional and Integrative Genomics 2002;2(4-5) 138-153.

[19] Chen P. Electrospray Ionization Tandem Mass Spectrometry in High-Throughput Screening of Homogeneous Catalysts. Angewandte Chemie - International Edition 2003;42(25) 2832-2847.

[20] Murphy RC, Barkley RM, Berry KZ, Hankin J, Harrison K, Johnson C, Krank J, McAnoy A, Uhlson C, Zarini S. Electrospray Ionization and Tandem Mass Spectrometry of Eicosanoids. Analytical Biochemistry 2005;346(1) 1-42.

[21] Iribarne JV, Dziedzic PJ, Thomson BA. Atmospheric Pressure Ion Evaporation-Mass Spectrometry. International Journal of Mass Spectrometry and Ion Physics 1983;50(3) 331-347.

[22] Schmelzeisen-Redeker G, Bütfering L, Röllgen FW. Desolvation of Ions and Molecules in Thermospray Mass Spectrometry. International Journal of Mass Spectrometry and Ion Processes 1989;90(2) 139-150.

[23] Wieser A, Schneider L, Jung J, Schubert S. MALDI-TOF MS in Microbiological Diagnostics-Identification of Microorganisms and Beyond (Mini Review). Applied Microbiology and Biotechnology 2012;93(3) 965-974.

[24] Dreisewerd K. The Desorption Process in MALDI. Chemical Reviews 2003;103(2) 395-426.

[25] Zenobi R, Knochenmuss R. Ion Formation in MALDI Mass Spectrometry. Mass Spectrometry Reviews 1998;17(5) 337-366.

[26] Knochenmuss R, Zenobi R. MALDI Ionization: the Role of in-Plume Processes. Chemical Reviews 2003;103(2) 441-452.

[27] Zhigilei LV, Garrison BJ. Velocity Distributions of Analyte Molecules in Matrix-Assisted Laser Desorption From Computer Simulations. Rapid Communications in Mass Spectrometry 1998;12(18) 1273-1277.

[28] Zhigilei LV, Garrison BJ. Velocity Distributions of Molecules Ejected in Laser Ablation. Applied Physics Letters 1997;71(4) 551-553.

[29] Benk AS, Roesli C. Label-Free Quantification Using MALDI Mass Spectrometry: Considerations and Perspectives. Analytical and Bioanalytical Chemistry 2012;404(4) 1039-1056.

[30] Reyzer ML, Caprioli RM. MALDI Mass Spectrometry for Direct Tissue Analysis: a New Tool for Biomarker Discovery. Journal of Proteome Research 2005;4(4) 1138-1142.

[31] Trimpin S, Inutan ED, Herath TN, McEwen CN. Matrix-Assisted Laser Desorption/Ionization Mass Spectrometry Method for Selectively Producing Either Singly or Multiply Charged Molecular Ions. Analytical Chemistry 2010;82(1) 11-15.

[32] Suckau D, Resemann A, Schuerenberg M, Hufnagel P, Franzen J, Holle A. A Novel MALDI LIFT-TOF/TOF Mass Spectrometer for Proteomics. Analytical and Bioanalytical Chemistry 2003;376(7) 952-965.

[33] Smith SA, Blake TA, Ifa DR, Cooks RG, Ouyang Z. Dual-Source Mass Spectrometer With MALDI-LIT-ESI Configuration. Journal of Proteome Research 2007;6(2) 837-845.

[34] Debois D, Smargiasso N, Demeure K, Asakawa D, Zimmerman TA, Quinton L, De PE. MALDI In-Source Decay, From Sequencing to Imaging. Topics in Current Chemistry 2012.

[35] Hillenkamp F, Karas M. The MALDI Process and Method. In: MALDI MS. Wiley-VCH Verlag GmbH & Co. KGaA; (2007). 1-28

[36] Tholey A, Heinzle E. Ionic (Liquid) Matrices for Matrix-Assisted Laser Desorption/Ionization Mass Spectrometry-Applications and Perspectives. Analytical and Bioanalytical Chemistry 2006;386(1) 24-37.

[37] Chang WC, Huang LC, Wang YS, Peng WP, Chang HC, Hsu NY, Yang WB, Chen CH. Matrix-Assisted Laser Desorption/Ionization (MALDI) Mechanism Revisited. Analytica Chimica Acta 2007;582(1) 1-9.

[38] March RE. Quadrupole Ion Traps. Mass Spectrometry Reviews 2009;28(6) 961-989.

[39] El-Aneed A, Cohen A, Banoub J. Mass Spectrometry, Review of the Basics: Electrospray, MALDI, and Commonly Used Mass Analyzers. Applied Spectroscopy Reviews 2009;44(3) 210-230.

[40] Hu Q, Noll RJ, Li H, Makarov A, Hardman M, Graham CR. The Orbitrap: a New Mass Spectrometer. Journal of Mass Spectrometry 2005;40(4) 430-443.

[41] Schaeffer-Reiss C. A Brief Summary of the Different Types of Mass Spectrometers Used in Proteomics. Methods in Molecular Biology (Clifton, N. J.) 2008;4843-16.

[42] Douglas DJ, Konenkov NV. Trajectory Calculations of Space-Charge-Induced Mass Shifts in a Linear Quadrupole Ion Trap. Rapid Communications in Mass Spectrometry 2012;26(18) 2105-2114.

[43] Paul W. Electromagnetic Traps for Charged and Neutral Particles. Reviews of Modern Physics 1990;62(3) 531-540.

[44] Ouyang Z, Gao L, Fico M, Chappell WJ, Noll RJ, Cooks RG. Quadrupole Ion Traps and Trap Arrays: Geometry, Material, Scale, Performance. European Journal of Mass Spectrometry (Chichester, England) 2007;13(1) 13-18.

[45] March RE. Quadrupole Ion Trap Mass Spectrometry: a View at the Turn of the Century. International Journal of Mass Spectrometry 2000;200(1ΓÇô3) 285-312.

[46] McAlister GC, Phanstiel D, Good DM, Berggren WT, Coon JJ. Implementation of Electron-Transfer Dissociation on a Hybrid Linear Ion Trap-Orbitrap Mass Spectrometer. Analytical Chemistry 2007;79(10) 3525-3534.

[47] Douglas DJ, Frank AJ, Mao D. Linear Ion Traps in Mass Spectrometry. Mass Spectrometry Reviews 2005;24(1) 1-29.

[48] Lee J, Chen H, Liu T, Berkman CE, Reilly PT. High Resolution Time-of-Flight Mass Analysis of the Entire Range of Intact Singly-Charged Proteins. Analytical Chemistry 2011;83(24) 9406-9412.

[49] Lee J, Reilly PTA. Limitation of Time-of-Flight Resolution in the Ultra High Mass Range. Analytical Chemistry 2011;83(15) 5831-5833.

[50] Croxatto A, Prod'hom G, Greub G. Applications of MALDI-TOF Mass Spectrometry in Clinical Diagnostic Microbiology. FEMS Microbiology Reviews 2012;36(2) 380-407.

[51] Bonk T, Humeny A. MALDI-TOF-MS Analysis of Protein and DNA. Neuroscientist. 2001;7(1) .

[52] Michalski A, Damoc E, Lange O, Denisov E, Nolting D, Muller M, Viner R, Schwartz J, Remes P, Belford M, Dunyach JJ, Cox J, Horning S, Mann M, Makarov A. Ultra High Resolution Linear Ion Trap Orbitrap Mass Spectrometer (Orbitrap Elite) Facilitates Top Down LC MS/MS and Versatile Peptide Fragmentation Modes. Molecular & Cellular Proteomics: MCP 2012;11(3) O111.

[53] Makarov A. Electrostatic Axially Harmonic Orbital Trapping: a High-Performance Technique of Mass Analysis. Analytical Chemistry 2000;72(6) 1156-1162.

[54] Makarov A, Scigelova M. Coupling Liquid Chromatography to Orbitrap Mass Spectrometry. Journal of Chromatography. A 2010;1217(25) 3938-3945.

[55] Kelstrup CD, Young C, Lavallee R, Nielsen ML, Olsen JV. Optimized Fast and Sensitive Acquisition Methods for Shotgun Proteomics on a Quadrupole Orbitrap Mass Spectrometer. Journal of Proteome Research 2012;11(6) 3487-3497.

[56] Hernandez P, Muller M, Appel RD. Automated Protein Identification by Tandem Mass Spectrometry: Issues and Strategies. Mass Spectrometry Reviews 2006;25(2) 235-254.

[57] Washburn MP, Wolters D, Yates JR. Large-Scale Analysis of the Yeast Proteome by Multidimensional Protein Identification Technology. Nature Biotechnology 2001;19(3) 242-247.

[58] Coon JJ, Syka JEP, Shabanowitz J, Hunt DF. Tandem Mass Spectrometry for Peptide and Protein Sequence Analysis. Biotechniques 2005;38(4) 519-523.

[59] Paizs B, Suhai S. Fragmentation Pathways of Protonated Peptides. Mass Spectrometry Reviews 2005;24(4) 508-548.

[60] Boersema PJ, Mohammed S, Heck AJR. Phosphopeptide Fragmentation and Analysis by Mass Spectrometry. Journal of Mass Spectrometry 2009;44(6) 861-878.

[61] Hunt DF, Yates JR, Shabanowitz J, Winston S, Hauer CR. Protein Sequencing by Tandem Mass Spectrometry. Proceedings of the National Academy of Sciences of the United States of America 1986;83(17) 6233-6237.

[62] Sleno L, Volmer DA. Ion Activation Methods for Tandem Mass Spectrometry. Journal of Mass Spectrometry 2004;39(10) 1091-1112.

[63] Shukla AK, Futrell JH. Tandem Mass Spectrometry: Dissociation of Ions by Collisional Activation. Journal of Mass Spectrometry 2000;35(9) 1069-1090.

[64] Palumbo AM, Smith SA, Kalcic CL, Dantus M, Stemmer PM, Reid GE. Tandem Mass Spectrometry Strategies for Phosphoproteome Analysis. Mass Spectrometry Reviews 2011;30(4) 600-625.

[65] Mikesh LM, Ueberheide B, Chi A, Coon JJ, Syka JE, Shabanowitz J, Hunt DF. The Utility of ETD Mass Spectrometry in Proteomic Analysis. Biochimica Et Biophysica Acta 2006;1764(12) 1811-1822.

[66] Wiesner J, Premsler T, Sickmann A. Application of Electron Transfer Dissociation (ETD) for the Analysis of Posttranslational Modifications. Proteomics 2008;8(21) 4466-4483.

[67] Miller K, Hao Z, Zhang T, Huhmer A. Alternating Real-Time Data Dependent ETD and CID for Improved Protein Coverage by LC/MS on a Linear Ion Trap Mass Spectrometer. Molecular & Cellular Proteomics: MCP 2006;5(10) .

[68] Zubarev RA. Electron-Capture Dissociation Tandem Mass Spectrometry. Current Opinion in Biotechnology 2004;15(1) 12-16.

[69] Kalli A, Hess S. Electron Capture Dissociation of Hydrogen-Deficient Peptide Radical Cations. Journal of the American Society for Mass Spectrometry 2012;23(10) 1729-1740.

[70] Zubarev RA, Haselmann KF, Budnik B, Kjeldsen F, Jensen F. Towards an Understanding of the Mechanism of Electron-Capture Dissociation: a Historical Perspective and Modern Ideas. European Journal of Mass Spectrometry 2002;8(5) 337-349.

http://dx.doi.org/10.5772/54484

[71] Simons J. Mechanisms for S-S and N-Cα Bond Cleavage in Peptide ECD and ETD Mass Spectrometry. Chemical Physics Letters 2010;484(20) 81-95.

[72] Kim MS, Pandey A. Electron Transfer Dissociation Mass Spectrometry in Proteomics. Proteomics 2012;12(4-5) 530-542.

[73] Syka JE, Coon JJ, Schroeder MJ, Shabanowitz J, Hunt DF. Peptide and Protein Sequence Analysis by Electron Transfer Dissociation Mass Spectrometry. Proceedings of the National Academy of Sciences of the United States of America 2004;101(26) 9528-9533.

Section 2

Molecular Characterization by Mass Spectrometry

Chapter 3

Contribution of Mass Spectrometry to the Study of Antimalarial Agents

Ana Raquel Sitoe, Francisca Lopes, Rui Moreira,
Ana Coelho and Maria Rosário Bronze

Additional information is available at the end of the chapter

http://dx.doi.org/10.5772/56225

1. Introduction

Mass spectrometry (MS) has become a powerful analytical tool for qualitative and quantitative applications, providing information about the structure and purity of compounds, and also about the chemical composition of complex samples.

The most recent applications of mass spectrometry are oriented towards biochemical applications such as proteome, metabolome and drug discovery. During the last decade, mass spectrometry has progressed rapidly and an evolution has been observed in the type of applications, software and equipments. Atmospheric pressure ionization sources are now used, an analyser based on a new concept (the orbitrap) was recently developed, existing ones were modified, and new hybrid instruments were developed using combinations of different analysers, depending on applications. One of the major trends was the transition to high resolution/accurate mass analysis, made routine by new MS instruments. The use of separation techniques as gas chromatography (GC), liquid chromatography (LC) and capillary electrophoresis (CE) coupled with mass spectrometry and tandem mass spectrometry, expanded the interest in this methodology.

In this chapter are presented general aspects related with characteristics of mass spectrometry equipments. The contribution of this technique to new discoveries concerning one of the major infectious diseases in man, malaria, is also discussed.

2. Basics of mass spectrometry

Mass spectrometry is a technique used to analyse from small inorganic molecules to biological macromolecules and relies on the formation of gas-phase ions (positively or negatively charged) that are isolated based on their mass-to–charge ratio (m/z). In order to achieve this state, the sample must be volatilized and this may become a problem to biological samples, as biomolecules have usually high molecular mass and high polarity, factors that limit their volatility.

All mass spectrometers share common components as an ionization source, a mass analyser and a detector (Fig. 1). As there are available equipments with different specifications, even from the same supplier, it is necessary to choose carefully the most adequate equipment for each type of application.

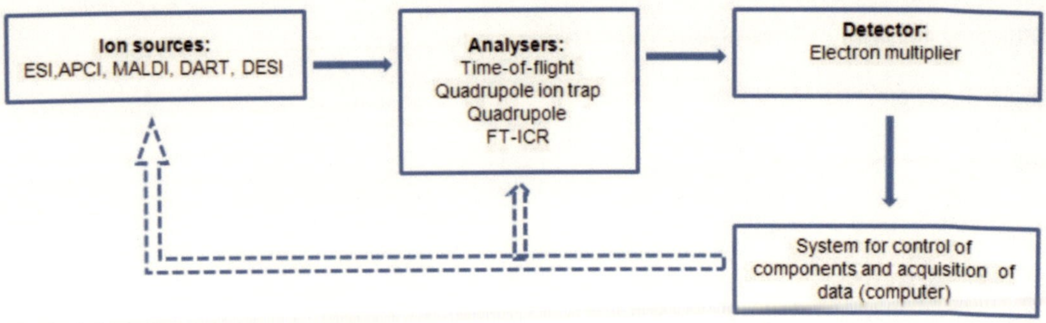

Figure 1. Basic components in a mass spectrometer. ESI, electrospray ionization, APCI, atmospheric-pressure chemical ionization; MALDI, Matrix-Assisted Laser Desorption ionization; DESI: Desorption Electrospray Ionization ; DART: Direct Analysis in Real Time; FT-ICR: Fourier transform ion cyclotron resonance (adapted from Glish & Vachet, 2003)

In order to achieve this state, the sample must be volatilized and this may become a problem to biological samples, as biomolecules have usually high molecular mass and high polarity, factors that limit their volatility.

Different ionization techniques may be used in mass spectrometry equipments, depending on the need of molecule disruption for the induction of ion formation. These techniques may perform strong and soft ionization processes. Soft ionization methods, like fast atomic bombardment (FAB), liquid secondary ion mass spectrometry (LSIMS), matrix-assisted laser desorption ionization (MALDI) and electrospray ionization (ESI) allow the detection of molecular ions and are more suitable for the analysis of biomolecules and non-purified analytes. The ions are generated by protonation, deprotonation or formation of adducts. In table 1 are summarized some of the main characteristics of the most used ionization methods.

The use of FAB is useful to assign the molecular ion peaks. The sample is dissolved in a suitable liquid matrix, with low vapour pressure (e.g. diethanolamine, triethanolamine, glycerol, thioglycerol or 3-nitrobenzyl alcohol), inserted into the mass spectrometer and bombarded with high energy argon or xenon atoms, providing efficient means to analyze polar, ionic, thermally labile, energetically labile, and high molecular mass compounds (El-Aneed et al., 2009).

Ionization method	Analytes	Sample introduction	Mass range	Type of ionization
FAB	Organometallic compounds	Direct injection, LC	<5000 Da	Soft
MALDI	Biomolecules	Sample co-crystallized with a matrix	500-500 000 Da	Very soft. Generates mainly single charged ions
ESI	Organic and inorganic compounds	Direct injection, LC	Large range	Softer than MALDI. Generates multiple charged ions
DESI	Small non-polar and large polar molecules (peptides and proteins)	Analysis of a surface	Large range	Generates single or multiple charged molecular ions from small or large analytes
DART	Low molecular mass compounds	Analysis of a surface	Less broad than DESI	Simple mass spectra (molecular ion)

Table 1. Characteristics of the most used ionization sources. FAB: Fast Atomic Bombardment; MALDI: Matrix Assisted Laser Desorption Ionization; ESI: Electrospray Ionization; DESI: Desorption Electrospray Ionization ; DART: Direct Analysis in Real Time

In MALDI, ions are produced by pulsed-laser irradiation (e.g. nitrogen lasers) of the sample co-crystallized with an organic matrix (e.g. gentisic, sinapic or ferulic acid) and operating in the vacuum or more recently, at atmospheric pressure. MALDI ionization uses a low amount of sample but low molecular mass molecules (below 500 Da) are difficult to analyse, due to strong interferences of the organic matrix ions.

The development of other soft ionization techniques has become crucial to the analysis of biomolecules dissolved in a mixture of water and a volatile organic solvent (e.g. methanol, acetonitrile). Techniques as ESI and MALDI make MS methodologies versatile as both techniques accomplish the conversion into gas-phase ions of non-volatile and thermally labile large molecules, allowing the study of biological compounds. Both techniques produce protonated peptide and protein ions, deprotonated deoxyribonucleic acids (DNA) and ribonucleic acids (RNA). Some reviews have been published on the covalent and non-convalent interactions between drug molecules with DNA and RNA, protein and enzyme targets for drug action and toxicity (Feng, 2004). When using ESI, proteins are ionized as they have several sites of protonation or deprotonation, and this multiple charging enables mass spectrometers with limited *m*/*z* ranges to analyse higher molecular mass molecules. However, ion suppression may occur when solutions contain high concentrations of salt, or when the target analytes are present in low concentration in matrices with high content of other analytes. Strategies based on the type of analyte, ionization reaction, ionization efficiency, analyte solution composition and pH, have been described for producing positive or negative ion modes when operating with an ESI source (Feng, 2004). APCI, is less susceptible to matrix interferences from salts, and is used for monitoring weakly polar compounds. However, labile compounds can be thermally decomposed, and due to its high sensitivity, the solvents used with this technique must have higher purity.

DART and DESI are well established open-air ionization techniques, as no sample preparation is required, making these techniques suitable for screening a large number of samples (Fernández et al., 2006). The DART ion source produces a heated stream of protonated reactant ions and the analytes in the sample are ionized, producing protonated molecules $[M+H]^+$ or deprotonated molecules $[M-H]^-$ in the open air of the laboratory environment, making possible the analysis of organic compounds directly, in real time, without time-consuming analytical protocols and destruction of the sample. The method may detect concentrations of analytes as low as femtomole (Arnaud, 2007). Due to these characteristics, DART has become an ionization method useful for rapid screening of pharmaceutical products. In DESI analysis, a high-speed charged liquid spray is directed to the sample (Takats et al., 2005). The DESI spray dissolves the material from the sample and the charged droplets are sampled downstream by a mass spectrometer. Desolvation and evaporation from these droplets creates ions that will generate a mass spectrum of the sample components.

Following the ionization process, the selected ions are extracted, accelerated, and analyzed. A mass analyser is characterized by its mass range limit, analysis speed, transmission, mass accuracy and resolution, expressed as full width at half maximum (FWHM). The most used analysers and their characteristics are summarized in Table 2.

Quadrupoles are widely used mass analysers, where ions are separated according to the stability of their trajectories in the oscillating electric fields applied between the four parallel rods. The QTOF, a hybrid quadrupole time of flight mass spectrometer, is a high-resolution mass spectrometer with MS/MS capability, and has been often used in drug studies (Nyunt et al., 2005). FT-ICR is also a high resolution and high mass accuracy analyser that enables the study of the binding of ligands (drugs) to RNA targets (Hofstadler et al., 1999; Masselon et al., 2000). The Orbitrap mass analyzer employs electrostatic trapping and it bears similarities to FT-ICR as both belong to the same Fourier Transform MS (FTMS) family of instruments. Orbitrap mass spectrometry is expected to provide maximum resolving powers of 100,000–200,000. A modified Orbitrap instrument has shown that this technology is capable of a resolution of 1,000,000 for $m/z < 300–400$, which makes it compatible to be used with chromatographic separation techniques (Denisov et al., 2012).

Tandem mass spectrometry (MS^n) development was crucial for the structural analysis of compounds. In tandem experiments, a molecular ion is selectively isolated and fragmented in a controlled environment. With this type of analysers, it is possible to perform different types of experiments (e.g. parent scan, daughter scan, neutral loss) and data obtained, will allow to identify or quantify the analytes, even in complex matrices (e.g. natural product extracts and biological fluids). Multiple Reaction Monitoring (MRM), has become an important tool, used for quantification purposes, allowing an increment of methods specificity and sensitivity.

Finally the signal obtained in the detector will produce a mass spectrum, the x-coordinate represents m/z values and the y-axis indicates total ion counts.

	Quadrupole	Ion Trap	Time-of-flight	Time-of-flight reflectron	Magnetic sector	Fourrier Transform ion cyclotron resonance	Fourrier Transform Orbitrap
Symbol	Q	IT	TOF	TOF	B	FT-ICR	FT-OT
Principle of separation	*m/z* (trajectory stability)	*m/z* (resonance frequency)	Velocity (flight time)	Velocity (flight time)	Momentum	m/z (resonance frequency)	m/z (resonance frequency)
Mass limit (Th)	4 000	6 000	>1 000 000	4 000	20 000	30 000	50 000
Resolution FWHM (m/z 1000)	2 000	4 000	5 000	20 000	100 000	500 000	100 000
Accuracy (ppm)	100	100	200	10	<10	<5	<5
Ion sampling	continuous	pulsed	pulsed	pulsed	continuous	pulsed	pulsed
Pressure (Torr)	10^{-5}	10^{-3}	10^{-6}	10^{-6}	10^{-6}	10^{-10}	10^{-10}
Tandem mass spectrometry	MS/MS Fragments Precursors Neutral loss Low-energy collision	MS^n Fragments Low-energy collision	-------	MS/MS Fragments Low-energy collision	MS/MS Fragments Precursors Neutral loss High-energy collision	MS^n Fragments Low-energy collision	-------

Table 2. Comparison of mass analysers (adapted from Hoffmann & Stroobant, 2002)

Liquid chromatography coupled to mass spectrometry (Triple Quadrupole TQ, QTOF, Linear ionTrap and Linear QTRAP analyzers) is today a well established methodology used due to its high sensitivity, speed, selectivity, versatility and ease of automation. Recently the advantages of using mass spectrometry in comprehensive liquid chromatography (LC X LC system) have been discussed and different applications have been described for pharmaceutical compounds (Donato et al., 2012).

3. An overview of malaria

Malaria is caused by *Plasmodium* parasites, which are transmitted through the bite of an infected female *Anopheles* mosquito, and remains one of the major infectious disease in man.

Five species from the genus *Plasmodium* namely: *P. falciparum*, *P. vivax P. ovale*, *P. malariae*, and *P. knowlesi* cause infection in humans. Of these, *P. falciparum* and *P. vivax* account for more than 95% of malaria cases in the world, with *P. falciparum*, being responsible for most of the deaths caused by malaria every year. The species of human malaria differ in the periodicity of their life cycle, as well as in the outcomes of the disease. Generally clinical manifestations can include fever, chills, prostration and anemia. Severe disease can include delirium, metabolic acidosis, cerebral malaria and multi-organ system failure, coma and death may ensue. (Kantele & Jokiranta, 2011)

The World Health Organization (WHO) estimated 225 million cases of malaria and about 800,000 deaths worldwide in 2010 (WHO, 2010). Due to the rapid evolution and spread of multi-resistant parasites to the current antimalarial drugs, both, chemotherapy and prophylaxis are at risk of impairment. Malaria is most prevalent in developing countries of tropical areas such as sub-Saharan Africa, East Asia and South America (Rodrigues et al., 2010; Eisenstein, 2012).

3.1. Life cycle of the malaria parasite

The malaria parasite exhibits a complex life cycle (Fig. 2) involving an insect vector (mosquito) and a vertebrate host (human). It includes an asexual cycle in humans, encompassing an asymptomatic liver-stage, a symptomatic blood-stage and a sexual cycle in a mosquito.

The liver or hepatic stage (A) is initiated when sporozoites injected through the bite of a mosquito travel to the liver and infect hepatocytes, where a clinically silent asexual multiplication takes place, generating thousands of merozoites. The release of merozoites into the bloodstream (B) marks the beginning of the erythrocytic stage of infection (C), during which parasites infect red blood cells, undergo repeated asexual replication cycles, and give rise to clinical illness. Some merozoites differentiate into gametocytes (D) that can be taken up by the mosquito during a posterior blood meal. Within the mosquito, gametocytes undergo a sexual development to form sporozoites that migrate to the salivary glands and can infect another host trough another bite (E).

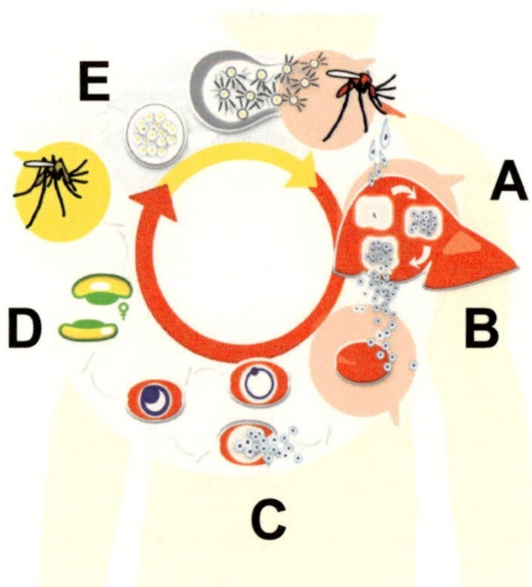

Figure 2. *Plasmodium* life cycle

3.2. Agents with antimalarial activity

The public health problem of malaria has been addressed by different approaches (Biot et al., 2012):

- use of insecticides to control the mosquito vector, but mosquitoes are developing resistance to insecticides;
- vaccines, but in spite of all the efforts there is yet not available a vaccine that effectively targets the parasite;
- chemotherapy to control malaria has relied mainly on a restricted number of chemically related drugs belonging to either the quinoline or the antifolate groups.

Increasing resistance of *P. falciparum* to the commonly used drugs is recognized as one of the major problems in eradication of the disease. The severe malaria situation underscores the continuing need of research for new classes of antimalarial agents with new mechanisms of action or re-utilization of the existing drugs with new types of therapies. The existing drug armamentarium is insufficient to answer the call for malaria eradication. The first line of treatment for malaria currently relies on a single class, the artemisinins. To overcome this problem scientists are exploring many approaches, targeting different stages of the parasite life cycle, to find agents that will prevent, cure or eliminate malaria. (Hobbs, C. & Duffy, P., 2011)

Many antimalarial agents contain a 4-aminoquinoline, 8-aminoquinoline or quinolone methanol scaffolds (Rosenthal, 2001). Chloroquine and amodiaquine are 4-aminoquinolines used to treat and prevent malaria, while primaquine is the single 8-aminoquinoline clinically approved to treat relapsing malaria caused by *P. vivax*. Mefloquine (Fig. 3) is a quinoline methanol antimalarial structurally similar to quinine, the first pure substance used to treat malaria and extracted from the bark of the cinchona tree. Other relevant classes of antimalarial agents include the antifolates (e.g. pyrimethamine and proguanyl), phenanthrene methanols (e.g. halofantrine), and naphthoquinones (e.g. atovaquone). More recently, artemisinin (Fig. 3), a sesquiterpene lactone isolated from the *Artemisia annua* chinese herb, and its analogues were a major breakthrough in malaria chemotherapy because they produce a very rapid therapeutic response, particularly against multidrug-resistant *Plasmodium falciparum* malaria.
With exception of primaquine, (Vale et al., 2009) most available antimalarials are active against the blood stage of the disease. However to achieve the eradication goal, new compounds with new modes of action are needed to block parasite transmission and eliminate the asymptomatic and latent hepatic forms. (Rodrigues et al., 2012) A strategy used to address this major goal is to combine two chemotypes - each one targeting a specific stage of the parasite's life cycle in a single chemical entity, to develop effective hybrid antimalarials capable of killing both the blood and liver-stage parasites with identical efficacy. (Capela et al., 2011)

4. Study of antimalarials agents by mass spectrometry

Structural and stability information is fundamental for any drug study, including antimalarials. In fig. 3 are presented currently available antimalarial drugs. Due to the rapid emergence and spread of resistant parasites to well-established antimalarial drugs, there is an urgent need for novel drugs. Studies performed on new antimalarial compounds using mass spectrometry are scarce but are useful for the elucidation of structures, also for prediction of compound stability and properties, isomer characterization, and detection of counterfeit products. Furthermore, studies using this technique coupled to chromatographic methods have been conducted for the evaluation of pharmacokinetics, metabolite identification, and detection of impurities.

4.1. Structural elucidation

One of the main applications of mass spectrometry is the structural elucidation of molecules. Based on the molecular ion peaks and their fragmentation patterns, the structure of compounds can then be proposed.

Among the different equipments that can be used for these purposes, FAB ion sources are frequently described. Applications can be found in the study of the oxidation products of primaquine, 5,5-di-[6-methoxy-8-(4-amino-1-butyl amino)] quinoline (PI), 6-methoxy-5,8-di-[4-amino-1-methyl butyl amino] quinoline (PII) and 5,5-di-[7-hydroxy-6-methoxy-8(4-amino-1-methyl butylamino)] quinoline (PIII) (Fig. 4) (Sinha & Dua 2004). The mass spectrum of PI with molecular formula $C_{30}H_{40}N_6O_2$ presents the molecular ion at *m/z* 517 confirming the molecular mass of the compound, and a fragment at *m/z* 500 is detected due to the presence of a terminal amino group at position 4′.

An LC-MS/MS method was developed for the analysis of bulaquine (BQ) 3-[1-[4-[(6-methoxy-8-quinolinylamino] pentylamino] ethylidene]dihydro-2 (3H)-furanone (Fig. 5) and its metabolite primaquine in monkey plasma. Protonated species at *m/z* 370 and 260 were detected for bulaquine and primaquine, respectively. MS/MS conditions were optimized generating product ions through fragmentation of the molecular ions. Based on the fragmentation spectra obtained from $[M+H]^+$ under the established analytical conditions, a fragmentation pattern was presented for these compounds. This type of study is important to establish analytical conditions for the quantification of drugs and their metabolites in biological fluids. (Nitin et al., 2003)

An ESI-Ion trap mass spectrometer was used to perform MS^n analyses, in the study of imidazolidin-4-one peptidomimetic derivatives of primaquine. (Vale et al., 2008a)

4.2. Pharmacokinetic studies

Pharmacokinetic (PK) studies provide a mathematical basis to assess the time course of drug in the body. It enables to quantify absorption, distribution, metabolism and excretion of the drug and their metabolites. The primary requirement to undertake a PK study, is to have an

http://dx.doi.org/10.5772/56225

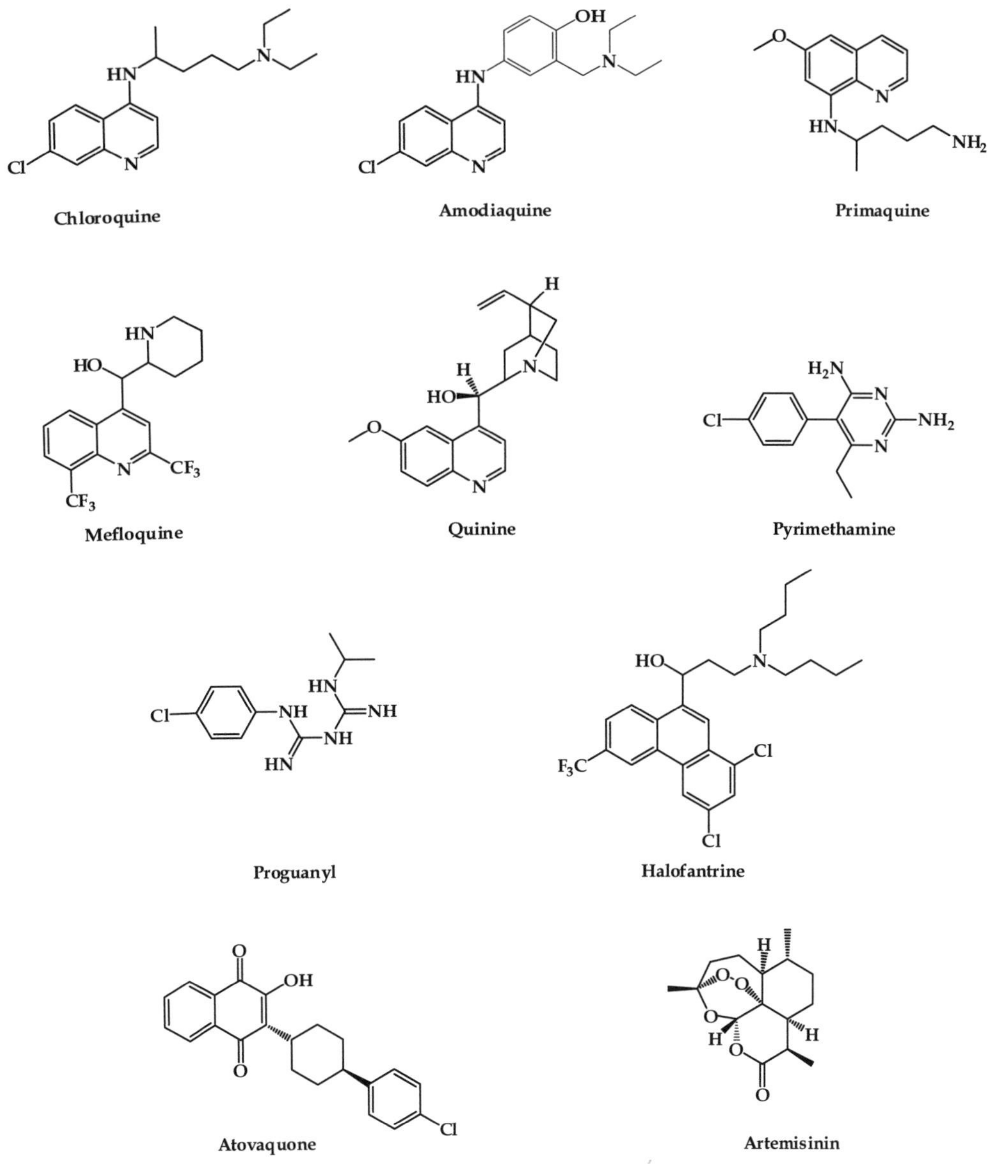

Figure 3. Currently available antimalarial drugs

analytical method which is reliable, reproducible, sensitive, selective, and if possible, compatible with high-throughput pharmacokinetic approaches.

Drug efficacy requires adequate drug concentration at the site of action. Monitoring drugs and their metabolites in biological samples (*in vivo* studies), is fundamental in order to control the intake of the antimalarials by the infected populations. Mass spectrometry has been successfully used for this purposes, coupled with liquid chromatography, and analytical methods

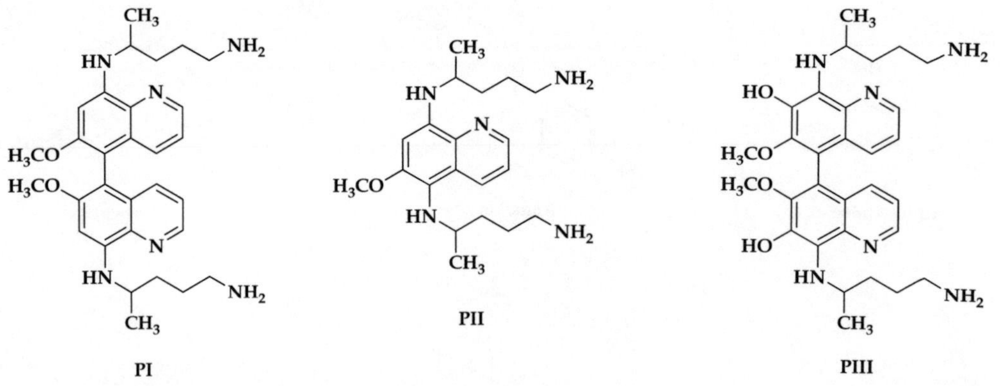

Figure 4. The oxidative antimalarial primaquine analogous (PI, PII and PIII)

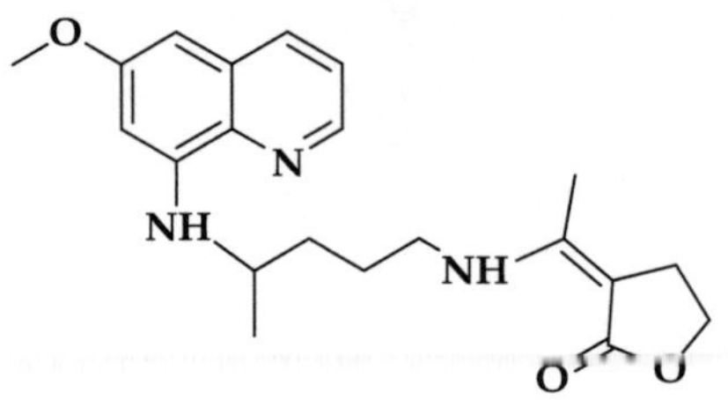

Figure 5. Bulaquine

have been optimized and validated for quantification of different drugs and metabolites in biological fluids.

A LC-MS/MS method was used to study 14 antimalarial drugs, which are the components of the current first-line combination treatments for malaria (artemether, artesunate, dihydroartemisinin, amodiaquine, N-desethyl-amodiaquine, lumefantrine, desbutyl-lumefantrine, piperaquine, pyronaridine, mefloquine, chloroquine, quinine, pyrimethamine and sulfadoxine). The best conditions for mass spectrometry analysis were optimized (Hodel et al., 2009) and the method developed was implemented, and used to analyse samples from an *in vivo* study with 125 Southeast Asian patients from two regions of Cambodia: one region with a high level of antimalarial drug resistance and another region with moderate levels of drug resistance (Hodel et al., 2010). The 14 antimalarial drugs were measured in plasma samples from the patients, and results showed that for half of them, an antimalarial drug was detected namely mefloquine, piperaquine, chloroquine or quinine. However all patients reported either not having taken any antimalarial before or not knowing to have taken. These results are important, as they show that it is urgent to ensure appropriate use of antimalarials among the populations.

Tafenoquine (8-[(4-amino-1-methylbutyl)amino]-2,6-dimethoxy-4-methyl-5-(3-trifluoromethyl-phenoxy) quinoline succinate) (Fig. 6) was measured in human plasma from patients and

http://dx.doi.org/10.5772/56225

healthy volunteers during a clinical efficacy trial, using a LC-MS/MS equipment.(Doyle et al., 2002)

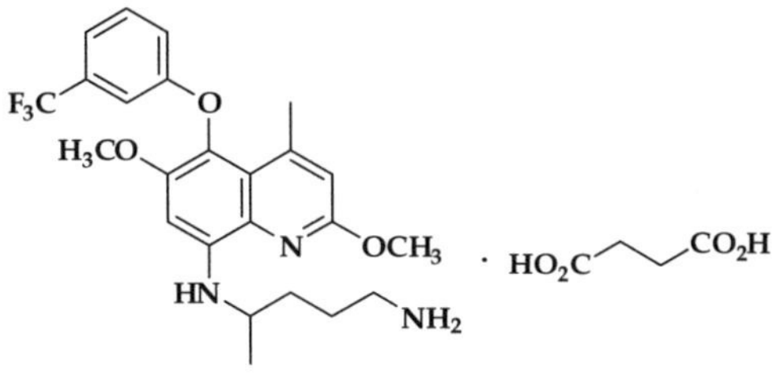

Figure 6. Tafenoquine

For NPC1161 (Fig. 7), an 8-aminoquinoline analog *(8-[(4-amino-1-methylbutyl)amino]-5-[3,4-dichloro-phenoxyl]-4-methyl-quinoline)* and their metabolites, a LC-MS method using an electrospray ionization source and a TOF analyzer, was implemented.

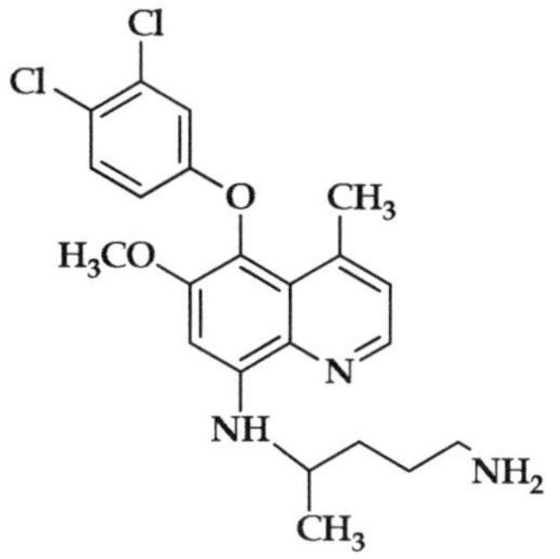

Figure 7. NPC1161, an 8-aminoquinoline analog

Using mass spectrometry other antimalarial molecules as α-/β-diastereomers of arteether (AE), sulphadoxine (SDX) and pyrimethamine (PYR) (Sabarinath et al., 2006) and three novel trioxane antimalarials (Fig. 8) (Singh et al., 2008) were determined in rat plasma. A *N*-alkylamidine compound, M64, and its corresponding bioprecursors were measured in human and rat plasma (Margout et al., 2011) (Fig. 9). Artemisinin class compounds and its active *in-vivo* metabolites were analysed in monkey plasma (Singh et al., 2009).

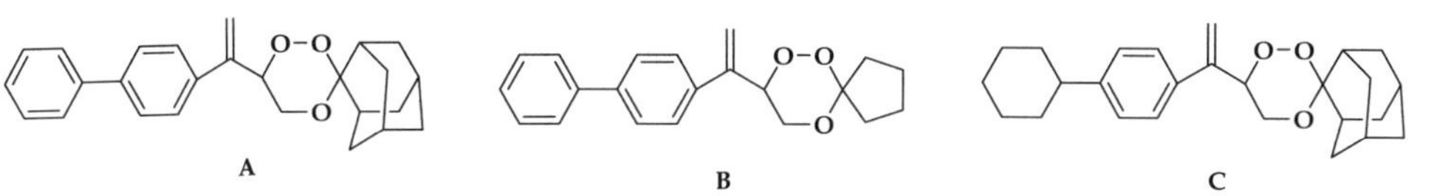

Figure 8. Chemical structures of three novel trioxane antimalarials

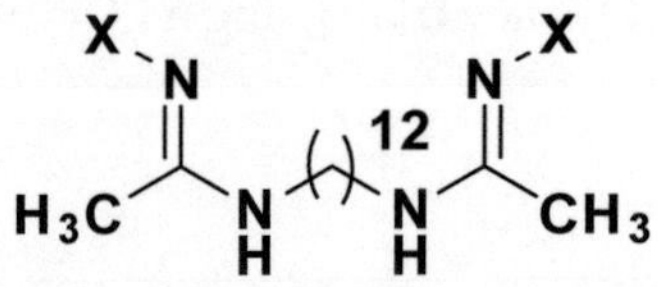

M64, X=H; M64AH, X=OH; M64-S-Me, X=OSO_2CH_3

Figure 9. Chemical structures of compound, M64, and its corresponding bioprecursors

A method was also developed and validated according to FDA guidelines for simultaneous determination of two mono-thiazolium compounds in plasma, whole blood and red blood cells from human and rat (Taudon et al., 2008). More recently a rapid (3 min analysis) and sensitive UPLC-MS/MS method using a triple quadrupole tandem mass spectrometer in positive ESI mode, has been implemented for the analysis of ARB-89 (7α-hydroxy artemisinin carbamate) (Fig. 10) in rat serum, for pharmacokinetics studies, (Pabbisetty et al., 2012).

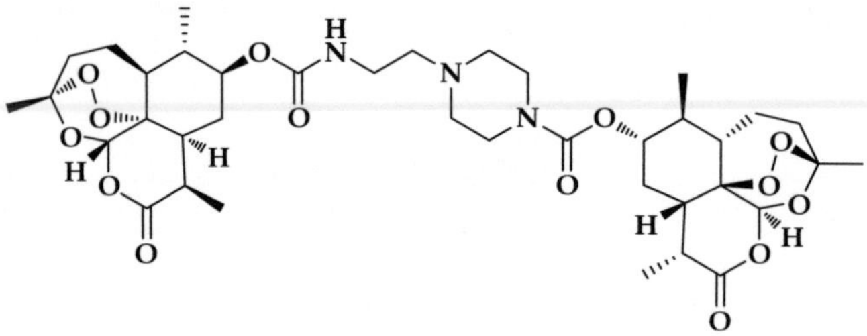

Figure 10. ARB-89 (7α-hydroxy artemisinin carbamate)

Mass spectrometry has proven to be particularly useful in identifying complex metabolites as those arising from phase I (e.g. those involving cytochrome P450 monooxygenases) and phase II (e.g. conjugation with glucuronic acid, sulfonates, glutathione or amino acids) reactions. In a study published by Liu et al., 2011, metabolites of artemisinin, also known as Qing-hao-su (QHS), and its active derivative dihydroartemisinin (DHA) were identified in *in vitro* and *in vivo* biological samples using a LTQ-Orbitrap mass spectrometer in tandem with H/D exchange. The authors were able to show that artemisinin drugs mainly undergo hydroxylation and loss of oxygen in the phase I metabolic pathway and can form glucuronides in the phase II processes, as shown in Fig. 11. Based on MS data it was proposed a metabolic pathway for these metabolites.

Piperaquine was synthesized for the first time about 50 years ago, but seems to be a suitable partner drug in artemisinin-based combination treatments. In a paper published by Tarning et al., 2006, the main metabolites of piperaquine were characterized in a 16-h human urine, after a single p.o. administration of a fixed combination of dihydroartemisinin-piperaquine, with a fatty meal. A LC method in tandem with a QTRAP system was used to analyse piperaquine and its metabolites and a FT-ICR/MS equipment was used to obtain mass spectra

http://dx.doi.org/10.5772/56225

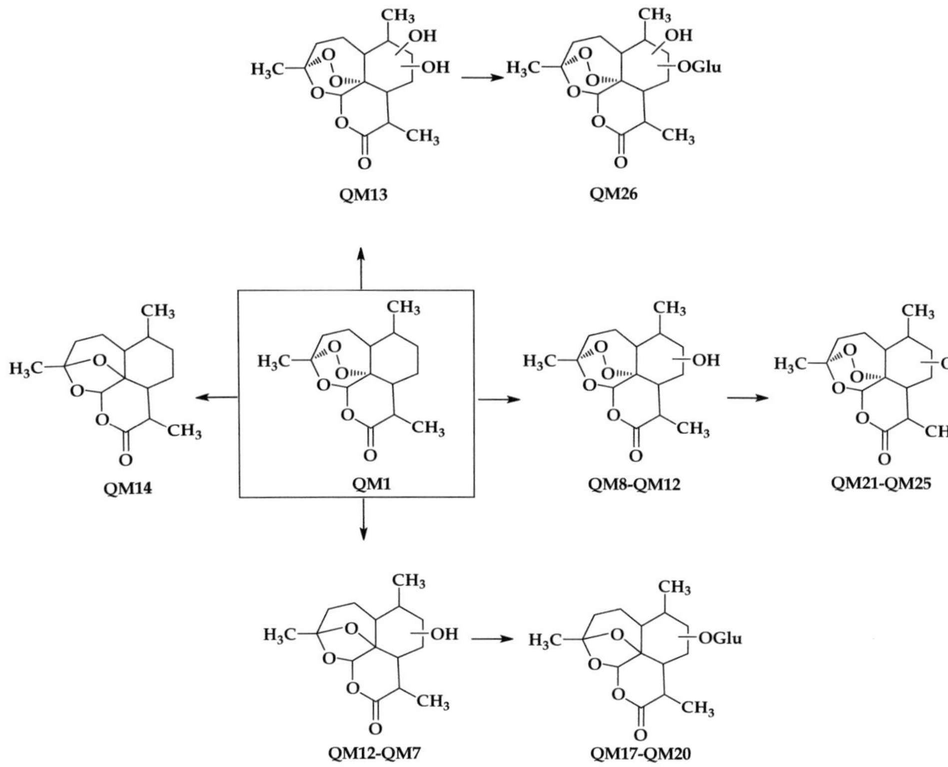

Figure 11. Proposed metabolic pathways for QHS *in vitro* and *in vivo* (Liu et al., 2011)

of the five metabolites of piperaquine in urine samples. Two of the metabolites (a carboxylic and a mono N-oxidated piperaquine metabolite) were considered as the most relevant as they were detected in the serum/plasma samples collected up to 93 days, and also in urine 123 days after administration of the drug. Other two monohydroxylated metabolites and a di-N-oxidized metabolite were also detected in urine samples.

4.3. Detection of impurities

A major impurity (8-(4-amino-4-methylbutylamino)-6 methoxyquinoline) associated with primaquine drug samples (Fig.12), obtained from European Pharmacopoeia and other commercial sources, was detected by gas chromatography-electron impact-mass spectrometry (GC–EI-MS) (Dongre et al., 2005).

4.4. Chemical stability studies

Mass spectrometry can also be conducted in order to contribute to study the properties of compounds, through knowledge of their stability and fragmentation mechanisms, under the gas-phase conditions of a mass spectrometer. This type of studies can have, in the future, important implications in drug analysis and development.

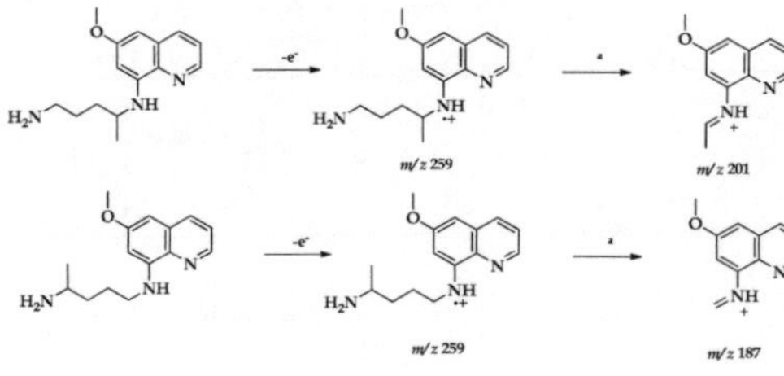

Figure 12. Fragmentation pattern of primaquine and the corresponding impurity

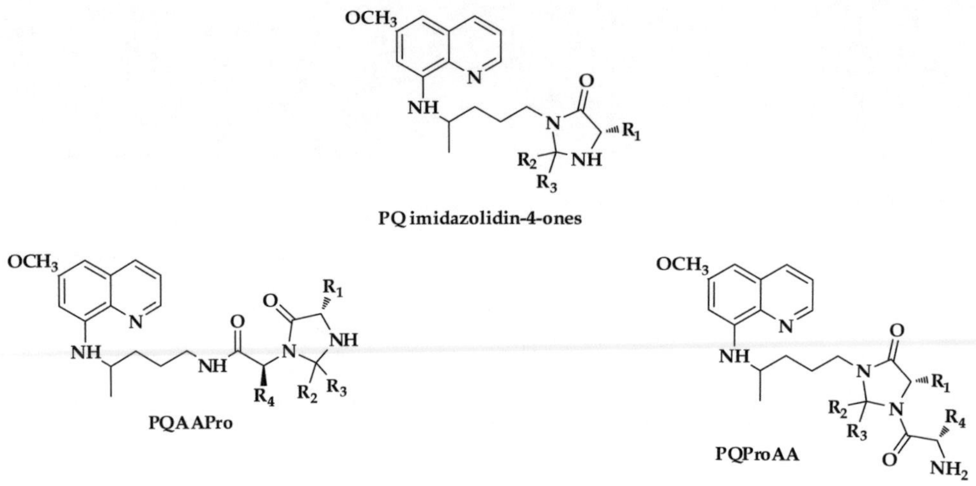

Figure 13. PQ imidazolidin-4-ones, PQAAPro and PQProAA mimetic derivatives of primaquine

Studies on primaquine derived imidazolidin-4-ones using an ESI-ion trap mass spectrometer have allowed to find a correlation between the stability of the ions in the nozzle-skimmer region during the CID (Collision Induced Dissociation) analyses and reactivity in both isotonic buffer and human plasma (Vale et al., 2008). The same authors (Vale et al., 2008a) studied imidazolidin-4-one peptidomimetic derivatives of primaquine, PQAAPro and PQProA (Fig. 13) and they also found the parallelism between compound reactivity to hydrolysis and stability during CID analysis. Using CID and MS/MS experiments to study the peptidomimetic imidazolidin-4-one derivatives of primaquine, it was possible to conclude that CID spectra reflected the reactivity of compounds under physiological conditions, and the relative abundances of MS/MS generated fragments were correlated with the Charton steric parameters associated to amino acid side chain in the molecule (Vale et al., 2009).

From the results obtained, ESI-MS proved to be a reliable tool for stability prediction of compounds towards hydrolysis at physiological pH and temperature although the mechanisms in water and in the gas-phase are not comparable. This type of studies were, for the first time, approached by these authors.

4.5. Detection of counterfeit drugs

The quality of commercially available drugs varies among countries. The WHO/International Medical Products Anti-Counterfeiting Taskforce estimates that in some less developed countries, the counterfeit drugs are up to 50% of the total drugs supplied to the populations(Hall et al., 2006). Due to the lack of regulations and poor quality control practices, the amount of the active ingredient may be incorrect, as a result of chemical degradation that occurs due to poor storage conditions, especially in warm and humid tropical environments. In some cases, expired drugs are repackaged with new expiration dates and put in the market. Also some drugs can be contaminated or replaced by other substances and people consume sawdust, paint and other toxic or inert substances (Kaur et al., 2009).

The report published by WHO in 2011, about the quality of antimalarial drugs in 6 countries of sub-Saharan Africa (Cameroon, Ethiopia, Ghana, Kenya, Nigeria and the United Republic of Tanzania) resumes the results obtained from the analysis of 935 samples and gives an idea about the quality and counterfeits that more often occur.

As an incorrect intake can result in a low bioavailability of the drug in the individual, leading to drug-resistance strains, provoking a therapeutic failure, reliable methods of analysis must be available to determine the quality of antimalarials commercialized, and LC coupled with mass spectrometry can be used. However this technique is expensive, requires training, technological support, and sample preparation. Actually, DART (Fernández et al., 2006) and DESI (Haiss et al., 2007) methodologies are often used, as they produce results rapidly, because they do not require sample preparation. Results obtained from a DESI MS method were used to validate Fourier-transform infrared imaging for characterization of counterfeit antimalarial pharmaceutical in tablets (Ricci et al., 2007). A DESI MS method was also applied for the quantitative screening of counterfeit antimalarial tablets containing artesunate (Nyadong et al., 2008), and more recently DESI and DART methods were used to validate results from the application of FT-Raman spectroscopy for *in situ* screening for potentially counterfeit artesunate antimalarial tablets (Ricci et al., 2008).

4.6. Rapid diagnosis of malaria

The rapid diagnosis of malaria infection can also be performed by mass spectrometry. Hemozoin, the malaria pigment, can be detected by laser desorption mass spectrometry (LDMS) in human blood. (Scholl et al., 2004) Detection of malaria in 45 asymptomatic pregnant Zambian women was performed by this technique. Detection of *Plasmodium falciparum* malaria during pregnancy is complicated by sequestration of parasites in the placenta reducing peripheral blood microscopic detection. LDMS was able to detect <10 parasites/uL cultured in human blood and provided a more rapid mean of screening for infection than the technique used currently for this purpose, light microscopy (Nyunt et al., 2005).

5. Conclusions

The information obtained from the use of mass spectrometry in the study of antimalarials agents is important, in order to understand all the mechanisms of the illness, malaria, and the way the different drugs interact in the human organism. Due to its characteristics (sensitivity, speed, possibility to be automated, possibility to combine with separation techniques) and diversity of equipments available, mass spectrometry can be used in the structural identification of new molecules, in the study of many phases of drug discovery, for assessment of compound stability, pharmacokinetic studies monitoring the concentrations of antimalarials and metabolites in biological matrices, the studies of cell permeability and plasma protein binding, and finally, in the quality control of commercial drugs.

The use of mass spectrometry to predict stability of compounds in physiological conditions may become an important tool.

Author details

Ana Raquel Sitoe[1], Francisca Lopes[1], Rui Moreira[1], Ana Coelho[2] and Maria Rosário Bronze[1,2]

1 Research Institute for Medicines and Pharmaceutical Sciences (iMed.UL), Faculty of Pharmacy, University of Lisbon, Portugal

2 Instituto de Tecnologia Química e Biológica, Oeiras, Portugal

References

[1] Arnaud, C. H. (2007). Taking mass spec into the open: Open-air ionization methods minimize sample pre and widen range odf mass spectrometry applications. Chemical & Engineering News , 85(41), 13-18.

[2] Biot, C, Castro, W, & Navarro, M. (2012). The therapeutic potential of metal-based antimalarial agents: Implications for the mechanism of action. Dalton Transactions , 41(21), 6335-6349.

[3] Capela, R, Cabal, G. G, Rosenthal, P. J, Gut, J, Mota, M. M, Moreira, R, Lopes, F, & Prudêncio, M. (2011). Design and Evaluation of Primaquine-Artemisinin Hybrids as a Multistage Antimalarial Strategy. Antimicrobial Agents and Chemotherapy , 55(10), 4698-4706.

[4] Denisov, E. Damoc; Lange, O. & Makarov, A. ((2012). Orbitrap mass spectrometry with resolving powers above 1,000,000. International Journal of Mass Spectrometry 325-327(0), 80-85.

[5] Donato, P. Cacciola; Tranchida, F.P.; Dugo, P. & Mondello, L. ((2012). Mass spectrometry detection in comprehensive liquid chromatography: basic concepts, instrumental aspects, applications and trends. Mass Spectrometry Reviews , 31(5), 523-559.

[6] Dongre, V. G, Karmuse, P. P, Nimbalkar, M. M, Singh, D, & Kumar, A. (2005). Application of GC-EI-MS for the identification and investigation of positional isomer in primaquine, an antimalarial drug. Journal of Pharmaceutical and Biomedical Analysis 39(1-2), 111-116.

[7] Doyle, E, Fowles, S. E, Summerfield, S, & White, T. J. (2002). Rapid determination of tafenoquine in small volume human plasma samples by high-performance liquid chromatography-tandem mass spectrometry. Jounal of Chromatography B Analytical Technologies Biomedical Life Sciences , 769(1), 127-132.

[8] Eisenstein, M. (2012). Drug development holding Holding out for reinforcements. Nature 484(7395): SS18., 16.

[9] El-Aneed, A, Cohen, A, & Banoub, J. (2009). Mass Spectrometry, Review of the Basics: Electrospray, MALDI, and Commonly Used Mass Analyzers. Applied Spectroscopy Reviews , 44(3), 210-230.

[10] Feng, W. Y. (2004). Mass spectrometry in drug discovery: a current review. Current Drug Discovery Technologies , 1(4), 295-312.

[11] Fernández, F. M, Cody, R. B, Green, M. D, Hampton, C. Y, Mcgready, R, Sengaloundeth, S, White, N. J, & Newton, P. N. (2006). Characterization of Solid Counterfeit Drug Samples by Desorption Electrospray Ionization and Direct-analysis-in-real-time Coupled to Time-of-flight Mass Spectrometry. ChemMedChem , 1(7), 702-705.

[12] Glish, G. L, & Vachet, R. W. (2003). The basics of mass spectrometry in the twenty-first century. Nature Reviews Drug Discovery , 2(2), 140-150.

[13] Haiss, W, Thanh, N. T, Aveyard, J, & Fernig, D. G. (2007). Determination of size and concentration of gold nanoparticles from UV-vis spectra. Analytical Chemistry , 79(11), 4215-4221.

[14] Hall, K. A, & Newton, P. N. Green, M.D; De Veij, M; Vandenabeele, P.; Pizzanelli, D.; Mayxay, M.; Dondorp, A. & Fernandez, F.M. ((2006). Characterization of counterfeit artesunate antimalarial tablets from southeast Asia. The American Journal Tropical Medicine and Hygiene , 75(5), 804-811.

[15] Hobbs, C, & Duffy, P. (2011). Drugs for malaria: something old, something new, something borrowed. F1000 Biology Reports, 3(24), 1-9.

[16] Hodel, E. M, Genton, B, Zanolari, B, Mercier, T, Duong, S, Beck, H. P, Olliaro, P, Decosterd, L. A, & Ariey, F. (2010). Residual antimalarial concentrations before treatment in patients with malaria from Cambodia: indication of drug pressure. Journal of Infectious Diseases , 202(7), 1088-1094.

[17] Hodel, E. M, Zanolari, B, Mercier, T, Biollaz, J, Keiser, J, Olliaro, P, Genton, B, & Decosterd, L. A. LC-tandem mass spectrometry method for the simultaneous determination of 14 antimalarial drugs and their metabolites in human plasma. Journal of Chromatography B , 877(10), 867-886.

[18] Hoffmann, E, & Stroobant, V. (2002). Mass Spectrometry: Principles and Applications, John Wiley & Sons, 3rd Edition, 978-0-47003-310-4HB), Great Britain.

[19] Hofstadler, S. A, Sannes-lowery, K. A, Crooke, S. T, Ecker, D. J, Sasmor, H, Manalili, S, & Griffey, R. H. (1999). Multiplexed screening of neutral mass-tagged RNA targets against ligand libraries with electrospray ionization FTICR MS: a paradigm for high-throughput affinity screening. Analytical Chemistry , 71(16), 3436-3440.

[20] Kantele, A, & Jokiranta, T. S. (2011). Review of Cases With the Emerging Fifth Human Malaria Parasite, Plasmodium knowlesi. Clinical Infectious Diseases , 52(11), 1356-1362.

[21] Kaur, H, Green, M. D, Hostetler, M. D, & Fernández, F. M. Paul N Newton ((2009). Antimalarial drug quality: methods to detect suspect drugs. Therapy , 7(1), 49-57.

[22] Liu, T, Du, F, Wan, Y, Zhu, F, & Xing, J. (2011). Rapid identification of phase I and II metabolites of artemisinin antimalarials using LTQ-Orbitrap hybrid mass spectrometer in combination with online hydrogen/deuterium exchange technique. Journal of Mass Spectrometry , 46(8), 725-733.

[23] Margout, D, Gattacceca, F, Moarbess, G, & Wein, S. Tran van Ba, C.; Le Pape, S.; Berger, O.; Escale, R.; Vial, H. J. & Bressolle, F. M. ((2011). Pharmacokinetic properties and metabolism of a new potent antimalarial N-alkylamidine compound, M64, and its corresponding bioprecursors. European Journal of Pharmaceutical Sciences 42(1-2), 81-90.

[24] Masselon, C, Anderson, G, Harkewicz, R, Bruce, J. E, Pasa-tolic, L, & Smith, R. D. (2000). Accurate Mass Multiplexed Tandem Mass Spectrometry for High-Throughput Polypeptide Identification from Mixtures. Analytical Chemistry , 72(8), 1918-1924.

[25] Nitin, M, Rajanikanth, M, Lal, J, Madhusudanan, K. P, & Gupta, R. C. (2003). Liquid chromatography-tandem mass spectrometric assay with a novel method of quantitation for the simultaneous determination of bulaquine and its metabolite, primaquine, in monkey plasma. Journal of Chromatography B , 793(2), 253-263.

[26] Nyadong, L, Late, S, Green, M. D, Banga, A, & Fernández, F. M. (2008). Direct Quantitation of Active Ingredients in Solid Artesunate Antimalarials by Noncovalent Complex Forming Reactive Desorption Electrospray Ionization Mass Spectrometry. Journal of the American Society for Mass Spectrometry , 19(3), 380-388.

[27] Nyunt, M, Pisciotta, J, Feldman, A. B, Thuma, P, Scholl, P. F, Demirev, P. A, Lin, J. F, Shi, L, Kumar, N, & Sullivan, D. J. (2005). Detection of Plasmodium falciparum in pregnancy by laser desorption mass spectrometry. The American Journal of Tropical Medicine and Hygiene , 73(3), 485-490.

[28] Pabbisetty, D, Illendula, A, Muraleedharan, K. M, Chittiboyina, A. G, Williamson, J. S, Avery, M. A, & Avery, B. A. (2012). Determination of antimalarial compound,

ARB-89 (7β-hydroxy-artemisinin carbamate) in rat serum by UPLC/MS/MS and its application in pharmacokinetics. Journal of Chromatography B 889-890(0), 123-129.

[29] Ricci, C, Nyadong, L, Fernandez, F. M, Newton, P. N, & Kazarian, S. G. (2007). Combined Fourier-transform infrared imaging and desorption electrospray-ionization linear ion-trap mass spectrometry for analysis of counterfeit antimalarial tablets. Analytical and Bioanaytical Chemistry , 387(2), 551-559.

[30] Ricci, C, Nyadong, L, Yang, F, Fernandez, F. M, Brown, C. D, Newton, P. N, & Kazarian, S. G. (2008). Assessment of hand-held Raman instrumentation for in situ screening for potentially counterfeit artesunate antimalarial tablets by FT-Raman spectroscopy and direct ionization mass spectrometry. Analytica Chimica Acta , 623(2), 178-186.

[31] Rodrigues, T, Moreira, R, & Lopes, F. (2010). New hope in the fight against malaria? Future Medicinal Chemistry , 3(1), 1-3.

[32] Rodrigues, T, Prudêncio, M, Moreira, R, Mota, M. M, & Lopes, F. (2012). Targeting the liver stage of malaria parasites: a yet unmet goal. J Med Chem , 55(3), 995-1012.

[33] Rosenthal, P. J. (2001). Antimalarial chemotherapy: mechanisms of action, resistance, and new directions in drug discovery, Springer-Science+Business Media, LLC, New Jersey.

[34] Sabarinath, S, Singh, R. P, & Gupta, R. C. (2006). Simultaneous quantification of α-/β-diastereomers of arteether, sulphadoxine and pyrimethamine: A promising anti-relapse antimalarial therapeutic combination, by liquid chromatography tandem mass spectrometry. Journal of Chromatography B , 842(1), 36-42.

[35] Scholl, P. F, Kongkasuriyachai, D, Demirev, P. A, Feldman, A. B, Lin, J. S, Sullivan, D. J, & Kumar, N. (2004). Rapid detection of malaria infection in by laser desorption mass spectrometry. The American Journal of Tropical Medicine and Hygiene, 71(5), 2004, 546-551.

[36] Singh, R. P, Sabarinath, S, & Gautam, N. Gupta, R. C & Singh, SK. ((2009). Liquid chromatographic tandem mass spectrometric assay for quantification of 97/78 and its metabolite 97/63: a promising trioxane antimalarial in monkey plasma. Journal of Chromatography B Analytical Technolologies and Biomedical Life Sciences , 877(22), 2074-2080.

[37] Singh, R. P, Sabarinath, S, Singh, S. K, & Gupta, R. C. (2008). A Sensitive and selective liquid chromatographic tandem mass spectrometric assay for simultaneous quantification of novel trioxane antimalarials in different biomatrices using sample-pooling approach for high throughput pharmacokinetic studies. Journal of Chromatography B, 864(1-2), 52-60.

[38] Sinha, S. N. & V. K. Dua (2004). Fast atom bombardment mass spectral analysis of three new oxidative products of primaquine. International Journal of Mass Spectrometry , 232(2), 151-163.

[39] Takats, Z, Wiseman, J. M, et al. (2005). Ambient mass spectrometry using desorption electrospray ionization (DESI): instrumentation, mechanisms and applications in forensics, chemistry, and biology. Jounal of Mass Spectrometry , 40(10), 1261-1275.

[40] Tarning, J, Bergqvist, Y, Day, N. P, Bergquist, J, Arvidsson, B, & White, N. J. Ashton, M & Lindegårdh, N. (2006). Characterization of human urinary metabolites of the antimalarial piperaquine. Drug Metabolism and Disposition , 34(12), 2011-2019.

[41] Taudon, N, Margout, D, Calas, M, Kezutyte, T, Vial, H. J, & Bressolle, F. M. (2008). A liquid chromatography-mass spectrometry assay for simultaneous determination of two antimalarial thiazolium compounds in human and rat matrices. Journal of Pharmaceutical and Biomedical Analysis , 48(3), 1001-1005.

[42] Vale, N, Matos, J, Moreira, R, & Gomes, P. (2008). Electrospray ionization-ion trap mass spectrometry study of PQAAPro and PQProAA mimetic derivatives of the antimalarial primaquine. Journal of the American Society for Mass Spectrometry , 19(10), 1476-1490.

[43] Vale, N, Moreira, R, & Gomes, P. (2008). Characterization of primaquine imidazolidin-4 ones with antimalarial activity by electrospray ionization-ion trap mass spectrometry. International Journal of Mass Spectrometry 270(1-2), 81-93.

[44] Vale, N, Matos, J, Moreira, R, & Gomes, P. (2009). Electrospray ionization mass spectrometry as a valuable tool in the characterization of novel primaquine peptidomimetic derivatives. European Journal of Mass Spectrometry , 15(5), 627-640.

[45] Vale, N, Moreira, R, & Gomes, P. (2009). Primaquine revisited six decades after its discovery. European Journal of Medicinal Chemistry , 44(3), 937-953.

[46] World Health Organization (2010). World Malaria Report 2010, WHO Press, Geneva, Switzerland.

[47] World Health Organization (2011). Survey of the quality of selected antimalarial medicines circulating in six countries of sub-Saharan Africa, Quality Assurance and Safety: Medicines Essential Medicines and Pharmaceutical Policies, WHO Press, Geneva, Switzerland.

Chapter 4

Mass Spectrometry Strategies for Structural Analysis of Carbohydrates and Glycoconjugates

Guilherme L. Sassaki and Lauro Mera de Souza

Additional information is available at the end of the chapter

http://dx.doi.org/10.5772/55221

1. Introduction

Carbohydrates are compounds rich in hydroxyl groups, being a monosaccharide a building block for complex carbohydrates. Beside the large amounts of hydroxyl groups, two chemical functions define the organic class, and even the simplest carbohydrate must contain either an aldehyde (polyhydroxyaldehyde) or ketone (polyhydroxyketone) functions (Fig. 1).

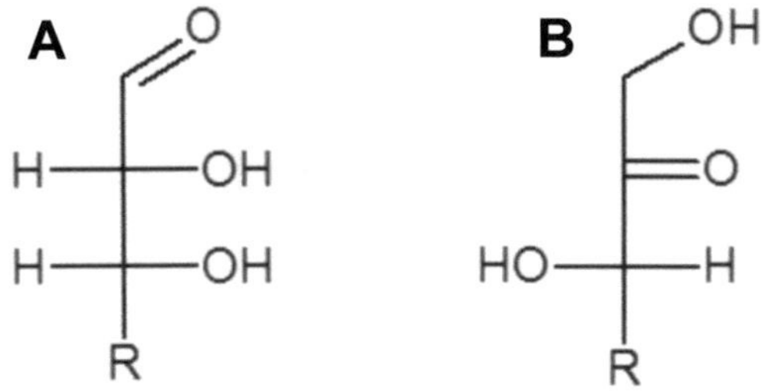

Figure 1. Functional groups defining carbohydrates (A) aldose (B) ketose

Carbohydrates can be naturally found as free monomers named monosaccharides (e.g. glucose, fructose), linked itself forming oligosaccharides such as the disaccharides sucrose and lactose, or larger structures containing hundreds of monosaccharides, the polysaccharides. Carbohydrates are the most abundant biomolecules worldwide, since they are found as structural matrix of plants (cellulose) and invertebrates (chitin). Other biological roles of carbohydrates are storage and transport of energy (e.g. starch, glycogen and sucrose). Despite many roles of carbohydrates are not well understood, it is well accepted that carbohydrates contain the codes for cell-cell recognition. To understand the importance of carbohydrates as code molecules it is important to emphasize that the blood typing results from different types of oligosaccharides on the surface of blood cells (Fig. 2).

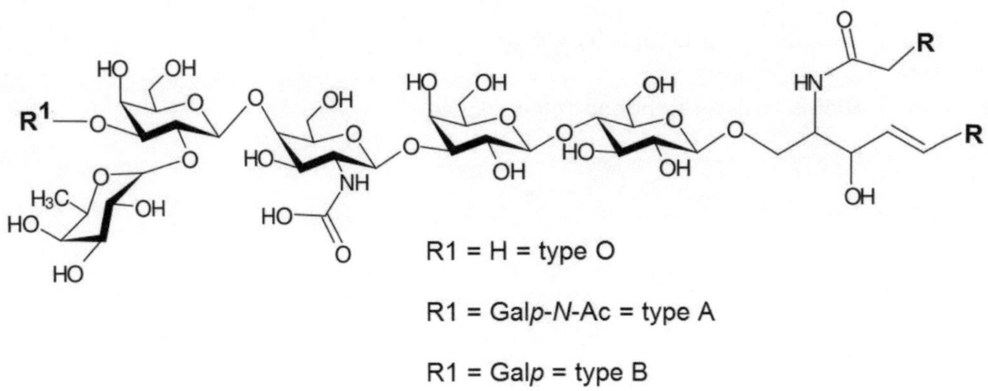

Figure 2. Oligosaccharides involved in the blood typing

Because of their constitution and architecture, each monosaccharide offers many linkage sites, for example a simple hexose such as glucose, in its cyclic form of glucopyranose, maintains four free hydroxyl groups (i.e. *O*-2, *O*-3, *O*-4 and *O*-6) and every one are available to be attached for other monosaccharides. Thus, different from other linear macromolecules, namely proteins and nucleic acids, the chemistry of carbohydrates is quite complex, considering the presence of several epimers, enatiomers, anomeric configurations and branches, with variable linkage possibilities. Also, their biosynthesis is considered extremely complex, since it lack any template. Nevertheless, carbohydrates can be found associated with virtually any other molecule being found linked to proteins, lipids, nucleobases, and several compounds from the secondary metabolism.

The diversity of the carbohydrates is firstly defined by the massive possibilities of monosaccharide hydroxyl configurations, producing many stereocenters, allowing different monosaccharides with same backbone, just alternating the hydroxyl configuration. In solution, the monosaccharides with carbon chains higher than tetroses tend to cyclize. For example, a simple monosaccharide (galactose, a hexose or arabinose, a pentose) is frequently found in two different ring configurations: galactopyranose (or arabinopyranose) and galactofuranose (or arabinofuranose), an analogy to pyran and furan rings. Nevertheless, when in the ring configuration, an additional stereocenter is formed on the C1, named the anomeric carbon (C1 for the aldoses or C2 for ketoses). In this case, two other configurations named as anomers α and β are possible and, according to ring configuration, the monosaccharide could be presented as α-galactopyranose, β-galactopyranose, α-galactofuranose and β-galactofuranose (Fig. 3).

http://dx.doi.org/10.5772/55221

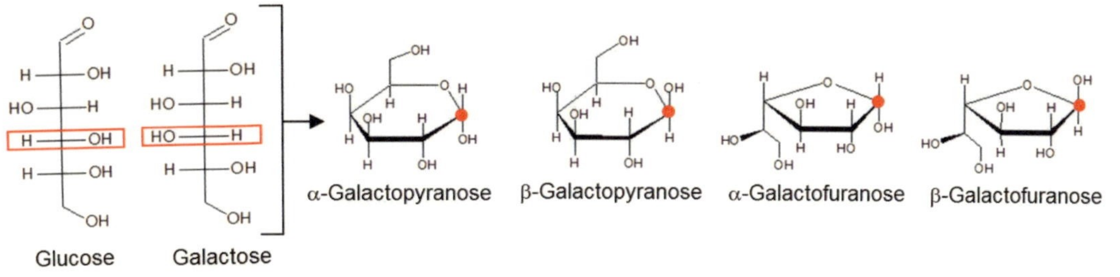

Figure 3. Monosaccharide epimers (glucose and galactose, epimers in C-4) and the diversity of configuration that can be assumed by a monosaccharide. Red circles indicate the anomeric carbons

1.1. Mass spectrometry in carbohydrate analysis

In the early of mass spectrometry development, the limitation of ionization modes avoided the carbohydrate analysis. Electron ionization (EI), formerly called electron impact, is one of the oldest ionization modes, developed by Dempster in 1918, this ionization is well used organic compounds [1-2]. Nevertheless, it requires volatile and thermally stable compounds hindering the carbohydrate analysis, because they are non volatile compounds. In 1963, Wolfrom and Thompson introduced a method to make monosaccharides suitable for the "in gas phase analysis", developed for gas chromatography (GC) [3-4]. It consisted to introduce acetyl radicals to any free hydroxyl making a non volatile monosaccharide in a volatile derivative at the GC conditions. A common problem in monosaccharide derivatization is the random formation of anomers (α and β) and ring configuration (furanose and pyranose). Since this hampers the GC analysis of monossacharides, an additional step was included, which consist into reduce the anomeric carbon with $NaBH_4$, yielding an aditol, which could be further acetylated [3-4]. These methods allowed monosaccharides to be analyzed by GC, but also met the requirements of the electron ionization for volatile compounds, making the hyphenated GC-MS a powerful tool for monosaccharide composition. Latter, these methods were combined with a previous alkylation of carbohydrates, becoming the main means for interglycosidic linkage analysis.

Considering that electron ionization promotes an extensive fragmentation of analytes, EI alone is not suitable for mixture analysis. Chemical ionization (CI) is able to make mixture analysis simpler than EI, however this is suitable only for mixtures containing compounds with different molecular mass. Therefore, for the monosaccharide analysis the coupling of gas chromatography with mass spectrometry was, actually, a perfect "wedding", considering that mass spectrometry (EI or CI) alone would not be able to describe their isomers but, on the other hand, the separation of gas chromatography can ensure the analysis.

After the 80s, when Baber and coworkers introduced a new ionization source [5], called "fast atom bombardment" (FAB), the oligosaccharides could be analyzed in their intact form. The method consists in to dissolve samples in a non volatile matrix, to which a bean of accelerated atoms is triggered. This produces lower fragmentation than EI, allowing to observe the ion of entire oligosaccharides, which can be post selected and fragmented individually. Currently, many types of ionization sources can be employed to carbohydrate analysis, but the main ones remains to be "matrix-assisted laser desorption ionization" (MALDI) and "electrospray ionization" (ESI). The later having a special advantage because it is easy for coupling with liquid chromatography systems, improving greatly the analytical potential of both.

1.2. Obtaining enriched saccharide extracts

Carbohydrates are essentially hydrophilic compounds, thus being extracted from their matrix in water. However, inter- and intramolecular interactions of some polysaccharides avoid their solubility in water. On the other hand, many glycans are found attached to different molecules, such as lipids, being insoluble in water, but well in organic solvents such as methanol-chloroform. For the most mass spectrometry analysis of carbohydrates, the entire polysaccharide is not suitable or not interesting to be analyzed, because unlike proteins which have a defined molecular mass, the polysaccharides are polydisperse. Thus, carbohydrates must be analyzed as oligosaccharides, which can be found as naturally occurring compounds, or then produced by controlled mild hydrolysis or enzymatic degradation. Most of glycoconjugates can be analyzed directly in its native composition, but oligosaccharides from glycoproteins should be released prior MS analysis.

1.3. Chemical releasing oligosaccharides

Chemical reactions for releasing oligosaccharides can be achieved by partial hydrolysis of polysaccharides, a nonselective process that lead to different oligosaccharides. There are many ways to get partial hydrolysis, but it is important to adapt the method for the polysaccharide of interest, considering that different polysaccharides will have different behaviors [6]. Acids such as trifluoroacetic acid or chloridric are always a good choice since they are easy to eliminate after hydrolysis. Another alternative to be considered is the controlled Smith degradation. This is of particular importance to degrade specific carbohydrates, those containing free vicinal hydroxyl. Thus depending on the overall polysaccharide backbone, it is possible to breakdown the main chain releasing the side chain oligosaccharides [7-8].

Oligosaccharides from glycoprotein can also be obtained by chemical releasing. This can be done by β-elimination, which consists in to submit the glycoproteins to alkali degradation under reductive condition, for example by adding $NaBH_4$. This process can release *O*-linked oligosaccharides only, converting the unit that was linked to the protein in its alditol [9]. Anhydrous hydrazine is a suitable reagent for releasing unreduced *O*- and *N*-linked glycans. The method introduced in 1993 by Patel an coworkers allows releasing selectively *O*- and *N*-linked glycans in dependence of temperature, 60 °C (5 h) for *O*-linked and 95 °C (4 h) for *N*-linked glycans [10-11].

1.4. Enzymatic releasing oligosaccharides

Unlike many chemical releasing methods, the enzymatic catalysis can be well controlled, are selective and reproductively. It consists in the use of enzymes to cleave specific glycosidic

http://dx.doi.org/10.5772/55221

linkages. The range of enzymes for polysaccharides cleavage is varied as well as the polysaccharides. Thus, some information about the structure is need, such as the monosaccharide composition and glycosidic linkage. Glycans from glycoproteins can also be released by enzymatic catalysis. This can be done by using endoglycosidases such as peptide *N*-glycosidase F (PNGase F) and peptide *N*-glycosidase A (PNGase A). Glycan from glycolipids can also be released with endoglycoceramidase, however this is not necessary, considering that most of glycolipids can be analyzed as entire structures [12-13].

2. Analysis of carbohydrates

2.1. Monosaccharide composition

The first step in the carbohydrate analysis is to know the type and amounts of monosaccharides that compose a particular structure of interest. The methods for it including complete hydrolysis that can be performed with chloridric acid, trifluoroacetic acid, sulfuric acid and so on, preferably with an easily removable acid. Mass spectrometry of carbohydrates gives new perspectives for their structural analysis and for the use of GC-MS, the chemical derivatization gave "wings" to non-volatile compounds, making possible to determine the chemical structure of native glycans, which can be constituted by oligosaccharide chains, fatty acid and amino acids. GC-MS can provide highly resolved chromatograms, providing the identification and quantification of compounds in fmol quantities. Carbohydrates are usually converted to derivatives by silylation, acylation and alkylation [14-16].

After hydrolysis, many derivatization methods can be applied, such as the silylation (Fig. 4A), which was firstly used for carbohydrates by Sweley and coworkers [17], becoming very popular because it is simpler, rapid and applicable for all carbohydrate, including monosacharides, alditols, uronic acids, deoxi-monosaccharides, amino sugars and can be extended to oligosaccharides [15-18]. The problem of silylation and fluoroacylation is the formation of many isomers from each monosaccharide, due the mutarotation and the glycosidation reaction (Fig. 4B). In order to resolve this problem, carbohydrates have been converted to alditols, dithiocetals, aldononitrile and other derivatives, these reactions are well described by Knapp (1979) [18] and Biermann & McGinnis (1989) [15].

A classical method for monosaccharide analysis by gas chromatography, introduced by Wolfrom and Thompson (1963) [3-4], includes a reduction step, which will avoid the mutarotation, consequently the α, β, pyranose and furanose isomers to each monosaccharide. This is followed by an acetilation (Fig. 4C) of hydroxyl groups that makes monosaccharides (as alditol acetate derivatives) suitable for gas chromatography and mass spectrometry with electron ionization. So the alditol-acetates are commonly used for identification and quantification [15,19]. Sassaki and coworkers (2008) provide modification in this method (Fig. 4D), creating the MAA (methyl-esters-alditol-acetates), which extended to lipid, amino acids and uronic acids [20]. Since some steps are needed to obtain the derivatized analytes, the follow schemes show the simplified pathway of some carbohydrates derivatives. The fragmentation profile from alditol acetates allows to easy distinguishing among monosaccharide class, i.e. a pentose from a hexose or deoxyhexose. However within the monosaccharide class, it is very difficult distinguish among them, being essential the chromatography separation.

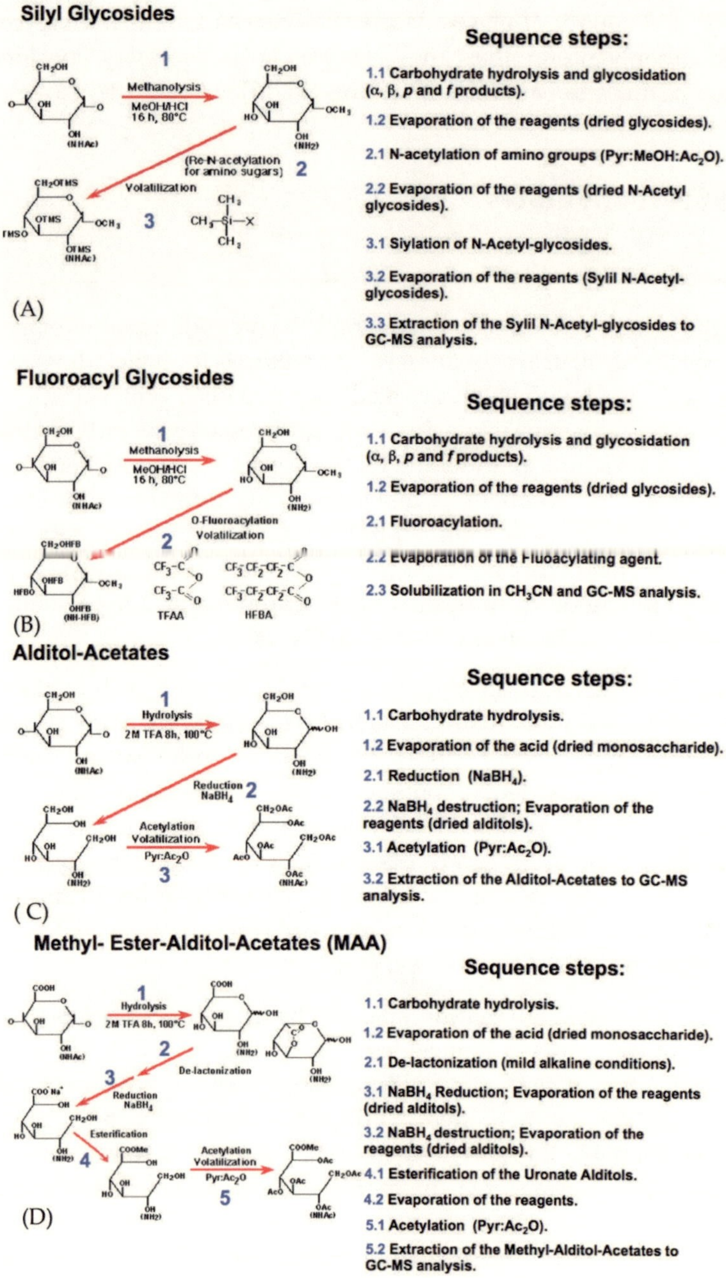

Figure 4. Schematic representation of monossacharide derivatization methods (A) sylilation, (B) fluoroacylation, (C) acetylation and (D) acetylation modified method.

The choice for a derivatizing procedure will depend of the nature of glycoconjugate. Generally, how much more complex is the structure, silylation and fluoroacylation are the desired procedures. However these procedures give rise to complex chromatograms and EI-MS profile, which normally led to misunderstand results. So, why to choose these procedures? Since both methods use glycosidation in mild conditions, avoiding carbohydrate degradation, mainly of ketosugars and also provide esterification of carboxylic groups on acidic sugars. By these properties, the high volatile the fluoracyl (HFBA, PFPA and TFA) and silyl (BSTFA and MBTFA) they are commonly used for structural analysis of complex sialyl glycans, although they are unstable and some cares should be done prior to analysis. So where is the field of application for the alditol-acetates? They are used for carbohydrate quantification and identification for heteropolysaccharides and non-degradable sugars. In the case of acidic ones they normally are carboxi-reduced by carbodiimide and $NaBH_4$ [21], which provide the correspondent alditol prior acetylation and GC-MS analysis, moreover it has been observed in our research laboratory that the alditol-acetates are cheap, easy and stable for ~30 years to date, which became an exceptional tool as unique standard and for quantification assays where stability and repetitions are need. Also the EI-MS profile aids to fit the monosaccharide classes, giving primary and secondary fragments that are key ions for identification and with lesser artefacts formation than the silyl and fluoracyl derivatives (Fig. 5-7 and Table 1) 15,19-20,22-23].

Since many derivatives could be prepared, each method has advantages and problems due the physical and chemical properties of the carbohydrates. In order to analyze the carbohydrates without formation of many isomers, the MAA had demonstrated robustness for qualitative and quantitative analysis of carbohydrates. The sylilated or fluoroacylated derivatives are a great option to obtain high volatile sugars, including oligosaccharides, however, they are not stable as the acetylated ones. Moreover, MAA use simple and less expensive reagents in comparison to the others.

2.2. Interglycosidic linkage analysis: partially methylated alditol acetates

Combined with NMR spectroscopy, methylation analysis is the most utilized method for determination of structure of complex carbohydrates, providing the linkage analysis and structure of monosaccharide units in oligo-, complex glycans. Per-*O*-methylation of carbohydrates has been carried out by several methods such as those of Haworth, Kuhn et al., Hakomori, and nowadays by Ciucanu and Kerek [24-27].

Per-*O*-methylated products can be converted to partially *O*-methylated alditol acetates (PMAAs) via successive hydrolysis, reduction/acetylation and identified by GC-MS using their characteristic GC retention times and EI-MS fingerprints [28]. The method is extremely sensitive, requiring low amounts as 50 μg of glycan. PMAAs were refined by Carpita and Shea by use of sodium borodeuteride in the reduction step [19], avoiding the problem of mass symmetry from different partially *O*-methylated aldoses (Fig. 8).

Usually, in glycan analysis more than one type of monosaccharide is present, which makes necessary to compare the retention times of the PMAAs, with standards. The common

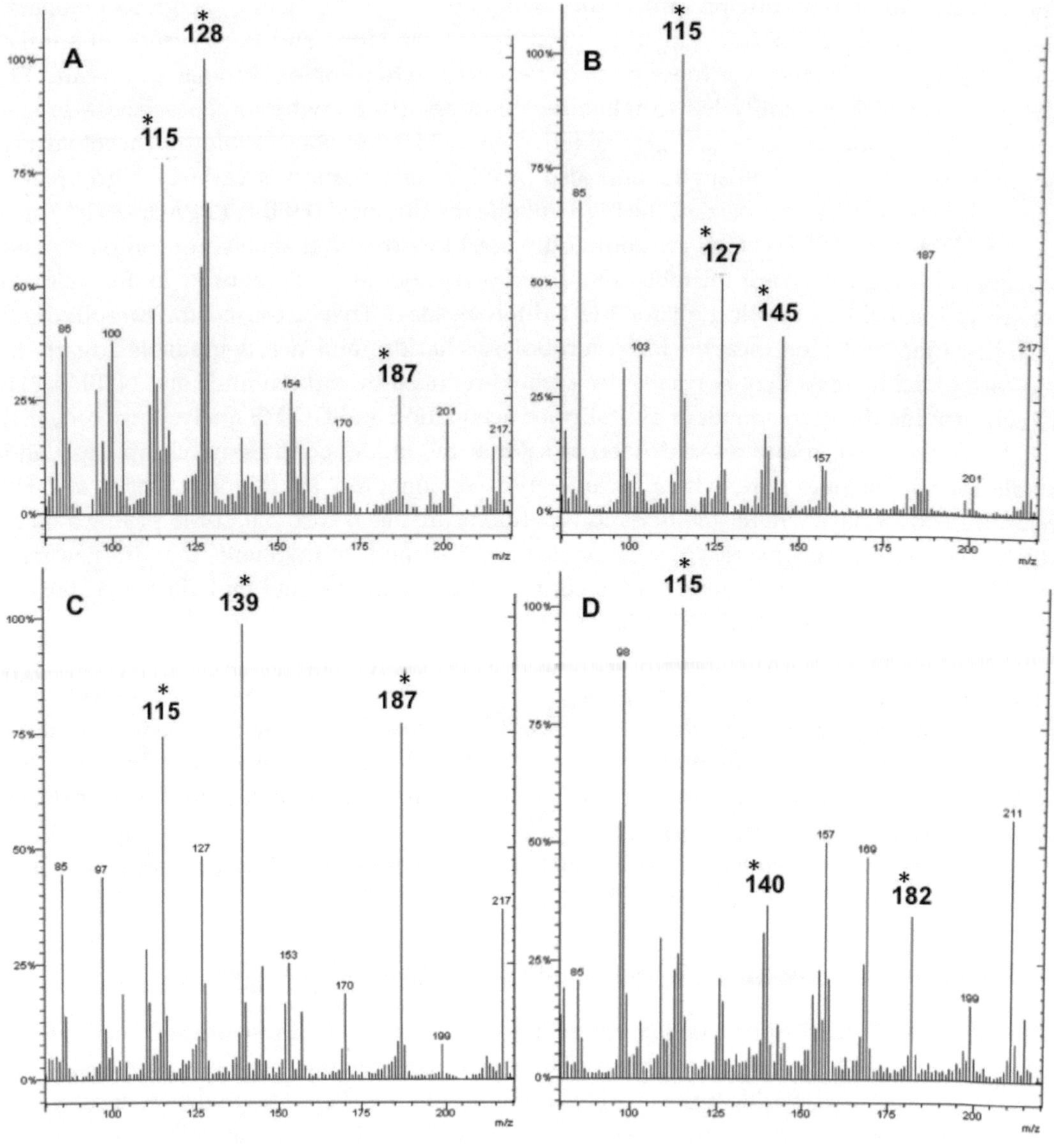

Figure 5. EI-MS profile of some alditol-acetates (80-220 *m/z*), key ions for identification are identified with (*) at the MS spectra. (A) 6-deoxi-hexitol; (B) pentitol; (C) hexitol; (D) non-reduced hexitol.

procedure is synthetize or acquire authentical standard for each monosaccharide. However this can be time consuming and expensive if it done individually. An alternative strategy was simultaneously provides partial *O*-methylation of each individual monosaccharide and convert it to a mixture of PMAAs. Recently, Sassaki et al. [29-30] produced series of PMAAs of Glc, Man, Gal, Ara, Xyl, Fuc, and Rha, and have identified them in the C-1 deuterated form and the EI-MS and retention time profile of the pyranosidic and furanosidic ring conforma-

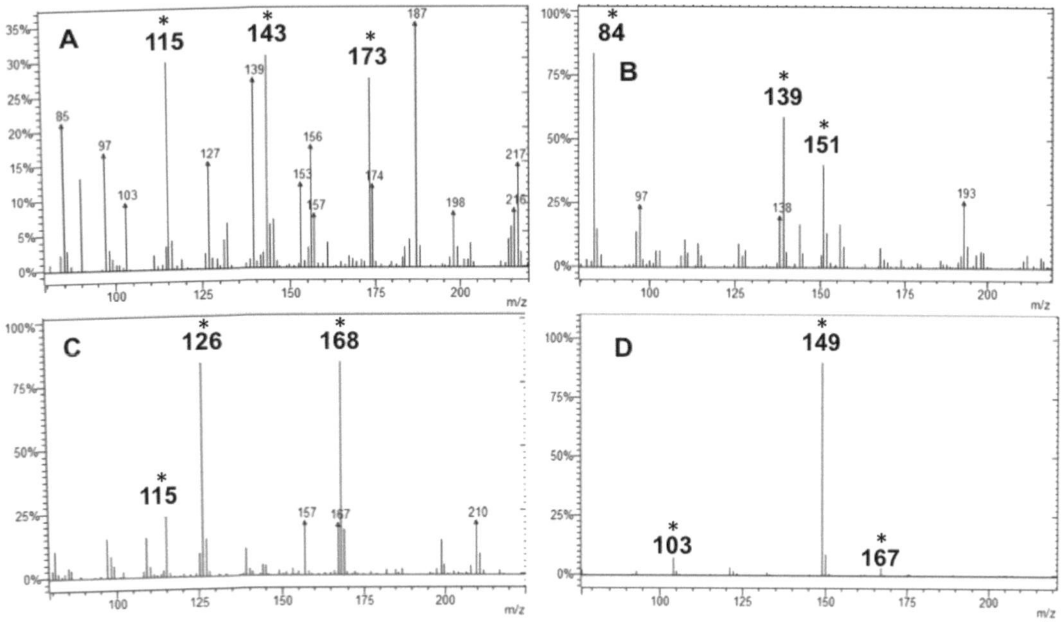

Figure 6. EI-MS profile of some alditol-acetates (80-220 *m/z*), key ions for identification are identified with (*) at the MS spectra. (A) Me-ester-hexitol; (B) Hexaminitol; (C) inositol; (D) ftalate.

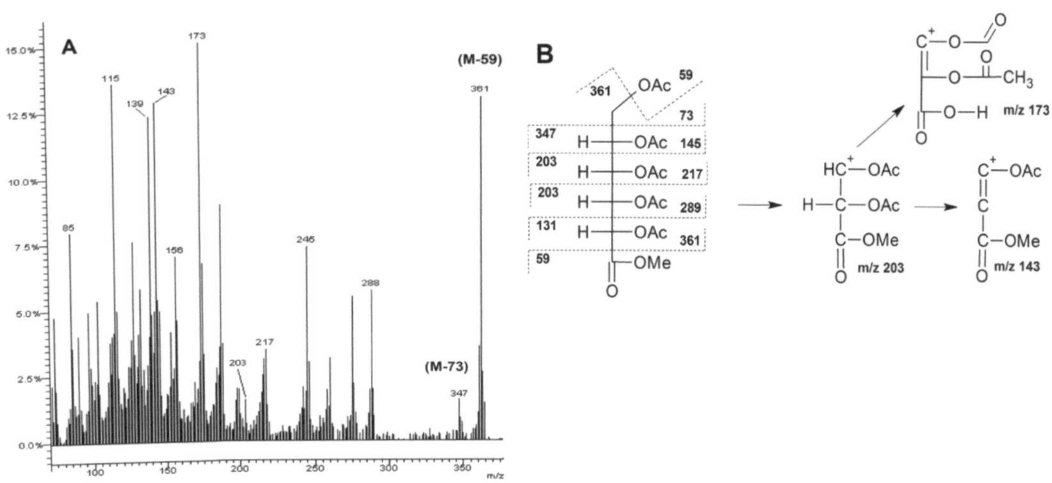

Figure 7. (A) EI-MS spectrum of 1-Me-ester-hexitol acetate (B). Primary and secondary fragmentations of the key ions on EI-MS spectrum.

tions, using the Purdie methylation (Ag_2O–MeI) [31]. So, what is the big advantage of the proposed work? The answer is a simple rationalization and rapid identification of the PMAA. Supposing that a glycan has the following monosaccharide composition: Xyl, Ara, Glc and Gal. Performing the methylation by Ciucanu and Kerek, you will have from EI-MS the following

Methyl-Esters-Alditol-Acetates	*Rt*	Reporter ions (m/z)
2-Deoxy-Rib	11.52	245-232-159-145-142-129-117-100-82-57
Rha	13.92	317-215-201-187-170-155-145-129-128-115-112-103-99-95
Fuc	14.17	317-215-201-187-170-155-145-129-128-115-112-103-99-95
Ara	14.27	303-217-187-145-140-127-115-103-98-95
Xyl	14.59	303-217-187-145-140-127-115-103-98-95
2-Deoxy-Glc	15.72	317-303-217-201-159-141-129-115-112-103-95
GalA	16.88	361-287-245-217-187-173-156-143-139-127-115-103-97
4-*O*-Me-GlcA	16.02	333-319-261-217-175-143-139-133-127-115-101-85
ManA	17.07	361-287-245-217-187-173-156-143-139-127-115-103-97
GulA	18.2	361-287-245-217-187-173-156-143-139-127-115-103-97
GlcA	17.13	361-287-245-217-187-173-156-143-139-127-115-103-97
IdoA	18.57	361-287-245-217-187-173-156-143-139-127-115-103-97
Man	17.91	375-289-273-259-217-187-170-153-145-139-127-115-103-97-85
Gal	18.15	375-289-273-259-217-187-170-153-145-139-127-115-103-97-85
Glc	17.98	375-289-273-259-217-187-170-153-145-139-127-115-103-97-85
m-Ins	17.62	375-211-199-168-157-139-126-115-109-97
Glc-HepA	20.23	433-420-359-317-275-259-217-197-187-173-169-143-139-127-115-103
Man-Hep	19.78	448-332-290-218-187-182-170-139-127-115-109-103-97-85
Glc-Hep	20.12	448-332-290-218-187-182-170-139-127-115-109-103-97-85
Perseitol	20.54	448-332-290-218-187-182-170-139-127-115-109-103-97-85
GalNAc	19.88	374-318-259-193-168-151-139-126-114-102-97-84
GlcNAc	19.74	374-318-259-193-168-151-139-126-114-102-97-84
ManNAc	19.93	374-318-259-193-168-151-139-126-114-102-97-84
NAc-Neu*	23.48	518-504-476-444-330-318-259-186-172-154-139-97
NAc-Neu*	24.05	518-504-476-444-330-318-259-186-172-154-139-97

GC-MS analysis of MAA on CP-Sil-8CB (DB-1) capillary column. [a]Retention time (R_t) in min, at 100 °C to 180 °C (10 °C min^{-1}, then held for 5min.) and to 320 °C (10 °C min^{-1}, then held for 5 min). NAc-Neu* derivatives formed during reduction of the ketone group. EI-MS were obtained using an Ion-trap at 220 °C, transfer line 320 °C and internal ionization.

Table 1. Retention times and EI-MS reporter fragments obtained by mass spectrometry from the MAA derivatives adapted from Sassaki et al. (2008)

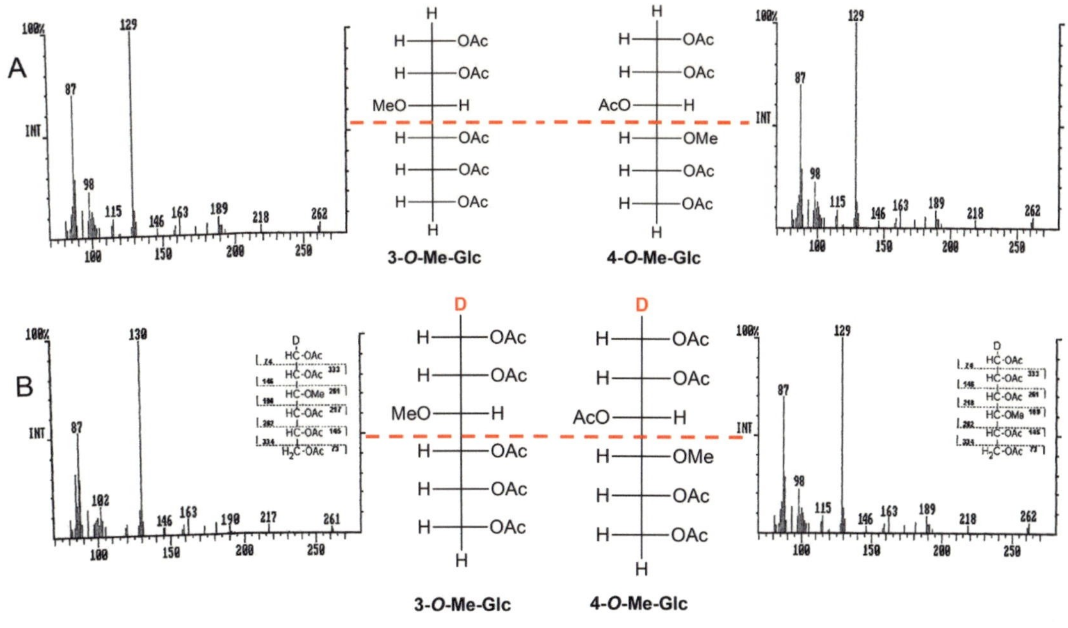

Figure 8. (A) Non deuterated PMAAs both derivatives have the same EI-MS pofile. (B) C-1 deuterated PMAA, the differentiation between the mass symmetrical derivatives is possible, the EI-MS profile are different.

answer: PMAAs-Hexitol and PMAAs-Pentitol, and their methylation distribution for linkage analysis. However, information of the type of monosaccharide is difficult to assign and normally misunderstood. Although, if you inject, individually, the mixtures of PMAAs from Xyl, Ara, Glc and Gal, the analysis will be easier, since now you have the Rt and the EI-MS profile of PMAA from each monosaccharide, an example for this application is demonstrate in Figure 9. From these PMAAs mixtures of individual monosaccharide is possible to create an EI-MS library for interglycosidic linkage (Fig. 10).

2.3. Oligosaccharide analysis

With the introduction of FAB-MS in early 80's [5], the analysis of carbohydrates swerved and oligosaccharides could be analyzed as entire structures, considering that FAB source, unlike EI, is able to transfer the entire oligosaccharides to the gaseous phase, ionizing then. Nowadays, the most used instrumentation are based on MALDI or ESI-MS ionization, considered soft ionization techniques that leads to formation of less unintended fragmentation during the ionization process, which are also called as in-source fragmentation.

Most of carbohydrates lacks acidic or basic functional groups, being lesser ionizable than peptides, for example. However, during the evolution of mass spectrometry of carbohydrates, many chemical reactions were developed to enhance the ionization and consequently the MS signal. Common derivatives processes included per-*O*-methylation or per-*O*-acetylation of entire oligosaccharides [33], these enhance their transfer to gaseous phase

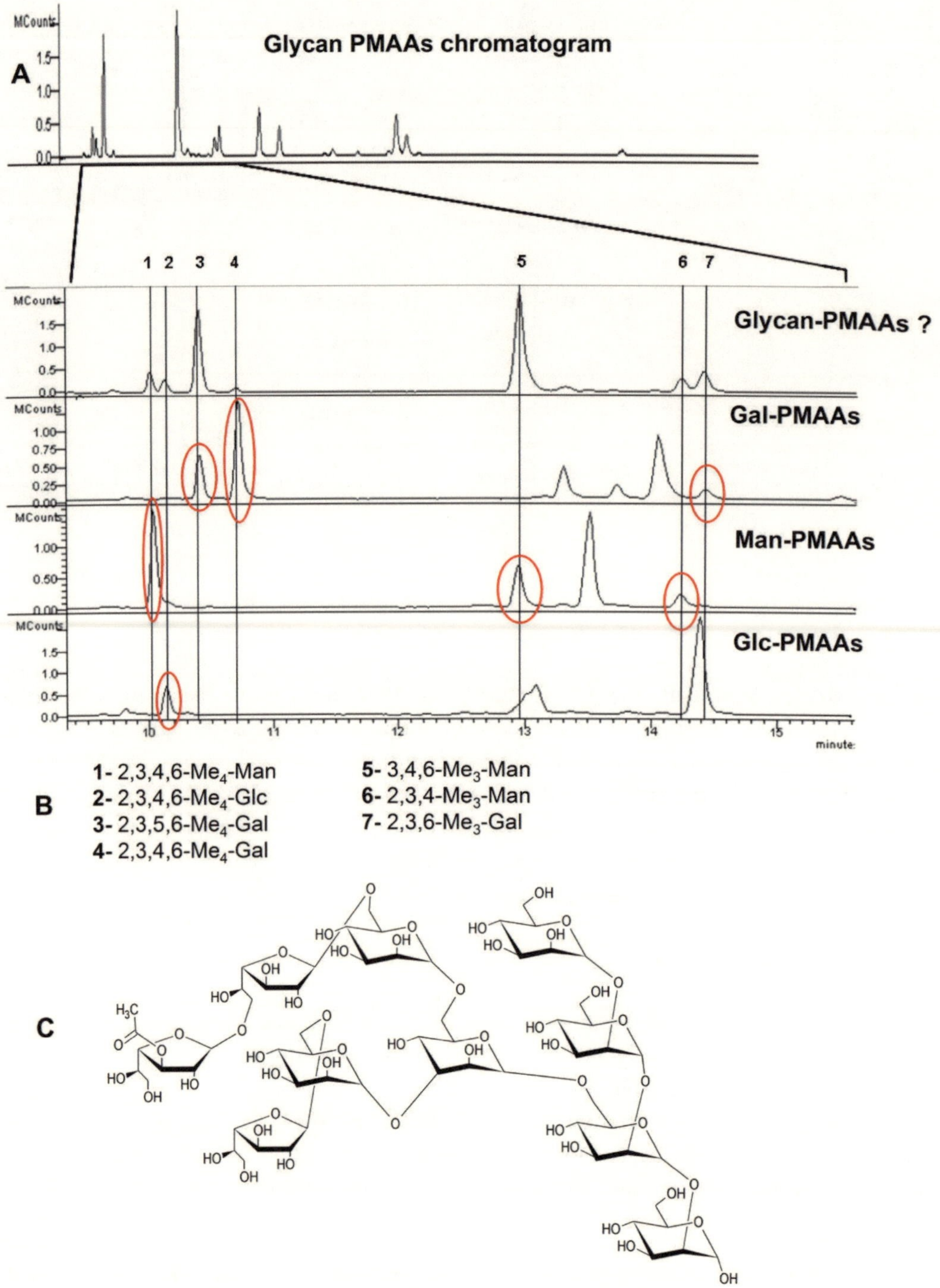

Figure 9. (A) GC-MS chromatogram of an exopolysaccharide obtained from *Exophiala jeanselmei* [32] (B) Identified PMAA from standard mixtures of Gal, Man and Glc, based on their Rt(s) and EI-MS profile (C). Hypothetical structure of the glycan based on methylation and NMR data.

during ionization and, also, per-O-methylation allows to easier detection of the branch sites via fragmentation.

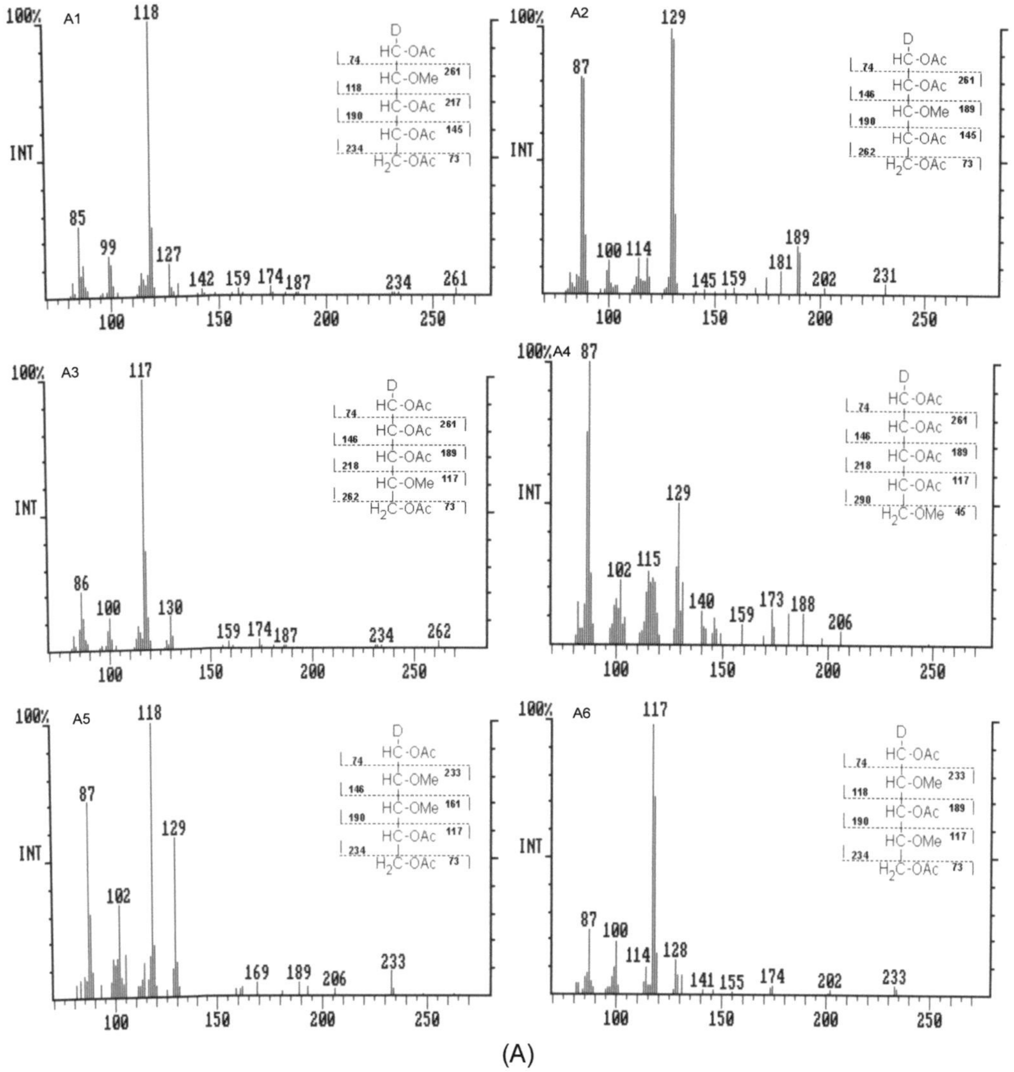

(A)

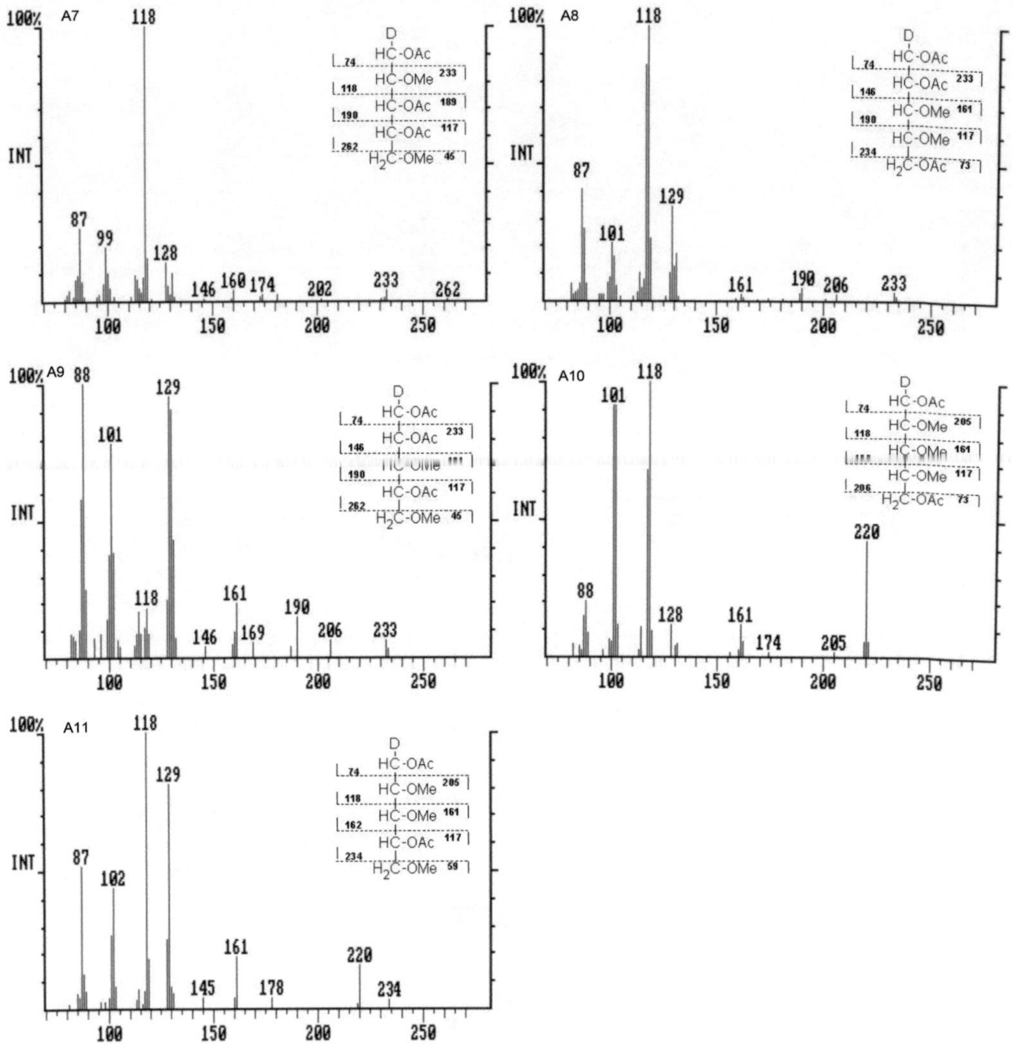

(B)

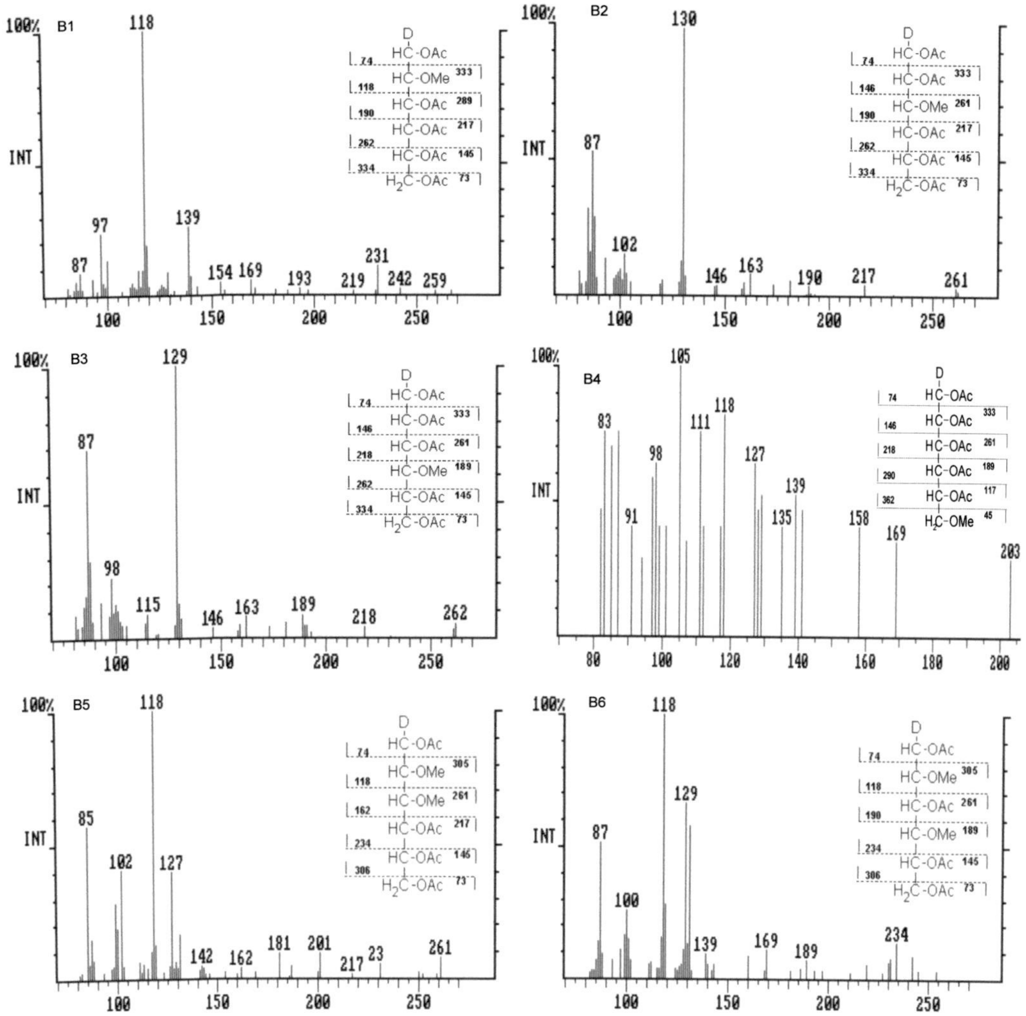

(C)

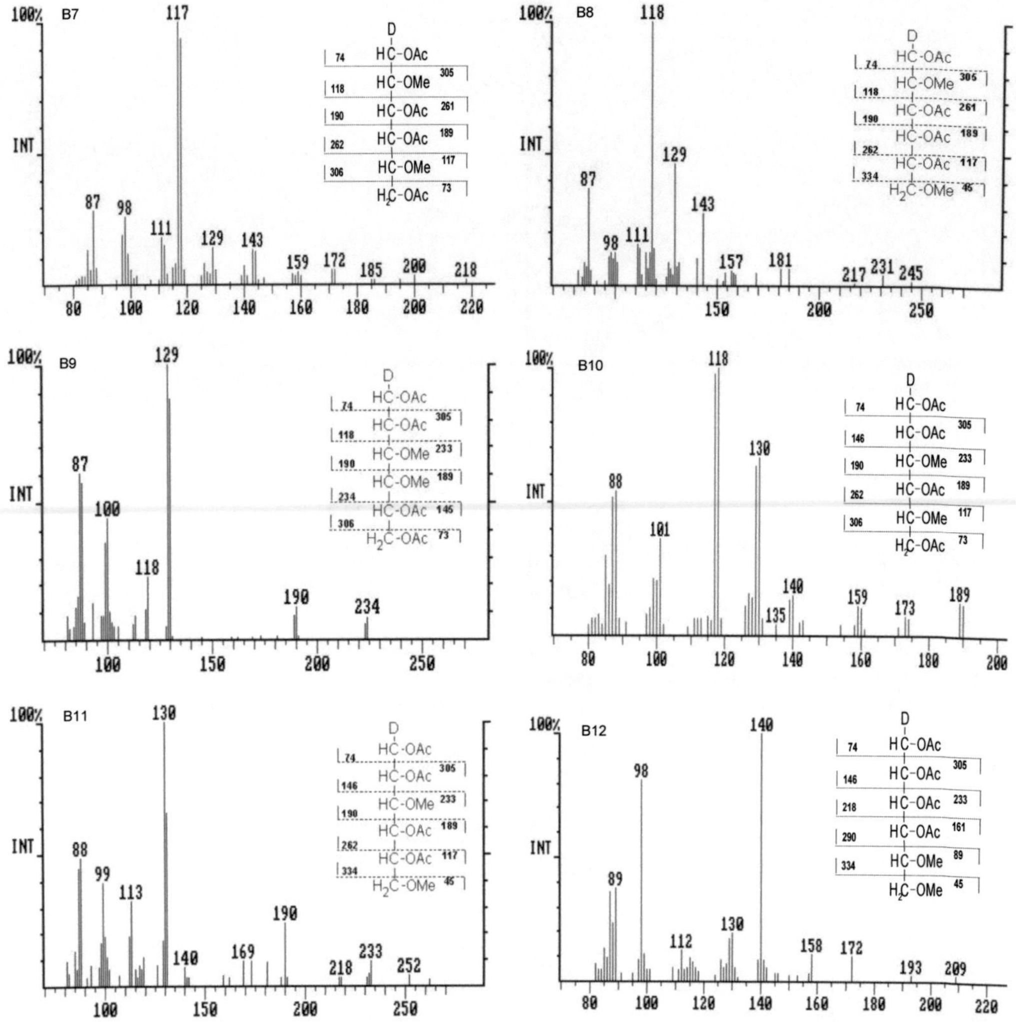
B7
100%
INT
117
87
98
111
129
143
159
172
185
200
218
D
HC-OAc
HC-OMe
HC-OAc
HC-OAc
HC-OMe
H2C-OAc
74
118
190
262
306
305
261
189
117
73
B8
118
87
98
111
129
143
157
181
217
231
245
HC-OAc
HC-OMe
HC-OAc
HC-OAc
HC-OAc
H2C-OMe
74
118
190
262
334
305
261
189
117
45
B9
129
87
100
118
190
234
HC-OAc
HC-OAc
HC-OMe
HC-OMe
HC-OAc
H2C-OAc
74
118
190
234
306
305
233
189
145
73
B10
118
88
101
130
135
140
159
173
189
HC-OAc
HC-OAc
HC-OMe
HC-OAc
HC-OMe
H2C-OAc
74
146
190
262
306
305
233
189
117
73
B11
130
88
99
113
140
169
190
218
233
252
HC-OAc
HC-OAc
HC-OMe
HC-OAc
HC-OAc
H2C-OMe
74
146
190
262
334
305
233
189
117
45
B12
140
98
89
112
130
158
172
193
209
HC-OAc
HC-OAc
HC-OAc
HC-OAc
HC-OMe
H2C-OMe
74
146
218
290
334
305
233
161
89
45

(D)

http://dx.doi.org/10.5772/55221

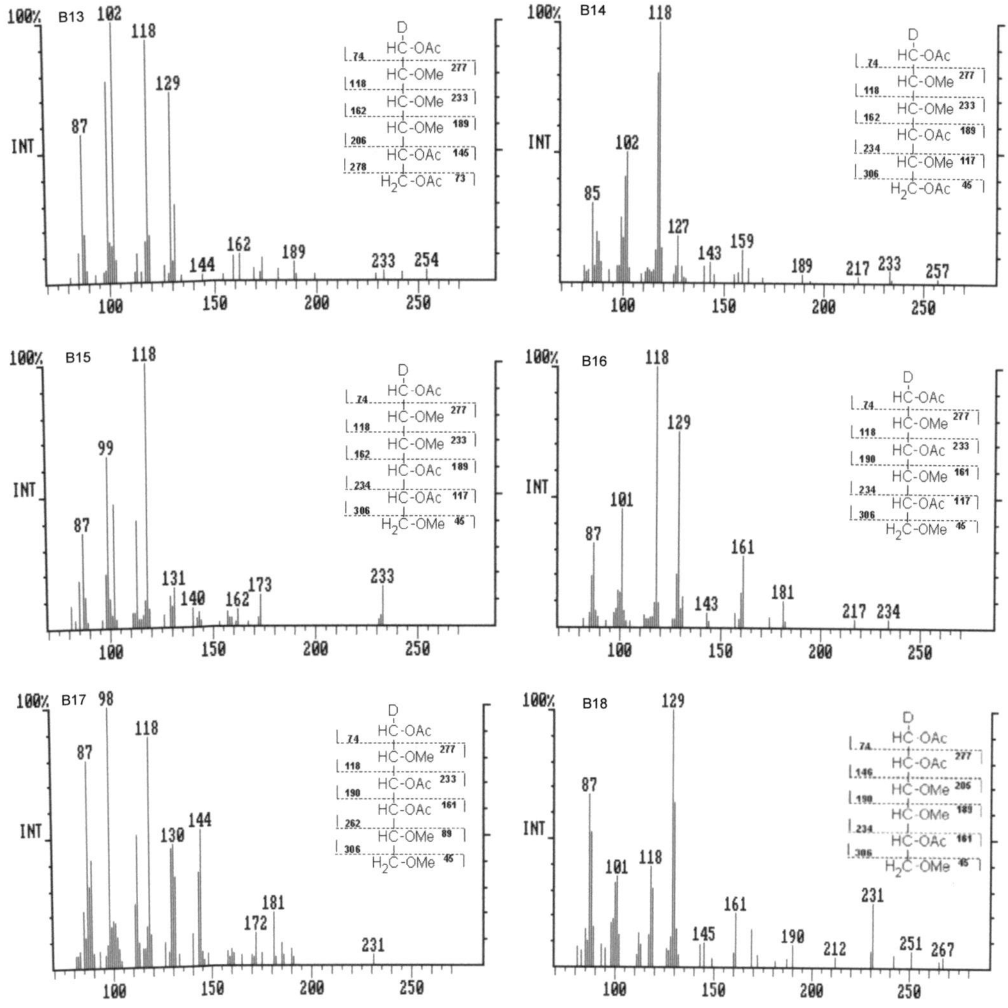

(E)

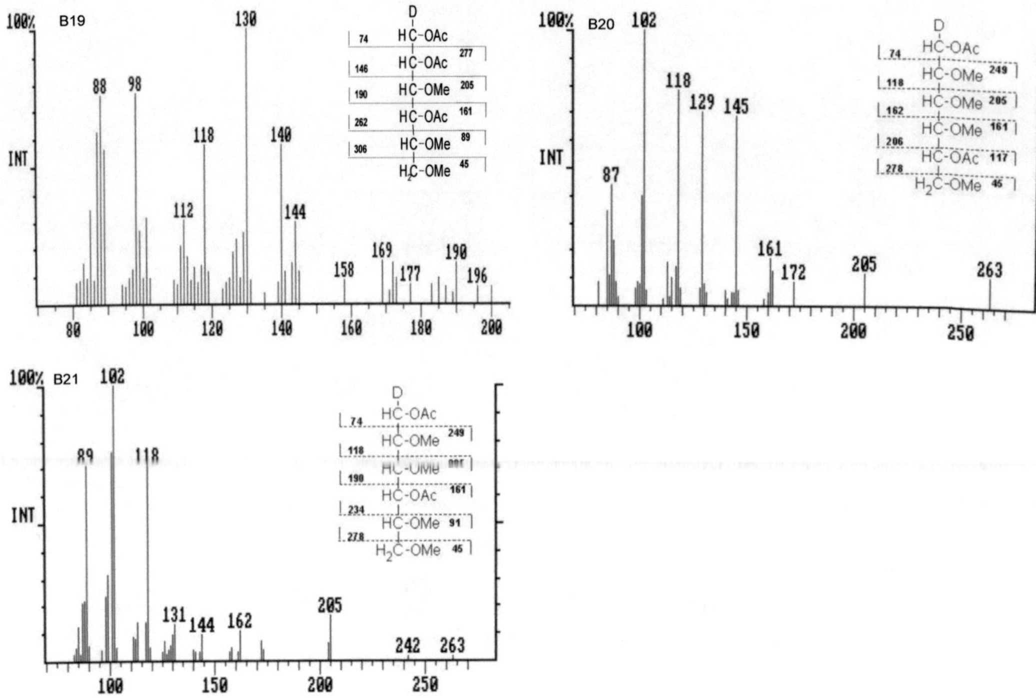

(F)

http://dx.doi.org/10.5772/55221

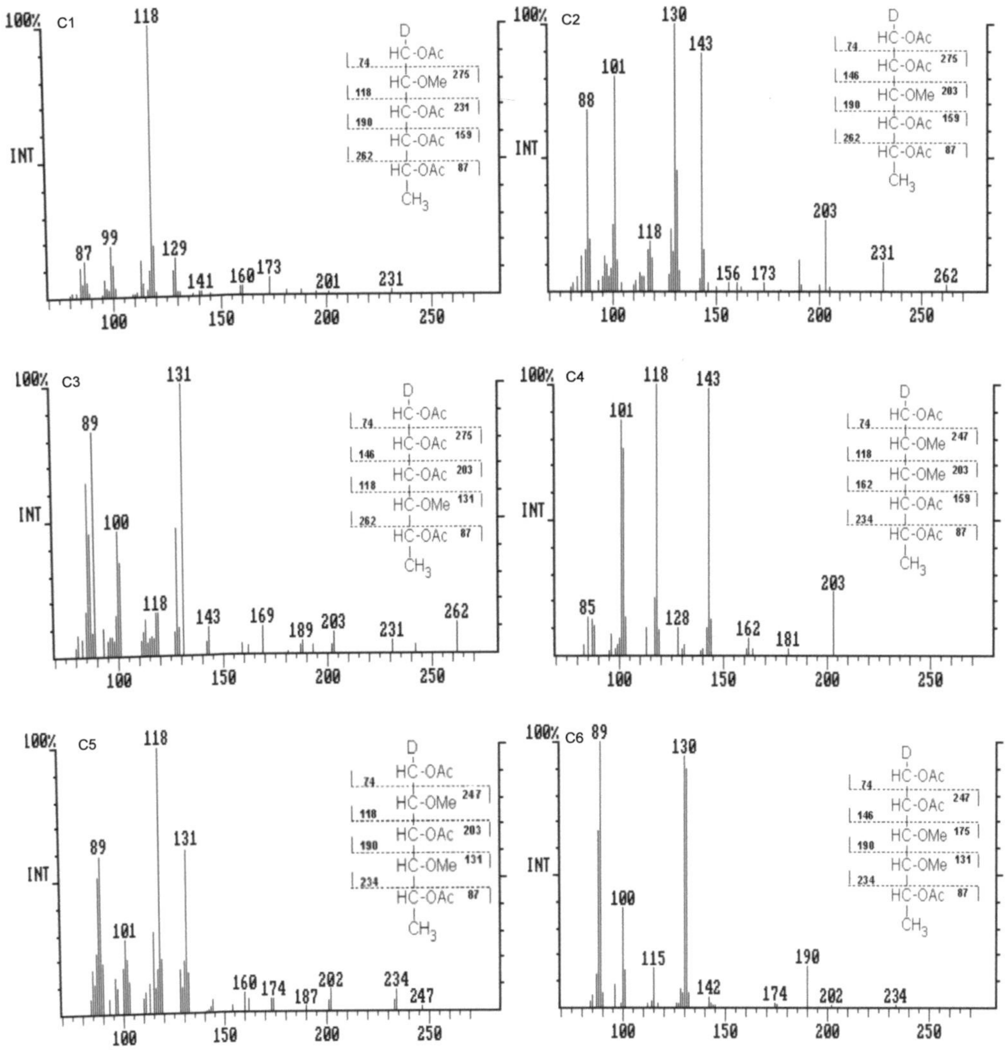

(G)

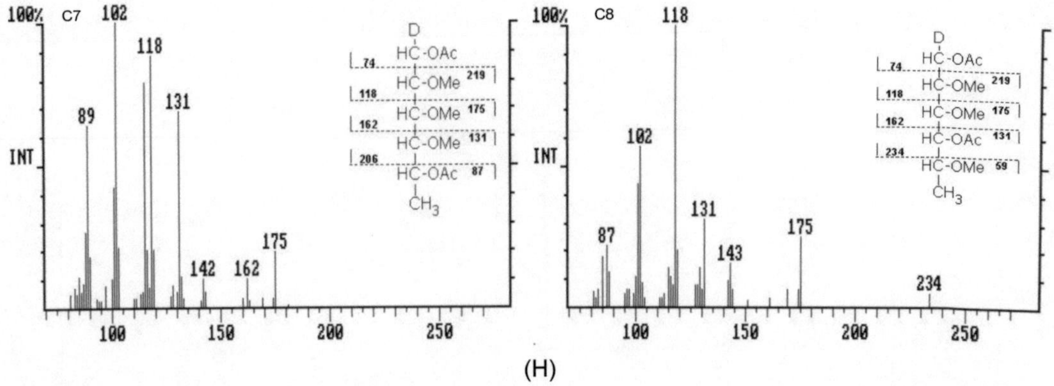

Figure 10. (A) – EI-MS patterns at *m/z* 80 to 270 of PMAA standards, deuterated at C-1: 2-MePentitol (A1), 3-MePentitol (A2), 4-MePentitol (A3), 5-MePentitol (A4), 2,3-Me_2Pentitol (A5), 2,4-Me_2Pent (A6), 2,5-Me_2Pentitol; (B) – EI-MS patterns at *m/z* 80 to 270 of PMAA standards, deuterated at C-1: 2-MePentitol (A7), 3,4-/2,3-Me_2Xyl (A8), 3,5-Me_2Pentitol (A9), 2,3,4-Me_3Pentitol (A10), 2,3,5-Me_3Pentitol (A11); (C) – EI-MS patterns at *m/z* 80 to 270 of PMAA standards, deuterated at C-1: 2-MeHexitol (B1), 3-MeHexitol (B2), 4-MeHexitol (B3), 6-MeHexitol (B4), 2,3-Me_2Hexitol (B5), 2,4-Me_2Hexitol (B6), 2,5-Me_2Hexitol; (D) – EI-MS patterns at *m/z* 80 to 270 of PMAA standards, deuterated at C-1: 2,5-Me_2Hexitol (B7) 2,6-Me_2Hexitol (B8), 3,4-Me_2Hexitol (B9), 3,5-Me_2Hexitol (B10) 3,6-Me_2Hexitol (B11), 5,6-Me_2Hexitol (B12); (E) – EI-MS patterns at *m/z* 80 to 270 of PMAA standards, deuterated at C-1: 2,3,4-Me_3Hexitol (B13), 2,3,5-Me_3Hexitol (B14), 2,3,6-Me_3Hexitol (B15), 2,4,6-Me_3Hexitol (B16), 2,5,6-Me_3Hexitol (B17), 3,4,6-Me_3Hexitol (B18); (F) – EI-MS patterns at *m/z* 80 to 270 of PMAA standards, deuterated at C-1: 3,5,6-Me_3Hexitol (B19), 2,3,4,6-Me_4Hexitol (B20), 2,3,5,6-Me_4Hexitol (B21); (G) – EI-MS patterns at *m/z* 80 to 270 of PMAA standards, deuterated at C-1: 2-Me6-Deoxy-Hexitol (C1), 3-Me6-Deoxy-Hexitol (C2), 4-Me6-Deoxy-Hexitol (C3), 2,3-$Me_2$6-Deoxy-Hexitol (C4), 2,4-$Me_2$6-Deoxy-Hexitol (C5), 3,4-$Me_2$6-Deoxy-Hexitol (C6); (H) – EI-MS patterns at *m/z* 80 to 270 of PMAA standards, deuterated at C-1: 2,3,4-$Me_3$6-Deoxy-Hexitol (C7), 2,3,5-$Me_3$6-Deoxy-Hexitol (C8).

A good option to insert an ionizable group on the oligosaccharides chains is the reductive amination. In this reaction, a reductive medium is enriched with a compound containing a primary amine. Virtually any amino-compound can be used, but especially those containing aromatic rings such as 2-aminoacridone, 2-aminobenzamide (2-AB), 2-aminopyridine, 2-aminoquinoline, 4-aminobenzoic among other are of peculiarly interesting, since the insertion of a chromophore also allows detection by ultra violet detectors, common in liquid chromatography. This reaction is considered quantitative, and in an elegant experiment, Xia and coworkers employed a glycan reductive isotope labeling (GRIL) methodology using conventional ^{12}C-anilin (called light) and $^{13}C_6$-anilin (called heavy) [34]. After the oligosaccharides being obtained from different sources, they were labeled via reductive amination using the heavy and light reagents. Then, the oligosaccharides from both sources could be combined and analyzed together by high performance liquid chromatography with mass spectrometry detection (HPLC-MS) and MALDI with time of flight (TOF) detector. Since the oligosaccharides were isotopically labeled, the difference of 6 mass units (m.u.) observed on MS, indicated the heavy- and light labeled oligosaccharides, allowing monitor any change in the amount of specific oligosaccharides (Fig. 11).

Reductive amination using a chiral reagent, such as 2-aminopropanol, has been employed to resolve enantiomeric monosaccharides. After being aminated with one of enantiomers (R or S) the amino-alditol formed is acetylated being suitable for GC-MS analysis, even without

http://dx.doi.org/10.5772/55221

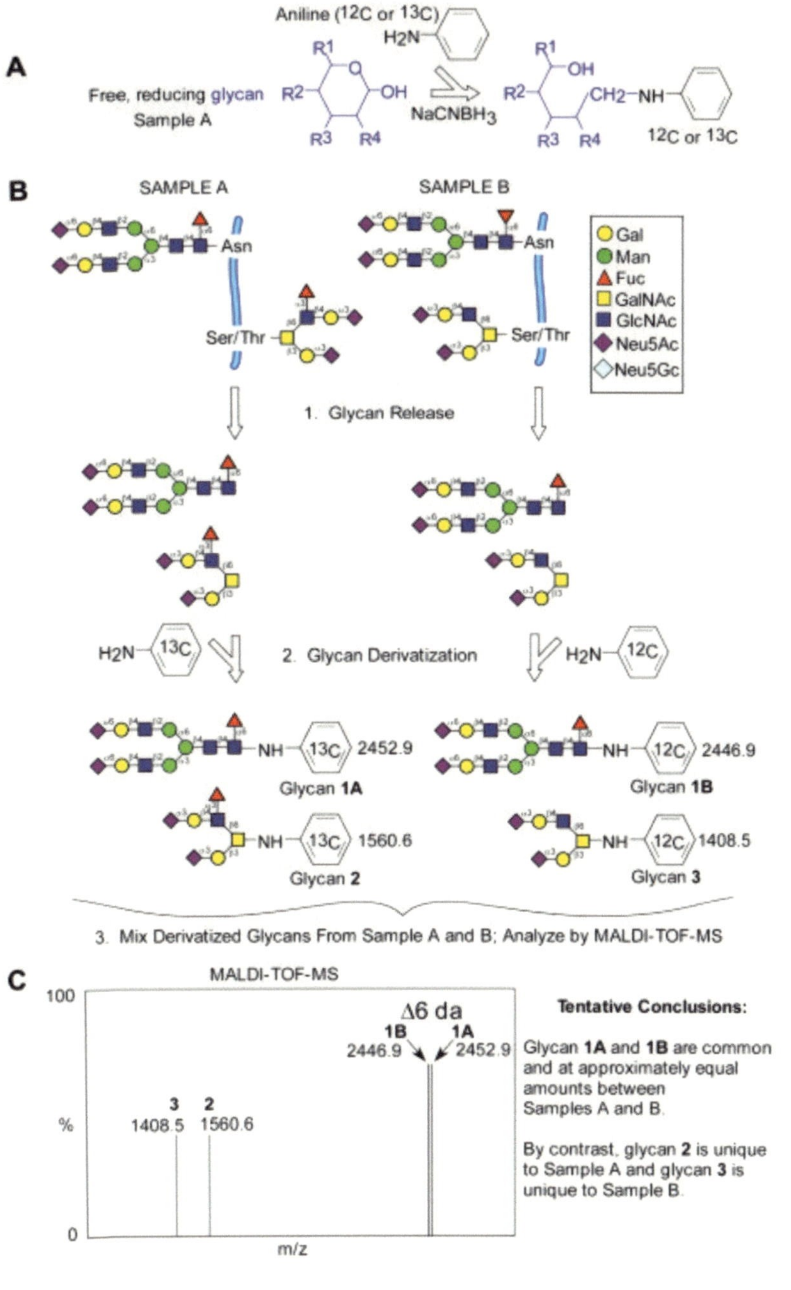

Figure 11. Schematic representation of the glycan reductive isotope labeling (GRIL). (A) Aniline labeling trough reductive amination, (B) Glycan release and derivatization with ^{13}C and ^{12}C aniline in different samples followed of sample mixture, (C) analysis of the glycan nixture. (Reproduced from Xia et al, Analytical Biochemistry, 387, 162-170, 2009)

using chiral columns. This is especially employed to determine the D/L-galactose ratio from algae agarans.

With the increase of sensitive of mass spectrometers, oligosaccharides do not need to be derivatized to become analyzable by MS. In several applications, neutral oligosaccharides from different sources are analyzed in their native structure. To aid the ionization procedures, the neutral oligosaccharides are cationized mainly by using adducts of alkaline metal, such as Na^+, K^+ and Li^+, other applications also use NH_4^+. The inconvenient of this method is to locate the reducing end of free oligosaccharides, since sometimes it is similar to non-reducing end(s). When possible a simple reduction will provide an increment of 2 m.u. and the terminus reduced site can be easily differentiated.

Another disadvantage of the method concerns the fragmentation process, considering that the cationization with the referred metals produces complex oligosaccharide-cation with lower stability than a protonation of an amino group, for example. This is well observed during the fragmentation of oligosaccharides complexed with K^+, since the complex is broken faster than glycosidic linkages, and the oligosaccharide fragments are lost as neutral loss (NL). However, Na^+ and Li^+ adducts provide good fragmentation, being Li^+ better than Na^+ for the most application (Fig. 12).

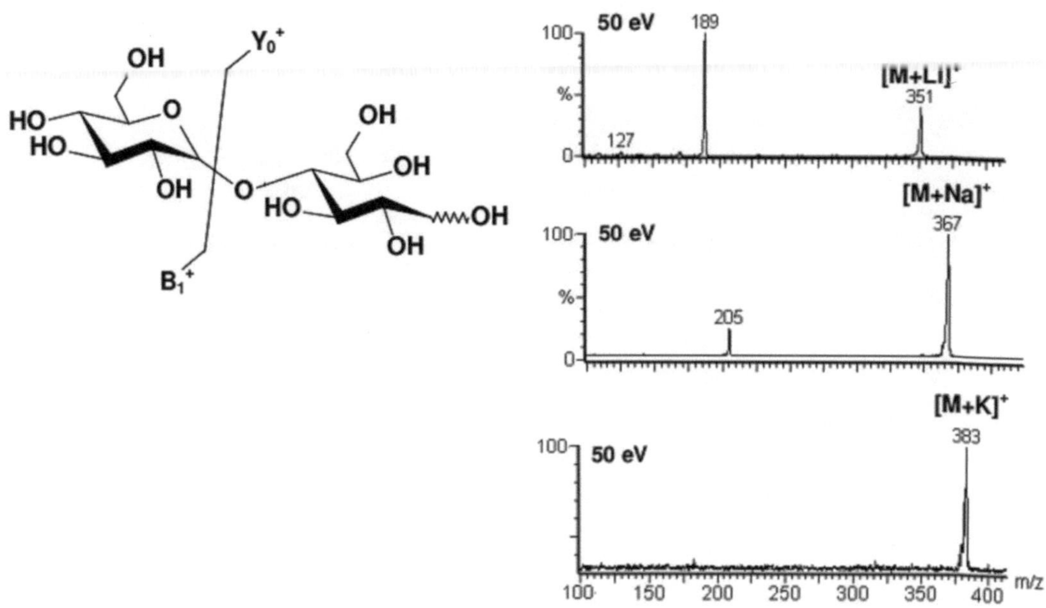

Figure 12. CID-MS (50eV) profile of a reduced disaccharide using Li^+, Na^+ and K^+ as aducts.

Na^+ is the main adduct naturally occurring in the samples, although vegetables have great amounts of K^+. This may causes severe misinterpretation mainly from low resolution MS-spectra, because the difference between both (Na^+ and K^+) is 16 m.u., similar to that observed from a hexose (e.g. glucose) and a deoxyhexose (e.g. rhamnose). Although not found naturally in the samples, Li^+ can be added to improve the MS detection, but it can also cause misinterpretation, since the mass Li^+ is 16 m.u. lower than Na^+ and 32 m.u. lower than K^+ (Fig 13). To avoid these erroneous interpretations, it is strongly recommend the use of a cation exchange resin to eliminate any residual Na^+ or K^+, and then the cation of interest can be added in lower amounts, avoiding the signal suppression. Using these simple steps, any neutral oligosaccharide or glycoconjugate can be easily analyzed by MS (data from our owner experience)

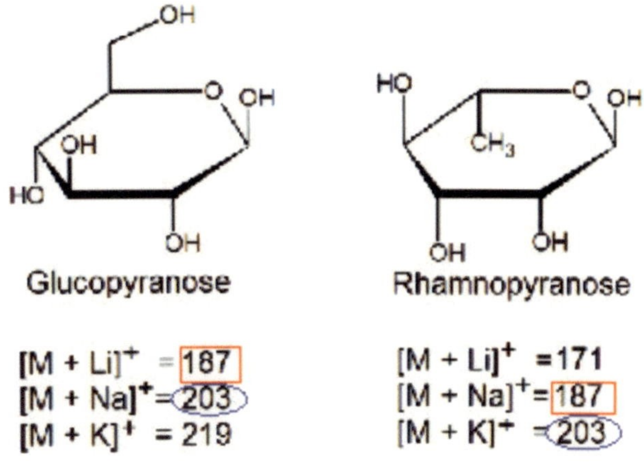

Figure 13. Common problems found in carbohydrate analysis with using alkali metals aducts.

Oligosaccharides or glycoconjugates containing acidic monosaccharides such as uronic and neuraminic acids can be directly analyzed by negative ionization mass spectrometry, since they will easily appear as deprotonated ions. Negative ions can also be formed during ionization of neutral carbohydrates, these can be formed by adduct with anions, such as Cl^- $[M+Cl]^-$, or then by deprotonation of some hydroxyl group to form $[M-H]^-$ or $[M-2H+Na]^-$.

2.4. Tandem-MS of oligosaccharides and glycoconjugates

Carbohydrates can complex with different adduct ions to produce charged molecules. However this complexation is, sometimes, not so stable to overcome the high energy events of fragmentation process, such as in collision induced dissociation (CID). Thus, the fragmentation pathway of carbohydrates is directly affected by ionization methods, but conserves similar characteristics; the fragmentation of carbohydrates occurs mainly on the glycosidic linkages, involving the dissociation of the two adjacent monosaccharides. Considering that the charge is not necessarily retained on a specific monosaccharide residue, this cleavage can releases fragment-ions from both sides, the reducing and non-reducing ends. These fragments can undergo to other fragmentation cycles giving rise the internal fragment-ions. Less abundant, the cross-ring fragmentation occurs with a double cleavage, in which the carbon-carbon or carbon-oxigen linkage is broken within the monosaccharide ring. Although not always observed, this kind of fragments may aid to describe the interglycosidic linkages.

To sort these different types of fragments observed in tandem-MS of glycoconjugates, Domon and Costello (1988) [35] proposed a nomenclature to assign them. Thus, following their nomenclature, when the charge is retained on carbohydrate non-reducing end, and the fragment-ions contain exclusively the glycan moiety, they are named *A*, *B* and *C*. But if the charge is retained on the aglycone (not carbohydrate) moiety, these fragments are termed *X*, *Y* and *Z* (Fig 14). The ions *B*, *C*, *Z* and *Y* are those produced by glycosidic cleavage, and they are accompanied by subscript numbers that refer to the number of monosaccharide residues that the fragment means (e.g. ion B_2 means a fragment containing two monosaccharide residues lacking aglycone, counted from the non-reducing end, whereas Y_2 means a fragment containing two monosaccharide residues linked to aglycone, counted from aglycone). Additional symbols α and β can be used to designate branched oligosaccharides. The fragment-ions *A* and *X* are those from the cross-ring cleavage, being accompanied by subscript numbers referring to the number of monosaccharide residues, preceding by the superscript numbers indicating the position from which bonds within monosaccharide rings were cleaved (e.g. a fragment assigned as $^{0,2}A_2$ indicates a cleavage occurring on bond positions 0 and 2, containing two monosaccharides residues, as shown on Fig. 14.

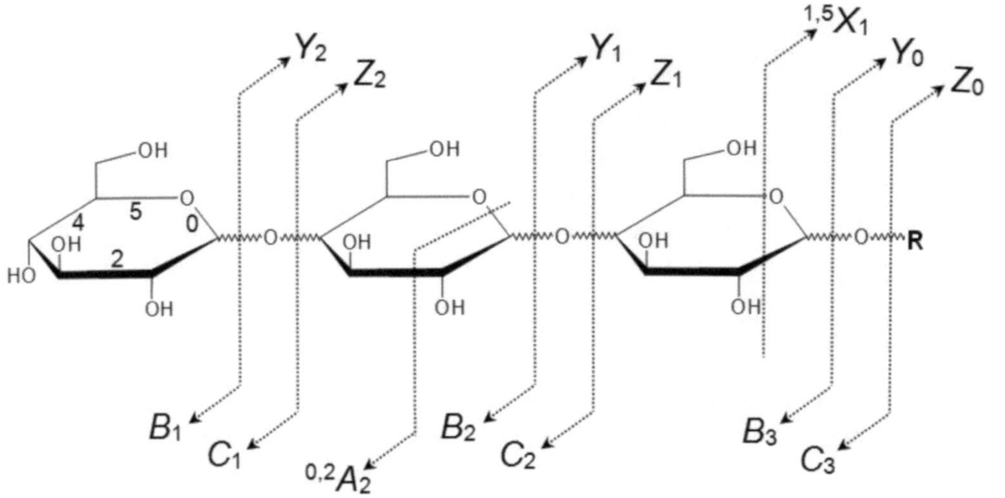

Figure 14. Cleavage profile of oligosaccharides and the fragment-ion nomenclature, R should be any compound different of a carbohydrate, named aglycone

For the most oligosaccharides and glycoconjugates Li^+ seems to be a good choice [36], because the complex [oligosaccharide or glycoconjugate + $Li]^+$ is not missed when undergoes the CID, allowing the use of less energy to produce good fragment-ions. Actually, not only oligosaccharide or glycoconjugates are better fragmented using Li^+ as adduct, even some stable ether bond can be broken.

Despite the large amounts of K^+ in samples from vegetables, Na^+ adducts are the most common ion in carbohydrate analysis and both can be used to produce $[M + Na]^+$ or $[M + K]^+$. However, K^+ adducts are lesser stable than Li^+ or Na^+, and the complexation is lost during CID, thus K^+ usually produces poor fragments or, they are missed. Although the varied cleavage possibilities, the fragments often observed for the oligosaccharide are those from glycosidic linkage cleavage, where the oxygen is retained on the fragment from reducing end, yielding mainly *B* or *Y* fragments, according to the place where the charge will remain lodged (Fig.15).

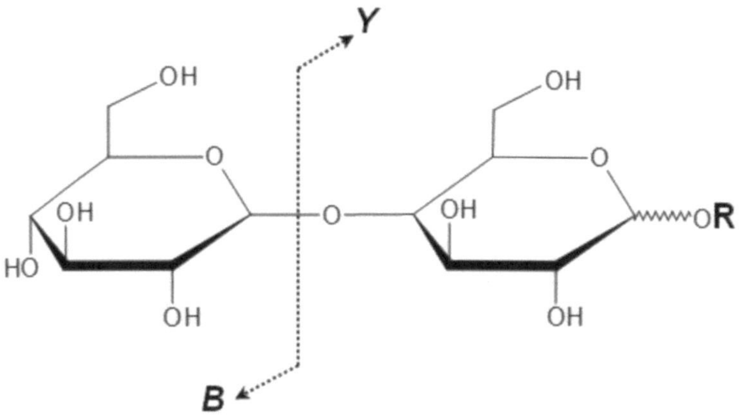

Figure 15. Typical cleavage site of oligosaccharides

In the oligosaccharides obtained by reductive β-elimination the reduced terminus seems to create a favorable environment to lodge metal adducts [34]. Also, the reduction gives an increment of 2 m.u., useful to differentiate both, non-reducing and the reduced ends. Additionally, with adduct placed on the reduced end all fragment-ions formed will be *Y*-type and no internal fragments will be produced, simplifying the spectrum interpretation (Fig. 16).

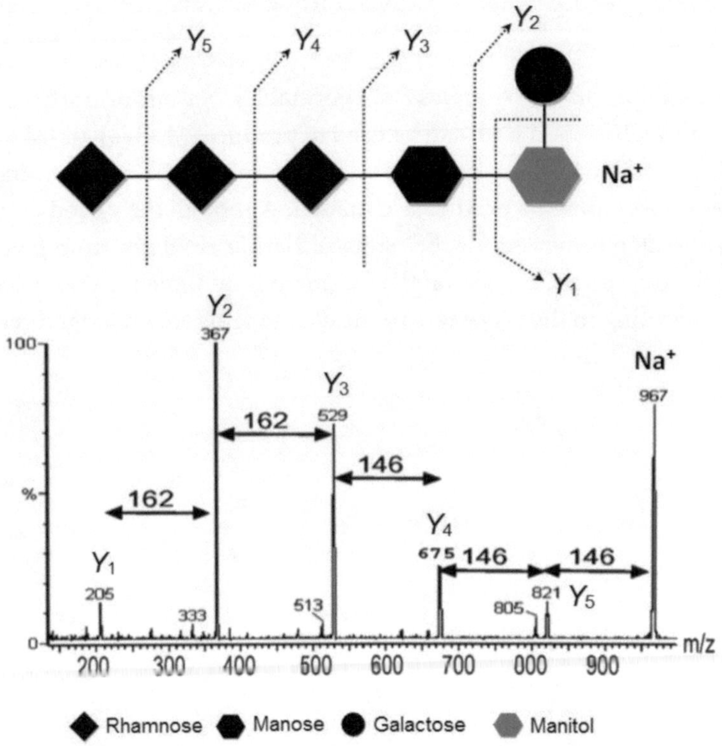

Figure 16. CID-MS profile of a reduced oligosaccharide from *Scedosporium prolificans* (Adapted from Barreto-Bergter et al., International Journal of Biological Macromolecules, 42, 93-102, 2008.)

The difference between the fragments indicates the type of monosaccharide, and for common non-derivatized oligosaccharides, a simple rule describes their monosaccharide sequence as follows: differences of 132 m.u. indicate a pentose, 146 m.u. indicates a deoxyhexose and 162 m.u. indicates a hexose (Fig.16). This occurs because the oxygen remains on the *Y*-type fragments, being recovered as a hydroxyl group via H^+ transfer from the adjacent unit which, on the other hand, appears as a dehydrated residue to give 150 – 18 = 132 Da for pentoses, 164 – 18 = 146 Da for dexoyhexoses and 180 – 18 = 162 Da for hexoses. This can be employed for de most monosaccharides even those complex. Since in the ionization with alkali metals, the complexation occurs randomly, *B*-type fragments is frequently observed, but not similar to classical formation of *B*-fragments that involves the oxonium formation via A_1-type cleavage pathway, instead the mechanism is similar to a β-cleavage with a double bond between C1 and C2 (Fig 17) [33].

For the negatively charged sulfonolipids, an alternative fragmentation pathway involving an epoxide formation between C1 and C2 are also described. To study this fragment, Zhang and coworkers [37] promoted a deuterium exchange on the free hydroxyl with an increment of 3 m.u. in the entire sulfonolipid, thus they were able to observe a lost of a deuterium during CID-MS (Fig 18).

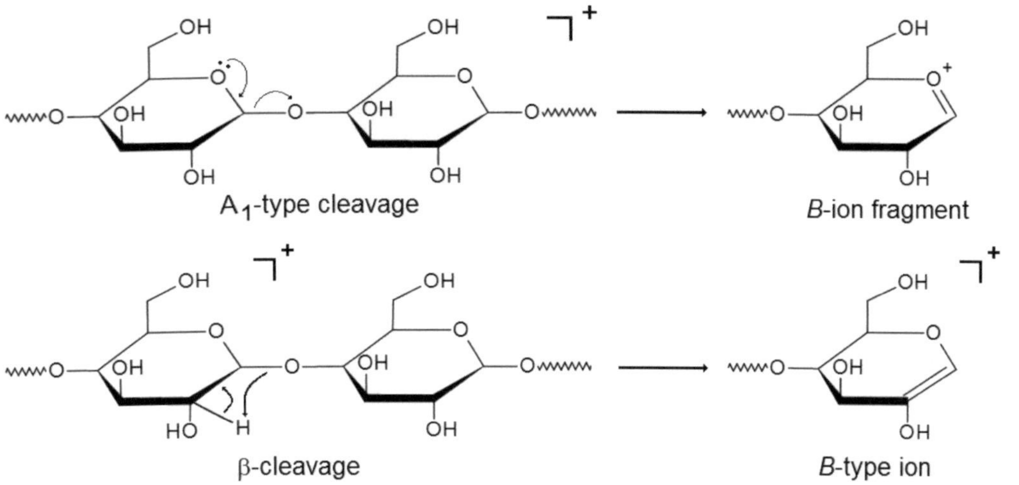

Figure 17. Typical cleavage mechanism observed in oligosaccharides leading to formation of *B* fragment-ions.

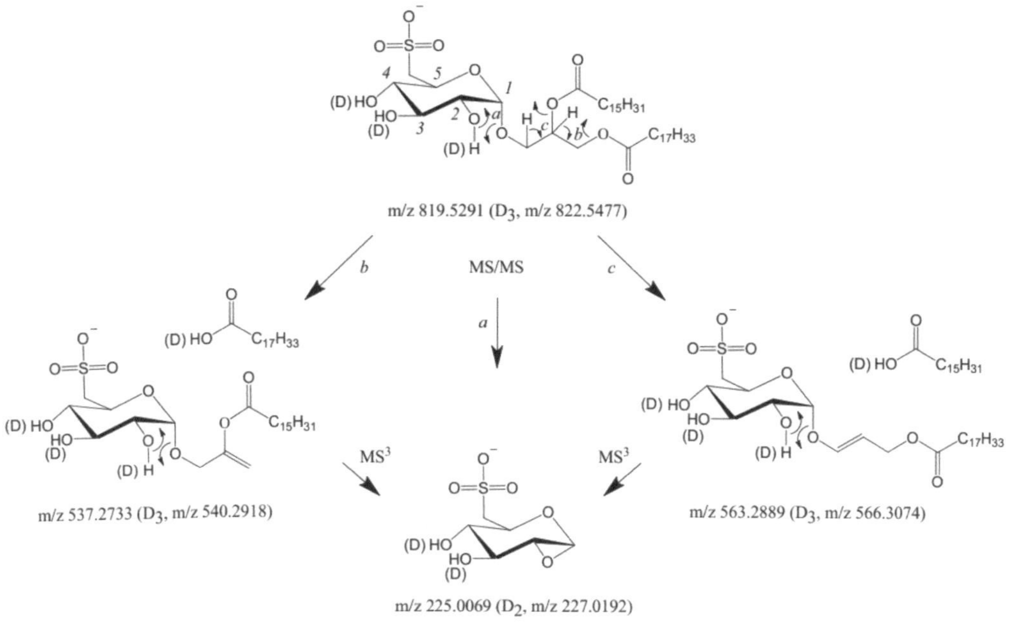

Figure 18. Cleavage mechanism observed for sulfoglycolipids that leads to formation of an epoxide between C-1 and C-2 (Reprduced from Zhang et al., International Journal of Mass Spectrometry, 316–318, 100-107, 2012.)

The ionization of glycoconjugates will vary according to the nature of aglycone moiety, but the glycan moiety enables ionization with the adducts cited above. Therefore, the choice for a specific ionization mode will constrain the fragmentation behavior. To exemplify, let's consider a glycoconjugate in which the charge is permanently retained on aglycone moiety. All the observed fragment-ions should be *X*, *Y* or *Z*, missing those of *A*, *B* and *C*. However, the *A*, *B*, *C* fragment-ions may be import to describe the structure. This occurs in glycosides from flavonoids, which can be ionized in the negative mode $[M-H]^-$ or positive mode $[M+H]^+$. In both situations, the charge is retained on the flavonoid (aglycone) and consequently only the fragment-ions X, *Y* and *Z* are produced. Considering that glycans can be attached in any hydroxyl group from flavonoid and sometimes in more than a single glycosilation site, the formation of *B* or *C* fragment-ions is critical to confirm the presence of the oligosaccharide structure, as shown in Fig. 19. To overcome this situation, the flavonoid-glycosides can be ionized with Na^+ or Li^+, since they have great affinity to the hydroxyl group from carbohydrates, they will provide mainly the fragments from the series *A*, *B*, *C*, complementing the information obtained from $[M+H]^+$ (Fig. 19) [38].

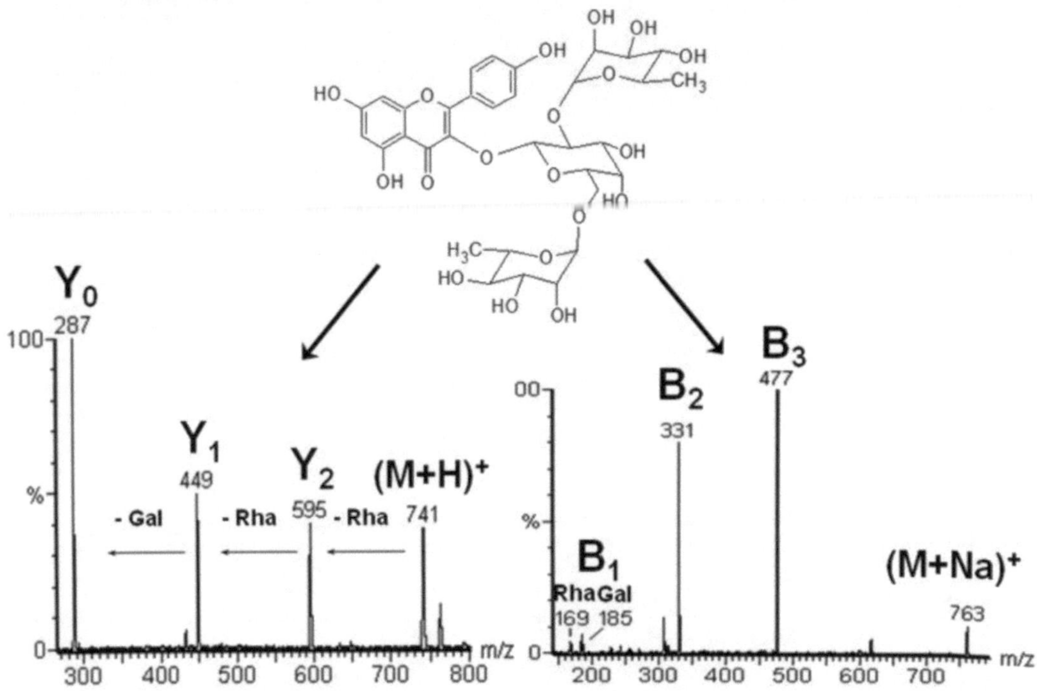

Figure 19. Changes in fragmentation behavior by using different adducts. The protonated ion gives rise to *Y*-type fragments whereas sodiated ion produces *B*-type fragments. The B_3 fragment confirms the presence of the trisaccharide moiety, being missed in protonated ion. (Adapted from Souza et al., Journal of Chromatography A, 1207, 101-109, 2008.)

As it was previously considered, Li^+ adducts produces better fragments from glycosides than other common alkali metals; though each situation must be evaluated as unique. It is well established that glycolipids produces good ionization and fragmentation as adduct of Li^+. However, Souza and Sassaki studying the fragmentation behavior of a glycolipid from *Haloarcula marismortui* [39], an Archaea, noted the absence of the series *A*, *B*, *C* in the fragmentation profile of a triglycosylarchaeol (TGA), when Li^+ was used, but these ions were well produce with Na^+ and all fragments were poorly produce with K^+ (not published data). Unlike acylglyceroglycolipids or sphingoglycolipids from other living cells, lipids from Archaea contain two branched chains in ether linkage with glycerol called archaeol. The ether linkages might create an environment to accommodate the charge $[M+Li]^+$ and thus allowing the formation of only *Y*-type fragment-ions (Fig. 20)

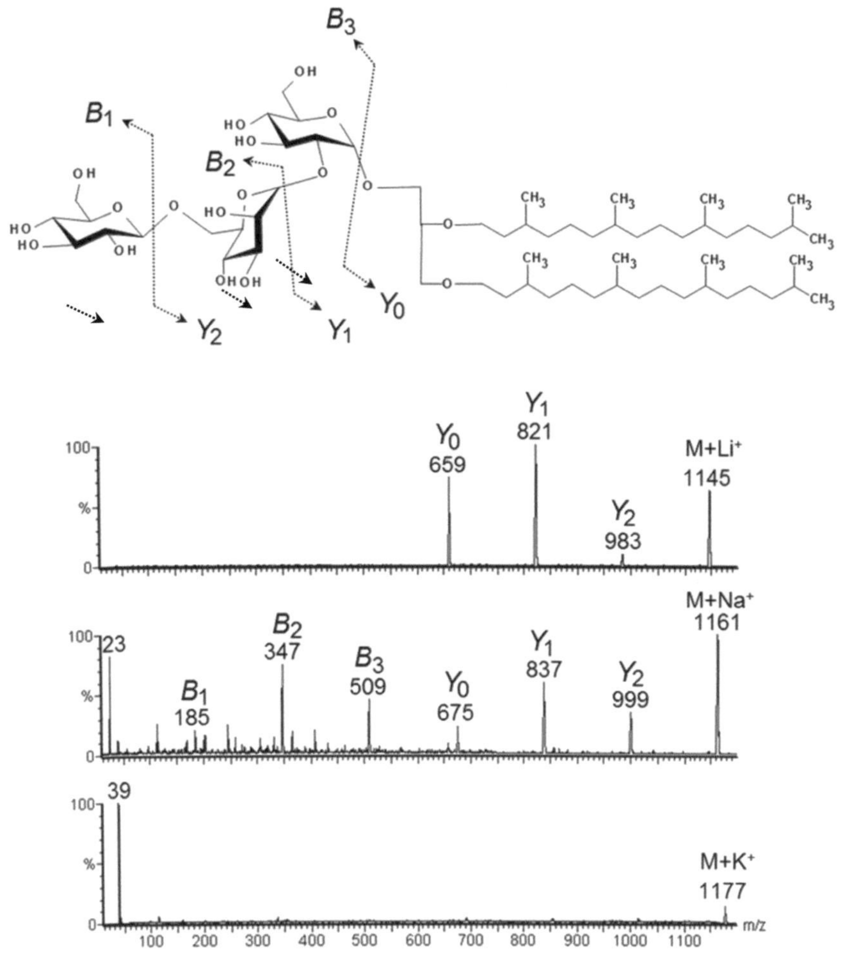

Figure 20. Fragmentation behavior of a triglycosylarchaeol from *Haloarcula marismortui* using different alkali metals as adducts. Not published data.

3. Tandem-MS of derivatized oligosaccharides and glycoconjugates

3.1. Per-O-methylation: Sequence and branching information

Per-*O*-methylation has dual importance in the carbohydrates analysis, the first was previously described, were the partially methylated alditol acetates allow determining the interglycosidic linkages via GC-MS analysis. However, permethylation for entire oligosaccharide analysis allows the using of more volatile solvents, which improves desorption and desolvation of the molecules in techniques such as ESI, enhancing the ion production and sensitive.

The fragmentation profile from per-*O*-methylated oligosaccharides also contains additional information about linear and branched oligosacchairde, barely observed from the native oligosaccharides. They can be well distinguished from per-*O*-methylated oligosacchairdes, due to the production of different fragment-ions from both chains. This occurs because each methyl radical added to a monosaccharide augment it mass in 14 m.u. thus, the *Y*-type fragment from the branched unit must have 14 m.u. lesser than other, due to the non methylated hydroxyl exposing (Figures 21 and 22). This is especially important in glycans from glycoproteins analysis. Another advantage of per-*O*-methylation concerns about the identification of internal fragments, since the reducing and non-reducing ends can be easily located by the mass increments, but those fragments from internal cleavage will appear with a mass depletion due to the non methylated hydroxyl exposing.

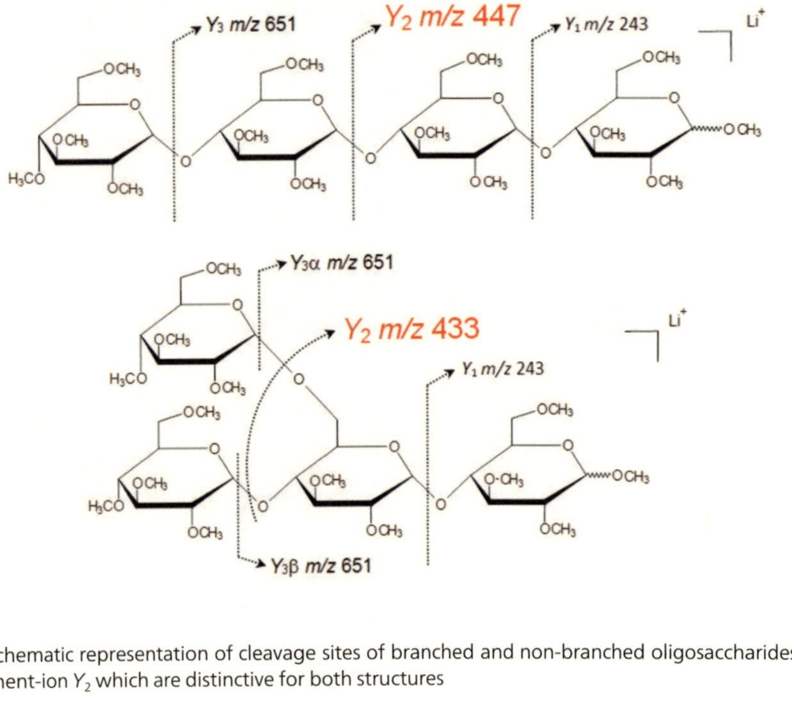

Figure 21. Schematic representation of cleavage sites of branched and non-branched oligosaccharides. It worth noting the fragment-ion Y_2 which are distinctive for both structures

http://dx.doi.org/10.5772/55221

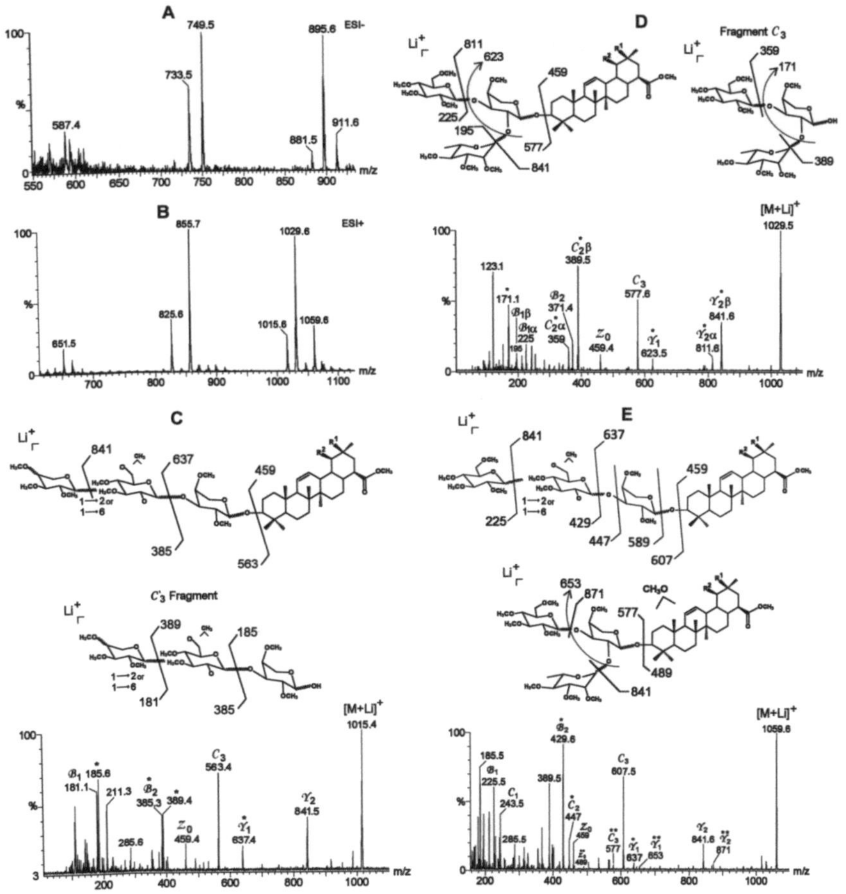

Figure 22. Application of per-*O*-methylation/CID-MS analysis for identification of matesapoins. (A) Non-derivatized saponins and (B) per-*O*-methylated. Fragments obtained from derivatized precursor-ions confirm if oligosaccharide chains are linear or branched, as mainly indicated by fragment Y_1, at *m/z* 637 (C), *m/z* 623 (D) and *m/z* 637/653 (E). (Reproduced from Souza et al., Journal of Chromatography A, 1218, 7307-7315, 2011).

3.2. Isopropylidene ketals: Interglycosidic linkage and monosaccharide information

The presence of several diastereomers from monosaccharides can cause many misinterpretation due to mass spectrometry cannot distinguished among spatial isomers. This situation is common in plant metabolites that contain a series of galactose and/or glucose glycosides. To overcome this, Souza et al (2012) developed a strategy based on ketal reactions to analyze a mixture of saponins [40]. Since the isopropylidene ketals are formed according to hydroxyl configuration, requiring free vicinal hydroxyl in *cis* configuration, they are selective formed in some monosaccharides. For example, galactopyranose (Gal*p*) has hydroxyl 3 and 4 in *cis* configuration suitable for the ketal formation, whereas glucopyranose (Glc*p*) does not. However, the ketal can be formed on Glc*p* if the hydroxyls 4 and 6 are not linked. Thus, even in mixtures many compounds could be well identified in terms of composition and interglycosidic linkages.

To describe the interglycosidic linkages from a mixture, it is appropriated to have a previous knowledge of the types of linkages that can be finding in the mixture, being easily accessed by PMMA/GC-MS analysis. Thus, with the amount of information obtained by previous analysis, the isopropylidene ketals will indicate exactly those glycosides are attached by galactose or glucose and the type of interglycosidic linkage that unit is involved (Fig 23). These methodologies are under recent development, but good prospects are glimpsed to be extended to other glycosides, including the direct identification of monosaccharides isomers (Fig. 23) employing multiple-stage tandem-MS.

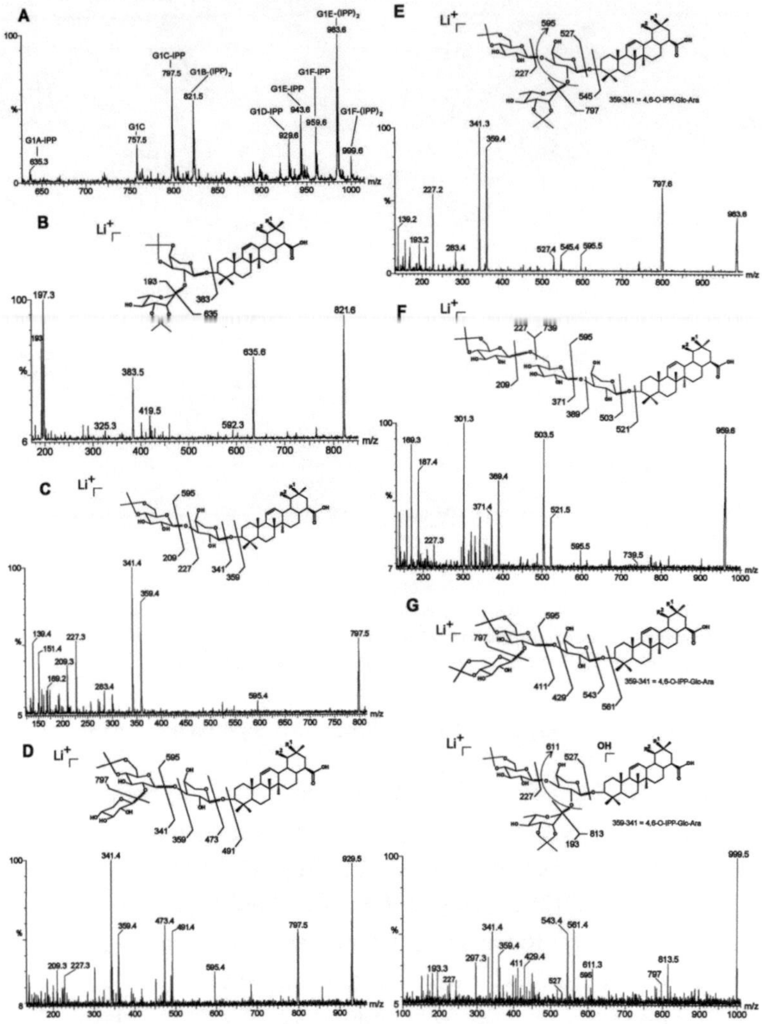

Figure 23. Application of isopropylidene ketals in matesapoins analysis (A). Ambiguous interglycosidic linkage observed on PMAA/GC-MS analysis of mixtures can be resolved by ketal formation (B-G). For more details consult Souza et al., Journal of Chromatography A, 1218, 7307-7315, 2011 (reproduction).

http://dx.doi.org/10.5772/55221

Author details

Guilherme L. Sassaki and Lauro Mera de Souza

Departamento de Bioquímica e Biologia Molecular, Universidade Federal do Paraná, Curitiba-PR, Brazil

References

[1] Dass, C. Fundamentals of contemporary mass spectrometry. John Wiley & Sons, Hoboken, New Jersey, 2007.

[2] Hoffmann, E.; Stroobant V. Mass Spectrometry: Principles and Applications. John Wiley & Sons, Chichester, UK. Third Edition 2007.

[3] Wolfrom, M. L., Thompson, A. *Meth. Carbohydr. Chem.*, v. 2, p. 65-67, 1963.

[4] Wolfrom, M.L.; Thompson, A. *Meth. Carbohydr. Chem.*, v. 2, p. 211-215, 1963

[5] Barber, M.; Bordoli, R. S.; Sedgwick, R. D.; Tyler, A. N. *J. Chem. Soc., Chem. Commun.*, p. 325-327, 1981.

[6] Galanos, C.; Lüderitz, O.; Himmelspach, K. *Eur. J. Biochem.* v. 8, p. 332-336, 1969.

[7] Hay, G.W.; Lewis, B.A.; Smith, F. *Methods Carbohydr. Chem.* (1965) 357-361.

[8] Goldstein, I.J.; Hay, G.W.; Lewis, B.A.; Smith, F. *Methods Carbohydr. Chem.* (1965) 361-370.

[9] Leitao, E. A.; Bittencourt, V. B.; Haido, R. M. ; Valente, A. P.; Peterkatalinic, J.; Letzel, M.; Souza, L. M.; Barreto-Bergter, E. *Glycobiology*, v. 13, n.10, p. 681-692, 2003.

[10] Kuraya, N.; Hase, S. *J. Biochem.* v. 112, p.122-126, 1992.

[11] Patel, T.; Bruce, J.; Merry A.; Bigge, C.; Wormald, M.; Parekh R.; Jaques A. *Biochem.* v. 32, p. 679-693, 1993.

[12] Tarentino, A.L.; Gomez, C.M.; Plummer, T.H.Jr. *Biochem.* v. 24, p. 4665-4671, 1985

[13] Altmann, F.; Paschinger, K.; Dalik, T.; Vorauer, K.; *Eur. J. Biochem.* v. 252, p. 118-123, 1998.

[14] Varki, A.; Freeze, H.H.; Manzi, A.E.; Coligan J.E. (Ed.), Current Protocols in Protein Science (1995), John Wiley & Sons, Hoboken, NJ (2001), p. 12.1.1

[15] Biermann, C.J.; Mcginnis, G.D. (Eds.), Analysis of Carbohydrates by GLC and MS, CRC Press, Boca Raton, FL (1989)

[16] Zanetta, J.P.; Timmerman, P.; Leroy, Y. Glycobiol. v. 9 p. 255, 1999.

[17] Sweley, C.C.; Bentley, R.; Makita, M.; Wells, W.W. *J. Am. Chem. Soc.*, v. 85, p. 2497, 1963.

[18] Knapp, D.R. 1979. Handbook of analytical derivatization reactions. New York: John Wiley & Sons.

[19] Carpita, N.C.; Shea, E.M.; Biermann, C.J.; Mcginnis, G.D. (Eds.), Analysis of Carbohydrates by GLC and MS, CRC Press, Boca Raton, FL (1989), p. 157.

[20] Sassaki, G.L.; Souza, L.M.; Serrato, R.V.; Cipriani, T.R.; Gorin, P.A.J.; Iacomini, M. *J. Chromatogr. A*, v. 1208, p. 215-222, 2008.

[21] Taylor, R. L.; Conrad, H. E. *Biochem.* v. 11, p. 1383-1388, 1972.

[22] Kochetkov, N.K.; Chizhov, O.S. *Adv. Carbohydr. Chem. Biochem.*, v. 21, p. 39, 1966.

[23] Lonngren. J.; Svensson, S. *Adv. Carbohydr. Chem. Biochem.* v. 29, p. 41, 1974

[24] Haworth, W.N. *J. Chem. Soc.* v. 107, p. 8–16, 1915.

[25] Kuhn, R.; Trischmann, H. *Löw Angew. Chem.* v. 67, p. 32, 1955.

[26] Hakomori, S.I. *J. Biochem.* v. 55, p. 205–207, 1964.

[27] Ciucanu, I.; Kerek, F. *Carbohydr. Res.* v. 131, p. 209–217, 1984.

[28] Jansson, P.E.; Kenne, L.; Liedgren, H.; Lindberg, B.; Lonngren, J. *Chem. Commun.* v. 8, p. 1-70, 1970.

[29] Sassaki, G.L.; Gorin, P.A.J.; Souza, L.M.; Iacomini, M. *Carbohydr. v. 340, p. 731-739, 2005.*

[30] Sassaki, G.L.; Iacomini, M.; Gorin, P.A.J. *Anais da Academia Brasileira de Ciências*, v. 77, p. 223-234, 2005.

[31] Purdie, T.; Irvine, J.C. *J. Chem. Soc.* v. 83, p. 1021-1037, 1903.

[32] Sassaki, G.L.; Czelusniak, P.A.; Vicente, V.A.; Zanata, S.M.; Souza, L.M.; Gorin, P.A.J.; Iacomini, M. Int. J. Biol. Macromol., v. 48, p. 177-182, 2011.

[33] Dell, A..Adv. Carbohydr. Chem. Biochem., v. 45, p. 19-72, 1987

[34] Xia, B.; Feasley, C.L.; Sachdev, G.P.; Smith, D.F.; Cummings, R.D. *Anal. Biochem.* v. 387, p. 162-170, 2009.

[35] Domon B, Costello CE. Biochemistry. 1988 Mar;27(5):1534-43 *Res.* v. 340, 731–739, 2005.

[36] Levery, S.B. *Met. Enzymol.* v. 405, p. 300-369, 2005

[37] Zhang, X.; Fhaner, C.J.; Ferguson-Miller, S.M.; Reid G.E. *Int. J. Mass Spectr.* v 316–318, p. 100-107, 2012.

[38] Souza, L.M.; Cipriani, T.R.; Serrato, R.V.; Costa, D.E.; Iacomini, M.; Gorin, P.A.J.; Sassaki, G.L. *J. Chromatogr. A*, v.1207, p. 101-109, 2008.

[39] Souza, L.M.; Muller-Santos, M.; Iacomini, M.; Gorin, P.A.J.; Sassaki, G.L. *J. Lipid Res.*, v. 50, p. 1363-1373, 2009.

[40] Souza, L.M.; Dartora, N.; Scoparo, C.T.; Cipriani, T.R.; Gorin, P.A.J.; Iacomini, M.; Sassaki, G.L. *J. Chromatogr. A*, v.1218, p. 7307-7315, 2011.

Chapter 5

Tandem MS and NMR: An Efficient Couple for the Characterization of Saponins

Rita Laires, Kamila Koci, Elisabete Pires,
Catarina Franco, Pedro Lamosa and Ana V. Coelho

Additional information is available at the end of the chapter

http://dx.doi.org/10.5772/56477

1. Introduction

1.1. Saponins are natural surfactants

Saponins are amphipathic glycosides that constitute a class of secondary metabolites found in natural sources, in particular abundance in various plant species and more recently found in marine organisms [1]. They were named by the soap-like foaming they produce when shaken in aqueous solutions, presenting surfactant properties, explained by their chemical and structural composition.

Saponins are constituted by one or more hydrophilic glycoside moieties combined with a lipophilic triterpene derivative. This aglycone part is termed sapogenin [2]. The number and length of oligosaccharide chains attached to the sapogenin core can vary. The chain lengths change from 1 to 11, with 2-5 residues of D-glucose, D-glucoronic acid or D-galactose being the most frequent, and with both linear and branched saccharides chain [3]. The lipophilic aglycone can be any one of a wide variety of polycyclic organic structures originating from the serial addition of 10-carbon (C10) terpene units to compose a C30 triterpene skeleton, often with subsequent alteration to produce a C27 steroidal skeleton [4].

2. Natural sources of saponins: Plants and marine animals

Many plants accumulate saponins in one or several organs, specifically in leaves, stems, roots, bulbs, blossom and fruit. The crushed leaves or roots of perennial herbs from the genus Saponaria were tradicionally used as soap. Particular types of saponins, like gypenosides and

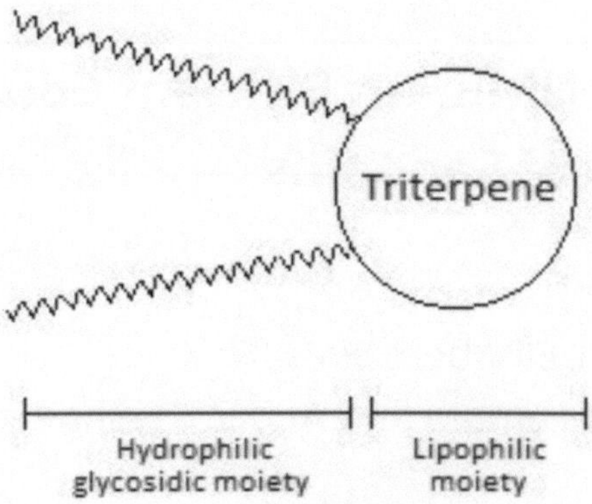

Figure 1. Schematic structure of a saponin, showing the hydrophilic glycosides moieties and the lipophilic triterpene derivative

ginsenosides, are heavily found in jiaogulan (a herbaceous climbing vine of the family Cucurbitaceae); and in ginseng (a slow-growing plant with fleshy roots, genus Panax), respectively [5].

There are several characteristics associated to saponins extracted from plants. These com pounds may serve as anti-feedants to protect the plant against microbes and fungi [2]. In addition, some plant saponins may enhance nutrient absorption and aid in animal digestion [6] and tea saponins can improve daily weight gain and feed efficiency in goats [7]. Many plant steroidal saponins have also been reported to exhibit antimicrobial activities, in particular by weakening the virulence of *C. albicans* and killing fungi by destroying the cell membrane [8]. Moreover, since some saponins are toxic to cold-blooded organisms, insects and fish, they were commonly used by indigenous tribes to obtain aquatic food sources [9].

Saponins were initially thought to be exclusive metabolites of plant origin but the world-wide development in the investigation of marine organisms as sources of new bioactive metabolites disclosed a wider distribution of these molecules also among marine animals [5]. Presently, saponins are recognized as the most common characteristic metabolites in two classes of the phylum Echinodermata (Holothuroidea and Asteroidea), where they occur as natural glycosidic surfactants. Furthermore, several steroid and triterpenoid oligoglycosides have been isolated from different species of marine sponges, more rarely *Anthozoans*, and also from fishes of the genus *Pardachirus*, where they have been shown to act as shark repellents [10].

3. Biomedical and pharmacological applications of saponins

Due to the surfactant properties of saponins they can be used to enhance penetration of macromolecules, e.g. proteins through cell membranes, making them useful as adjuvants in vaccines [11]. A wide range of pharmacological applications, such as antiplatelet, hypocholesterolemic, antitumoral, anti-HIV, immunoadjuvant, anti-inflammatory, antibacterial, insecticide, fungicide and anti-leishmanial agents have been also described for saponins [2]. Seven triterpenoid saponins from the plant Gypsophila paniculata have been shown to increase the cytotoxicity of immunotoxins and other targeted toxins directed against human cancer cells [12][13].

Holothurins, saponins isolated from sea cucumber, have displayed a wide spectrum of biological effects such as hemolytic, cytostatic, antineoplastic, anticancer and antitumor activities [14]. These glycosides are also frequently studied in the research of chemical constituents and activities of starfish, with considerable clinical interest, since they showed several physiological, pharmacological and immunological activities, such as cytotoxic, hemolytic, antifungal, antiviral, anti-inflammatory or ichthyotoxic. In particular, sulfated steroidal glycosides (asterosaponins) are one of the bioactive secondary metabolites from starfish, responsible for the toxicity of these marine organisms [15].

Concerning the commercial formulations of plant-derived saponins, these compounds are available via controlled manufacturing processes by Sigma-Aldrich (St. Louis, USA), which make them of use as chemical and biomedical reagents.

4. Saponins from asteroidea

The echinoderms (phylum Echinodermata) are exclusively marine invertebrates and, with some exceptions, are all benthic organisms (bottom-dwellers) and are one of the closest living relatives to vertebrates (phylum Chordata), since they both belong to the superphylum Deuterostomia. Asteroidea (starfishes) is one of the five classes of echinoderms, with about 1,500 living species [16] The surface of their body is often brightly coloured and is generally spiny or warty. All starfishes possess five-part radial symmetry around a central disk. This means that each of their arms has an exact replica of all internal organs. They are also characterized by a unique water vascular system, consisting of a set of water-filled canals branching from a ring canal and leading to tube feet, involved in locomotion, respiration, sensation and feeding [17].The body cavity of echinoderms is filled with coelomic fluid, which bathes the internal organs and forms the fluid medium, where the coelomocytes (the echinoderm immune cells) are suspended. The composition of coelomic fluid is similar to sea water in dissolved salts and other minerals [18]. Since the coelomic fluid bathes all the internal organs, it is extremely rich in secreted molecules, like growth factors, hormones, neuropeptides and glycosides, which are involved in cell signaling and immunity processes.

According to their most relevant structural features, glycosides from starfish were subdivided into three main groups: glycosides of polyhydroxy steroids, cyclic steroidal glycosides and asterosaponins.

The glycosides of polyhydroxy steroids consist of a polyhydroxylated steroidal aglycone and a carbohydrate portion that is usually composed of several monosaccharide units. The most common glycosylation position is C(24), but sometimes glycosides carry the sugar moiety at C(3) and C(26). In starfish they occur as sulfonylated and free hydroxy forms, with few examples of phosphorylated ones. The OH groups are usually found in positions 3β,6α (or β), 8β,15α (or β), 16α (or β).

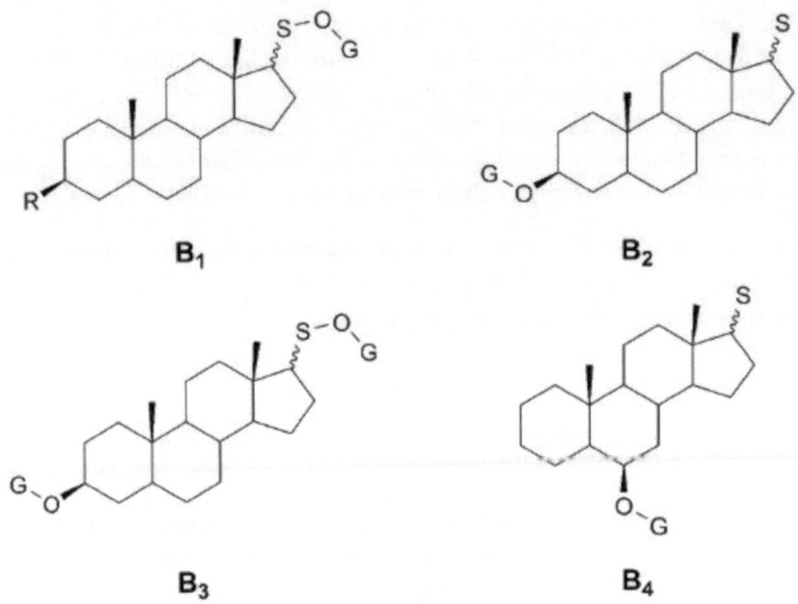

Figure 2. Main groups of glycosides of the polyhydroxy steroids from starfish. The first group (B1) are 3β-OH steroids with glycosylation on the side chain. The second group (B2) contains 3β-O-glycosylated steroids. The third group (B3) contains 3β-Oglycosylated steroids with additional glycosylation on the side chain. The fourth group (B4) are 6β-O-glycosylated steroids. G represents a glycosylation component. Adapted from [15].

The cyclic steroidal glycosides occur in few starfish. An anionic charge is due to the presence of a glucuronic acid unit. The 7,8-dehydro-3b,6b-dihydroxy steroidal nucleus is unprecedented, and the most remarkable feature is the trisaccharide chain, which is cyclized between C(3) and C(6) of the aglycone giving rise to a macrocyclic ring reminiscent of a crown ether.

Asterosaponins are constituted by an aglycone with 9,11-didehydro- 3β,6α-dihydroxy steroidal nucleus; a sulfate group at C(3); and generally a side chain with the 20β-OH and 23-oxo functions. The oligosaccharide chain, commonly made up of five or six sugar units with β-oriented structure, and sometimes containing also three or four sugar units, is always glycosidically linked at C(6). The sugar units can be xyloses, galactoses, fucoses or quinovoses. Most of the structural diversity is confined to the substitution pattern of the side chain [15].

Four asterosaponins from *M. glacialis* have been scrutinized to date [15]. Their structures are illustrated in Figure 5 and Figure 6.

http://dx.doi.org/10.5772/56477

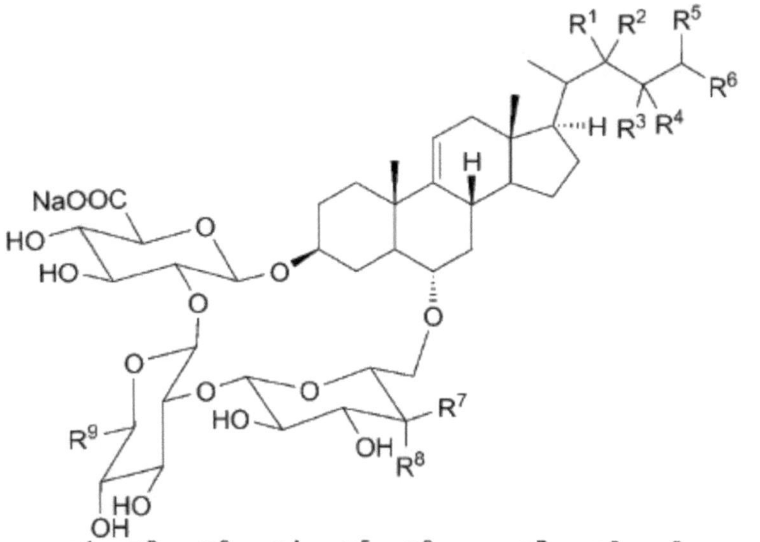

R¹	R²	R³	R⁴	R⁵	R⁶	R⁷	R⁸	R⁹
H	H	=O		H	$CHMe_2$	OH	H	HO–CH_2

Figure 3. Structure of cyclic steroidal glycoside sepositoside A, found in two starfish species, *Echinaster sepositus* and *E. luzonicus*. Adapted from [15].

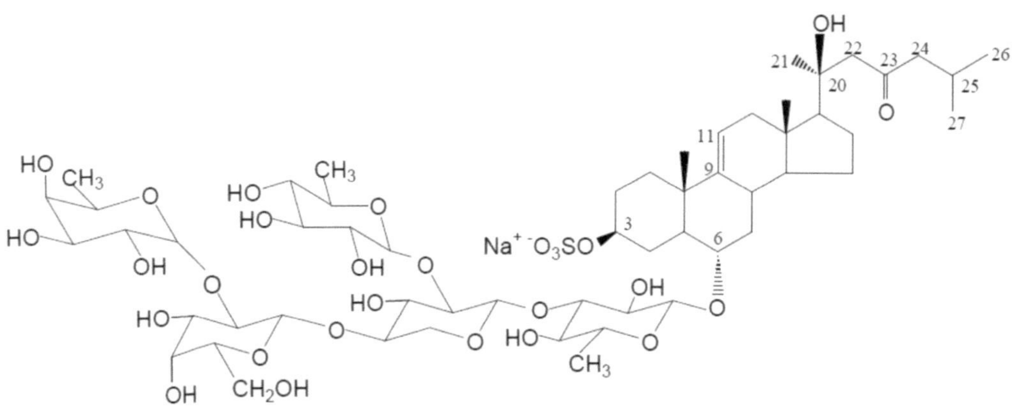

Figure 4. A sulfated steroidal glycoside (asterosaponin) typical structure. Adapted from [19].

Marthasterosides A1 and A2 (see Figure 5) differ only in the identity of one sugar residue, while marthasterosides B and C (see Figure 6) differed only in the steroidal side chain.

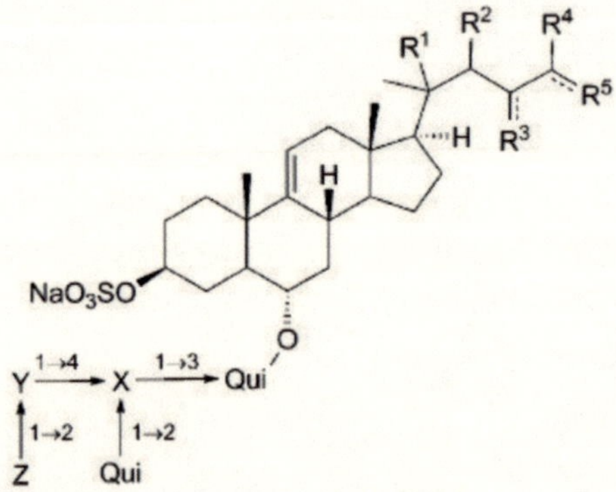

	X	Y	Z	—R¹	—R²	⋯R³	—R⁴	⋯R⁵
A1	Xyl	Gal	Fuc(1→3)Fuc	—OH	—H	=O	—H	—$CHMe_2$
A2	Xyl	Qui	Fuc(1→3)Fuc	—OH	—H	=O	—H	—$CHMe_2$

Figure 5. Asterosaponins marthasterosides A1 (A1) and A2 (A2) structures. Adapted from [15].

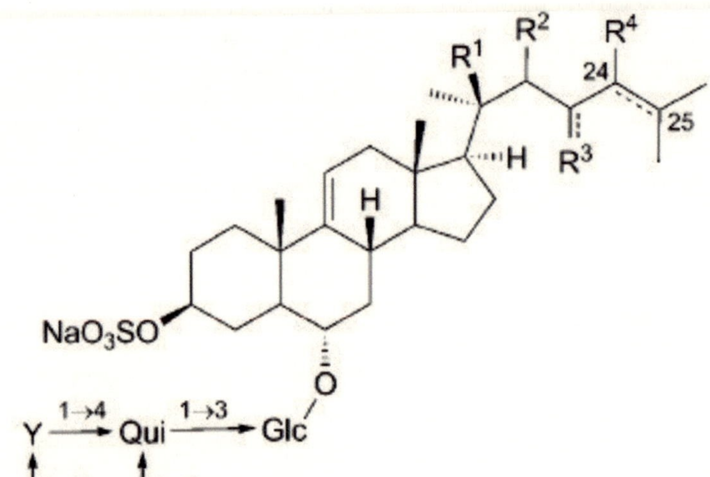

	Y	R¹	—R²	⋯R³	—R⁴	
B	Fuc	H	—H	=O	—H	C(24)=C(25)
C	Fuc	H	—H	=O	—H	C(24)–C(25)

Figure 6. Asterosaponins marthasterosides B (B) and C (C) structures [15]. Adapted from [15].

So far, studies performed with asterosaponins from starfish indicated that they possess several bioactive properties such as: cytotoxic to tumor cells and viruses; hemolytic activity toward erythrocytes of various origins; and anti-inflammatory and antifungal activities [20]. Additionally, cytotoxic asterosaponins from the starfish *Culcita novaeguineae* were reported to promote polymerization of tubulin [21]. Agents that promote tubulin polymerization exhibit anticancer activity by disrupting normal mitotic spindle assembly and cell division as well as inducing apoptosis (programmed cell death) [22].

5. Methods to extract asterosaponins

Usually, the purification/isolation of steroidal glycosides from a sample mixture, extracted from starfish, is not an easy task [23]. The extraction of the crude sample material with organic solvents often takes several hours and is frequently followed by a series of preparation steps such as gel chromatography, counter current chromatography or preparative column chromatography [24].

Currently, it is common to collect steroidal glycosides from *n*-BuOH extracts of entire animals or arms and central disks of starfish [25]. The animals are chopped in small pieces, homogenized in EtOH, filtered and then the extraction is performed with *n*-BuOH. Each *n*-BuOH extract is chromatographed and the enriched fraction separated by HPLC on RP-C18 columns typically with MeOH:H_2O (2:1) and eluted to give fractions containing mixtures of sulfated saponins [21], [26]. These fractions are analyzed by ESI-MS/MS to infer about the molecular masses and structures of these compounds, as will be discussed in the next section.

The investigation conducted in our group with *Martasterias glacialis* showed that asterosaponins can be found in the coelomic fluid as well (unpublished results). The used method includes a first step of ultrafiltration, to obtain a low molecular mass fraction; and then a step of desalination/concentration in Solid Phase Extraction (SPE) cartridges, where the compounds can be eluted in an increasing order of acetonitrile with 5% (v/v) formic acid (unpublished results). Each SPE elution fraction was analyzed by direct infusion in ESI-MS/MS.

6. MS to characterize asterosaponins

Mass spectrometry has been playing an important role in the structural analysis of complex natural products mainly due to its high sensitivity, rapid analysis time and selectivity [27]. It has the potential ability to rapidly detect the bioactive compounds in mixtures and give information on their structures as well as their molecular masses [28]. Over the last decade, the development of the so-called soft ionization techniques such as electrospray ionization (ESI) allowed the transfer of the analyte into the gas phase without extensive degradation. This led to a rapid and direct analysis of polar, non-volatile and thermally labile classes of compounds [29], e.g., polypeptides, carbohydrates and natural glycosides.

Initially, previous studies of saponins were performed using electron impact (EI) MS but this technique requires derivatization. The development of desorption chemical ionization (DCI) MS allowed analysis of saponins without derivatization, but only for saponins with ether glycosidic linkages [30]. Field desorption was also employed to analyze native saponins. However, due to the instability of ion currents dependent on the temperature of the emitter, the mass spectra were not reproducible [31]. Fast atom bombardment (FAB) ionization combined with tandem mass spectrometry (MS/MS) was employed to analyze native saponins as well, and some useful structural information was obtained. Unfortunately, the sensitivity of FAB was not satisfactory due to the chemical noise from the matrix background [23]. As a consequence, the ESI technique replaced FAB by the end of the 1990s. Moreover, nuclear magnetic resonance (NMR) spectroscopy is generally used to provide detailed structural information for saponins (as described in Chapter 8), but milligram quantities of high-purity samples are usually needed [27].

There is a lack of information concerning the fragmentation pattern of asterosaponins in MALDI-TOF/TOF. In our experience, using α-cyano-4-hydroxycinnamic acid as a MALDI matrix (unpublished results), this fact is related with some ionization difficulties of these compounds by MALDI.

Recent studies have reported the use of ESI-MS for determination of saponins with higher sensitivity and better reproducibility than the other types of ionization [30]. Moreover, the possibility of using electrospray tandem mass spectrometry (ESI-MS/MS) presents great advantages for the characterization of these compounds, by providing more information of their structure. Based on each fragmentation spectra obtained from MSn experiments, the molecular structures of the compounds can be estimated by the identification of the mass losses between successive fragmentation peaks.

In fact, ESI-MS/MS has been shown to provide high sensitivity for steroidal glycoside analysis. In particular, this technique seems to be a fast and suitable screening method for the structural information of sulfated steroidal glycosides extracted from starfish. It can provide information about their molecular mass and oligossacharide sequence by cleavage of glycosidic bonds [31].

7. MS spectra characteristic for asterosaponins

Asterosaponins can be detected in the ESI-MS spectra in the form of $[M+Na]^+$ (due to the presence of sodium ions during the process of sample preparation and the strong affinity of sugar to sodium ions in the gas phase) and $[M-Na]^-$ ions, in positive and negative ion modes, respectively (see an example of a full MS spectrum in Figure 7).

Full scan MS spectra in negative ion mode, usually show characteristic peak series with two or more peaks located in a higher mass range (*m/z* 1000-1400), increasing their value of the same mass difference, typically 14 Da. The mass difference of 14 Da can be attributed to the presence of a methoxy group in one of their sugar residues. This structural feature is very common in asterosaponins isolated from starfishes [19]. More structural information of these compounds can be easily achieved by ESI-MS/MS, as previously mentioned.

http://dx.doi.org/10.5772/56477

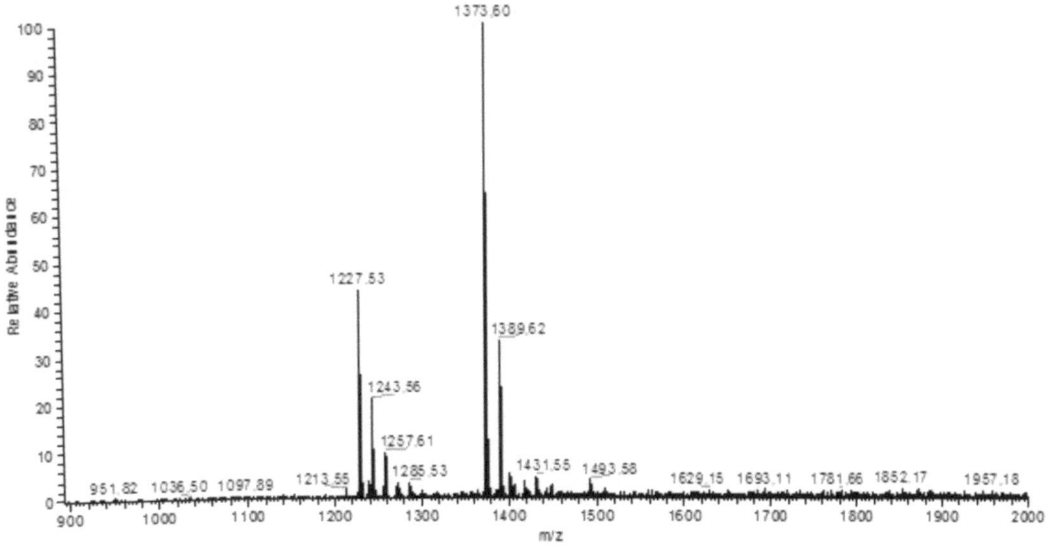

Figure 7. Example of a full ESI-MS spectrum, in negative mode, of the SPE fraction eluted with 75% acetonitrile extracted from coelomic fluid of the starfish *Marthasterias glacialis*, showing some major precursor ions. The precursor ion *m/z* 1389.6 [M-Na]$^-$ is asterosaponin masthasterosides A1 ($C_{62}H_{101}NaO_{32}S$).

There are several typical mass losses between the precursor and the fragment ions, detected in the MS^n spectra, which are characteristic for asterosaponins. Specifically, the typical mass losses detected in the ESI-MS^n spectra are related to the aglycone, the sulphate group or the oligosaccharide chain losses, which are structural features of asterosaponins. The most common sugars found in asterosaponins are xyloses, fucoses, quinovoses, galactoses and glucoses.

In the ESI-MS/MS spectra, it is common to detect a mass loss of 100 Da between the precursor and the more intense fragment ion (see an example in Figure 8). This corresponds to the loss of a $C_6H_{12}O$ molecule arising from C(20)-C(22) bond cleavage and 1H transfer (known as a retro aldol cleavage), characteristic for asterosaponins containing an aglycone with a 20-hydroxy-23-oxo side chain [19]. Additionally, it is possible to detect a fragment ion of *m/z* 97, which indicates the dissociation of the HSO_4^- group.

As mentioned before, it is possible to perform MS^n experiments to infer about the structure of compounds. As long as the signal intensity of the precursor ion is strong enough, the fragmentation process can be repeated. As so, in the ESI-MS^n spectra, ions arising from the cleavages of the glycosidic bonds from the terminal sugar moieties of the oligosaccharide chain of asterosaponins can be detected (see an example in Figure 9). In particular, the mass difference of 146 Da between two fragment ions indicates a loss of a terminal deoxyhexose residue (attributable to isomeric fucose or quinovose). In addition, the mass differences between two fragment ions of 132 and 162 Da are attributable to the losses of a pentose and of a hexose residue, respectively [25].

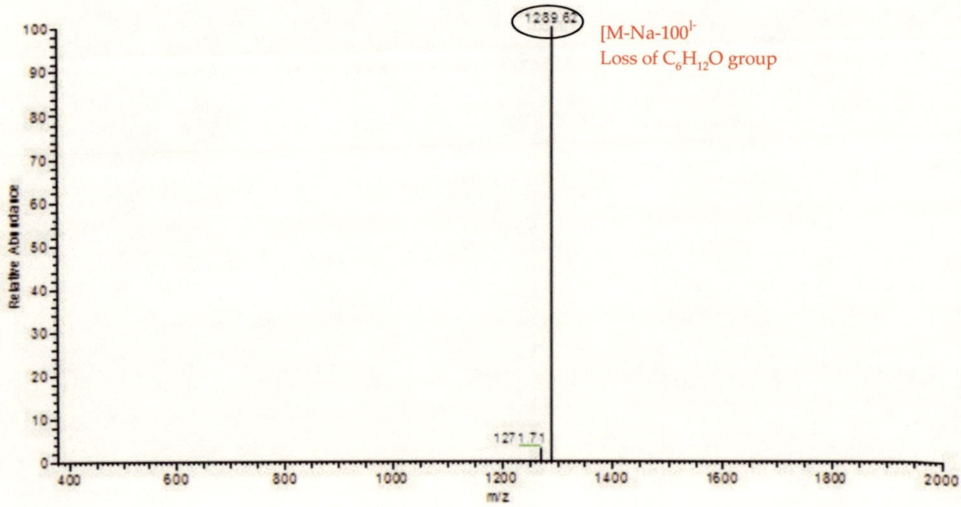

Figure 8. Example of a ESI-MS^2 spectrum, in negative mode, obtained for precursor ion *m/z* 1389.6. In this figure it is possible to detect a mass difference of 100 Da between the precursor and the fragment ion *m/z* 1289.6.

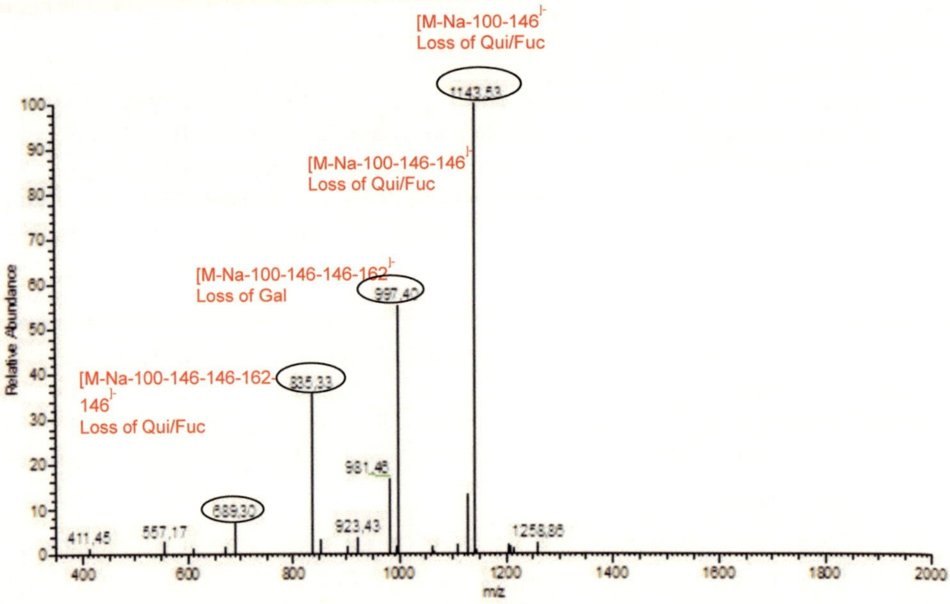

Figure 9. Example of a ESI-MS^3 spectrum, in negative mode, obtained for the precursor ion *m/z* 1289.6 generated from the molecular ion *m/z* 1389.6. In this figure it is possible to detect ions arising from the cleavages of glycosidic bonds. It can be detected a mass difference of 146 Da between precursor and fragment ion *m/z* 1143.5, attributable to the loss of isomeric fucose (Fuc) or quinovose (Qui). The same mass difference of 146 Da can be detected between fragment ions *m/z* 1143.5 and *m/z* 997.4. Also, a mass difference of 162 Da can be detected between fragment ions *m/z* 997.4 and *m/z* 835.3, which is consistent with a loss of one unit of galactose (Gal).

http://dx.doi.org/10.5772/56477

Figure 8 and Figure 9 show the fragmentation spectra of precursor ion *m/z* 1390, illustrating the typical asterosaponin mass losses of 100 (loss of a $C_6H_{12}O$ molecule), 146 and 162 Da. This precursor ion ([M-Na]$^-$) corresponds to masthasterosides A1 ($C_{62}H_{101}NaO_{32}S$), an asterosaponin that has been described for the starfish *Marthasterias glacialis*. Furthermore, the losses of three units of 146 Da (fucose or quinovose) and one unit of 162 Da (galactose) are consistent with the molecular structure of this asterosaponin (see Figure 10). An illustration of the fragmentation of masthasterosides A1 (precursor ion *m/z* 1390) can be seen in Figure 11, where the typical asterosaponin mass losses are represented.

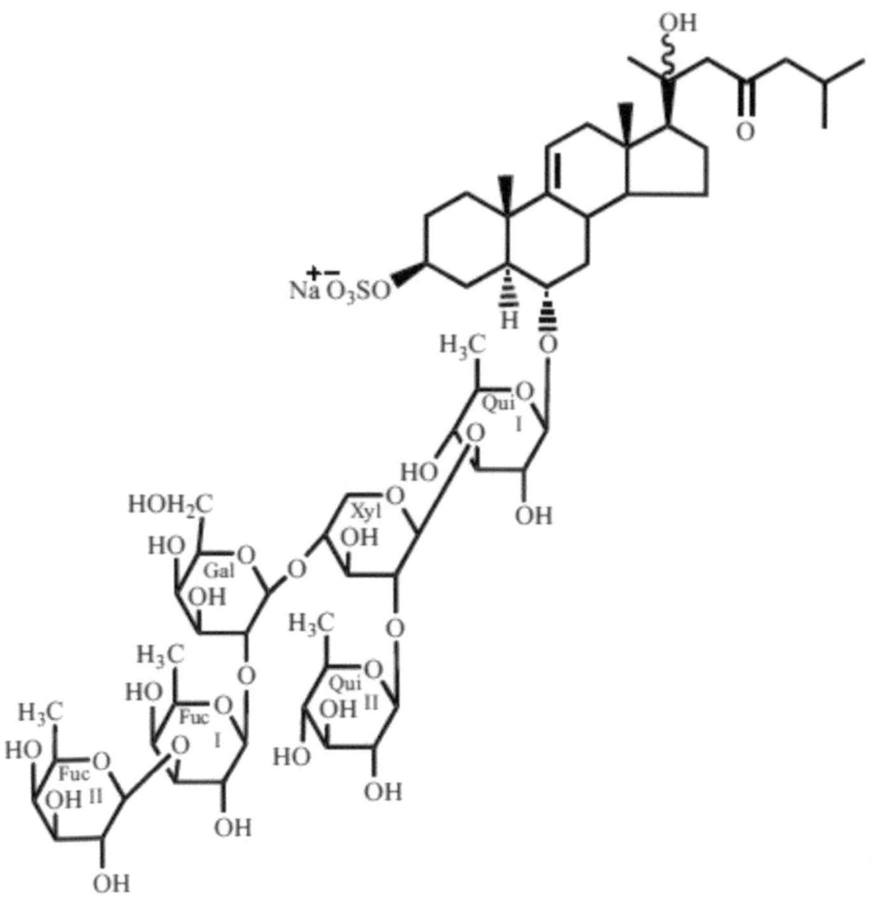

Figure 10. Structure of asterosaponin masthasterosides A1 ($C_{62}H_{101}NaO_{32}S$), indicating the fucose (Fuc), quinovoses (Qui), galactoses (Gal), xyloses (Xyl) units. [32].

ESI-MS and ESI-MS^n seem to be essential techniques to study saponin mixtures. The isolation of pure saponins is a time and/or material consuming tasks, and for this reason, these techniques are important tools to obtain information on the complexity of a saponin mixture, with the objective of finding new structures. However, only a partial characterization of asterosaponins is possible using ESI-MS^n approach since the information obtained is limited on the presence of sugar residues, the sulfate groups and the aglycone. As so, NMR spectroscopy and chemical reactions are required in order to complete characterize these molecules [19].

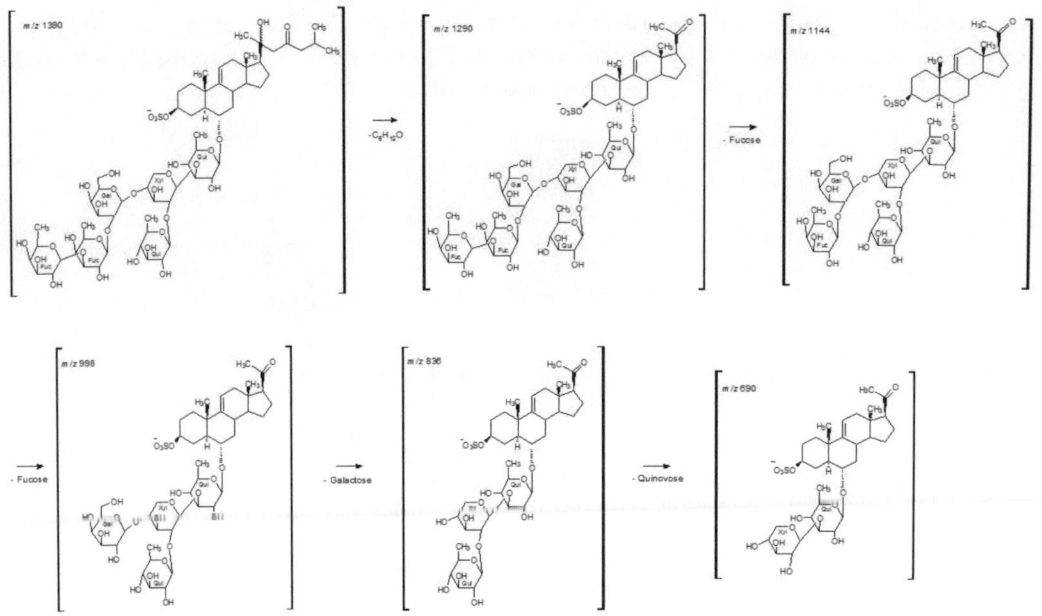

Figure 11. Scheme of the fragmentation of precursor ion *m/z* 1390, showing typical asterosaponin mass losses: $C_6H_{12}O$, fucose, quinovose and galactose.

8. Limitations of MS: Future NMR spectroscopy work (both ^1H and ^{13}C)

Nuclear Magnetic Resonance (NMR) is a very powerful tool in the study of natural compounds in general, insofar as this technique provides a wealth of structural information in the form of chemical shifts, coupling constants and coupling patterns. While the chemical shift values inform us of the nature of the chemical group in which a particular nucleus is involved, the coupling constants inform us about the structural relationship between pairs of atoms, their magnitude and splitting patterns depending on the shape and density of the electronic clouds surrounding them. To this information, two-dimensional correlation techniques, allow us to follow the resonating spins along the molecular structure, assigning them to confirm the identity of a known compound or establish the molecular structure of a new molecule. These general features of the NMR technique are perfectly applicable to the study of saponins and in particular to asterosaponins, and especially suited to determine the molecular structure of a newfound saponin or asterosaponin.

http://dx.doi.org/10.5772/56477

The general procedure is based on ^{1}H and ^{13}C NMR and consists in acquiring a one-dimensional ^{1}H spectrum and a series of five 2D spectra: COSY, TOCSY, NOESY, HSQC and HMBC.

The COSY (or COrrelation SpectroscopY), is a proton-proton spectrum, which relies on the existence of coupling constants between pairs of nuclei, and so, correlates signals belonging to geminal or vicinal hydrogen nuclei, i.e. two or three bonds apart in the molecule. This is a very important tool, since it allows the sequential assignment of the signals within the molecule.

The TOCSY (or TOtal Correlated SpectroscopY), is a proton-proton spectrum that allows to detect the signals belonging to the same spin system, i.e. with sequential coupling constants between them. This spectrum can be of vital importance in overcoming signal overlap, its use being, not restricted, but most obvious, in the assignment of the sugar resonances (see below).

The NOESY (or Nuclear Overhauser Effect SpectroscopY), is a proton-proton spectrum that allows to establish proximity in space. This spectrum allows to overcome regions in the structure for which there is no proton-proton coupling (quaternary carbons, ester or ether bonds, glycosidic bonds, etc), and thus, among other features, establish acetilation or glycosilation sites.

The HSQC (or Heteronuclear Single Quantum Coherence spectrum), is a proton-carbon spectrum that correlates carbon signals with directly bond protons. It is a very robust experiment that relies on the existence of relatively large one bond J coupling ($^1J_{CH}$~145 Hz) between ^{13}C nuclei and directly bound ^{1}H. As the signal acquisition in this spectrum is done on the ^{1}H frequency, it is much more sensitive than the experiments that observe carbon directly, and allows obtaining ^{13}C information with ^{1}H sensitivity. One drawback of this experiment is that quaternary carbons are not detected.

The HMBC (Heteronuclear Multiple Bond Correlation spectrum), is a proton-carbon spectrum in which the $^1J_{CH}$ correlations (one bond) are suppressed and the sequence is optimized for long range smaller couplings, two, three and sometimes four bonds apart. Like the HSQC, the HMBC also provides ^{13}C information with ^{1}H sensitivity, but because it is optimized for smaller values of J coupling (one order of magnitude smaller) it is a much more time consuming and less sensitive experiment. The HMBC and the HSQC experiments work as a pair in the sense that the HSQC carries very little structural information (each carbon is only correlated with its own hydrogen), while the HMBC can carry a large amount of information regarding neighboring chemical groups but it is very difficult to interpret without the HSQC information. Taken together, these experiments allow, in most cases, to follow the molecular structure through its carbon backbone.

The main drawback of NMR is its relative insensitivity, in fact, in order to record a ^{1}H spectrum the compound of interest must be present in the milimolar concentration range. Using state of the art equipment, like high field spectrometers equipped with cryogenically cooled probes this value can be reduced to 0.1 mM or less, but in general a 1 mM (or higher) concentration sample is required to acquire all the necessary information. When available, the highest field machine is always the better choice. This is not only because of the increase in sensitivity provided by the higher field but also, and most importantly, because of the higher resolution between signals that can be obtained. In fact, the main difficulty in analyzing NMR spectra is signal overlap. Because of the structural similarities between different saponins, this also means that when characterizing a new saponin, the sample has to be purified prior to analysis.

As previously described, asterosaponins, like saponins in general, are composed of an aglycone polycyclic structure and one or more sacharide or polisacharides with possible several modifications. The aglycone structures contain, in most of the cases, several chemical groups resonating in very different chemical shift ranges (see Table 1). This dispersion facilitates spectral interpretation and assignment. However, the carbon and hydrogen nuclei of the sacharide structures have chemical shifts in relatively narrow regions of the spectrum (65-75 ppm in ^{13}C and 3.0-4.5 ppm in ^{1}H, with the exception of position one of hexoses (the anomeric position), which resonate between 90 and 105 ppm in ^{13}C and 4.0 to 5.5 ppm in ^{1}H).

Type of chemical group	^{13}C chemical shift range (ppm)
Primary alkane carbons	12-24
Secondary alkane carbons	20-41
Tertiary alkane carbons	35-57
Quaternary alkane carbons	27-43
Alcohol carbons	65-91
Olefinic carbons	119-172
Carbonyl carbons	177-220
Carbons bearing fluoride atoms	88-102

Table 1. Typical ^{13}C chemical shift ranges of chemical groups found in saponins. Adapted from [33].

Since all sacharides have one anomeric position with characteristic carbon and proton resonances, these can be used as "handles" to discover the type of sacharide and its glycosidic linkage to the rest of the molecule. Starting on the anomeric position and using the COSY information one could follow the sequential assignment of each of the sugar signals, but because the rest of the sugar moiety is chemically very similar, this task becomes difficult due to signal overlap. If more than one sugar unit is present, the task becomes daunting. This problem, however, can be solved with the assistance of the TOCSY spectrum. Since all the hydrogen signals in the sugar ring are linked via J couplings to their vicinal partners, they constitute a spin-system, which will appear as a correlating unit in a TOCSY spectrum (see Figure 12)

With the sugar signals identified, their chemical shifts and J coupling patterns allow their identification. The value of the $^{3}J_{H1,2}$ (the coupling constant between protons at positions 1 and 2) of an hexose can be indicative of its configuration. In hexoses where the hydroxyl at position 2 is in the equatorial configuration (like glucose or galactose), values of $^{3}J_{H1,2}$ around 3 or 7 Hz

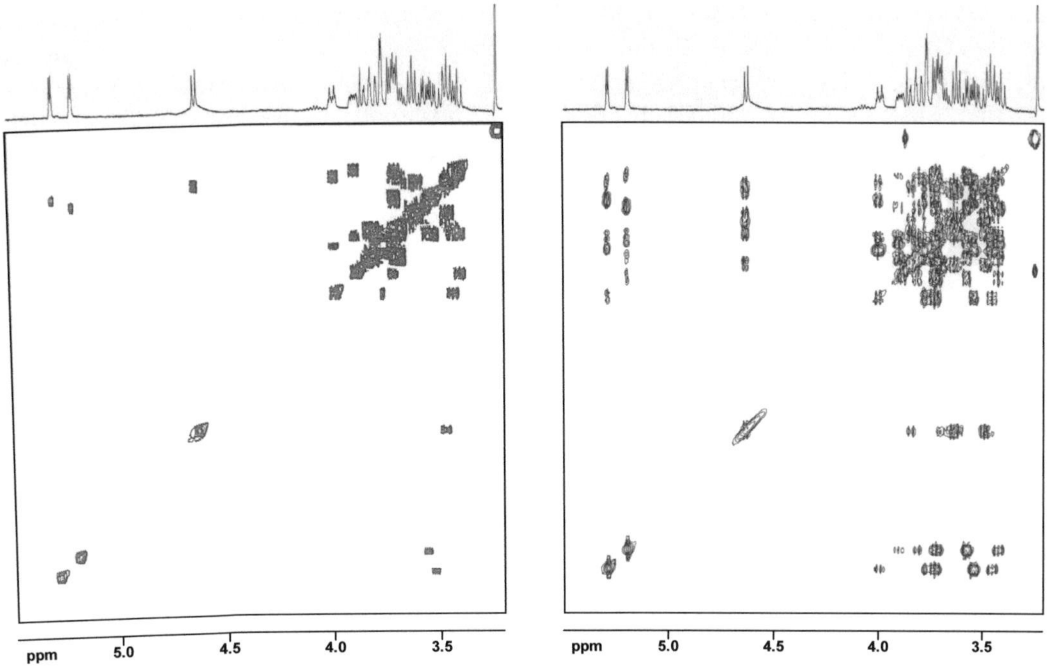

Figure 12. COSY (on the left-hand side) and TOCSY (on the right) spectra of a trisacharide (α-glucopyranosyl-(1-3)-β-glucopyranosyl-(1-1)-α-glucopyranose) acquired at 500 MHz. In the TOCSY, the spin systems of all the resonances belonging to each sacharide unit are clearly visible at the anomeric frequencies

are indicative of the α or β configuration, respectively. In the case of hexoses where the hydroxyl at position 2 is in the axial configuration (like mannose or talose), both anomers produce couplings at position 1 of around 1.5 Hz, and the distinction can only be made by measuring the $^{1}J_{C,H1}$ (the one bond coupling constant between the carbon at position 1 and its directly attached proton); α anomers displaying values around 170 Hz, while β anomers display values around 160 Hz [34]. Since the anomeric position is involved in the glycosidic linkage, these signals can also be used to establish the glycosylation sites using NOESY (that detects proximity in space and therefore can correlate signals across the glycosidic bond) or using a combination of HSQC/HMBC to follow the carbon backbone resonances and the correlation of the anomeric carbon of the sugar and a proton resonance of the aglycone structure.

NMR cannot distinguish between optical isomers, but it can detect differences between diastereoisomers. These differences are not apparent in the 2D correlation maps, since the distance in terms of bonds between the several atoms of diastereoisomeric structures is always the same, but are manifested in different chemical shift and J coupling values. The most obvious example of how NMR can be used to solve diastereoisomeric structures is the identification of sugars and their configuration (see above) but, in certain cases, it can also be used to solve other chiral centers by comparison of the acquired data and the published literature.

Also, in the case of other modifications, like phosphorylation or sulforilation, NMR can provide the site of those modifications. In the case of phosphorylation, the answer can be readily obtained by recording a $^{31}P/^{1}H$ HSQC spectrum that will correlate the phosphorus resonances with the ^{1}H signals closest in the molecule (3 or 4 bonds apart). In the case of sulfate groups, as sulfur is not very amenable to NMR studies, a different approach is taken that requires chemical modification. A desulfation procedure, like the one described in Tang et al. (2009), is applied to produce the desulfated saponin. A direct comparison of HSQC spectra before and after desulfation will detect a large chemical shift perturbation (usually a 10 ppm decrease in the ^{13}C chemical shift values) in some signals providing the modification sites.

9. Concluding remarks

Saponins are glycosides isolated from plant and marine organisms with several promising biomedical and pharmacological applications. Due to their structural complexity and diversity their characterization requires combination of results from different methodologies, namely of mass spectrometry and NMR. ESI-MS/MS analysis appears to be more suitable mass spectrometry approach to study these compounds, since it allows some structural elucidation using MSn experiments. Although, there are several structural features like sugar identity, sugar linkage pattern or site of attachment of sulfate groups, that mass spectrometry cannot address readily and that NMR spectroscopy can solve unambiguously. So, in the full structural characterization of a new saponin or asterosaponin, studies on the pure compounds using several NMR techniques (eventually in combination with specific chemical modifications) are of fundamental importance.

Author details

Rita Laires, Kamila Koci, Elisabete Pires, Catarina Franco, Pedro Lamosa and Ana V. Coelho*

Instituto de Tecnologia Química e Biológica, Universidade Nova de Lisboa, Oeiras, Portugal

References

[1] G. Francis, Z. Kerem, H. P. S. Makkar, and K. Becker, "The biological action of saponins in animal systems: a review," *British journal of nutrition*, vol. 88, pp. 587–605, 2002.

[2] A. C. a Yendo, F. de Costa, G. Gosmann, and A. G. Fett-Neto, "Production of plant bioactive triterpenoid saponins: elicitation strategies and target genes to improve yields.," *Molecular biotechnology*, vol. 46, no. 1, pp. 94–104, Sep. 2010.

[3] J. D. C. Codée, A. E. Christina, M. T. C. Walvoort, H. S. Overkleeft, and G. A. van der Marel, "Uronic Acids in Oligosaccharide and Glycoconjugate Synthesis," in *Reactivity Tuning in Oligosaccharide Assembly*, B. Fraser-Reid and J. C. López, Eds. Springer Berlin Heidelberg, 2011, pp. 253–289.

[4] R. A. Hill and J. D. Connolly, "Triterpenoids," *Natural Product Reports*, vol. 29, no. 7, pp. 780–818, 2012.

[5] B. Dinda, S. Debnath, B. C. Mohanta, and Y. Harigaya, "Naturally Occurring Triterpenoid Saponins," *Chemistry & biodiversity*, vol. 7, pp. 2327–2580, 2010.

[6] E. Wina, S. Muetzel, and K. Becker, "The impact of saponins or saponin-containing plant materials on ruminant production--a review.," *Journal of agricultural and food chemistry*, vol. 53, no. 21, pp. 8093–105, Oct. 2005.

[7] J.-K. Wang, J.-A. Ye, and J.-X. Liu, "Effects of tea saponins on rumen microbiota, rumen fermentation, methane production and growth performance--a review.," *Tropical animal health and production*, vol. 44, no. 4, pp. 697–706, Apr. 2012.

[8] M. Saleem, M. Nazir, M. S. Ali, H. Hussain, Y. S. Lee, N. Riaz, and A. Jabbar, "Antimicrobial natural products: an update on future antibiotic drug candidates.," *Natural product reports*, vol. 27, no. 2, pp. 238–54, Feb. 2010.

[9] L. Randriamampianina, A. Offroy, L. Mambu, R. Randrianarivo, D. Rakoto, V. Jeannoda, C. Djediat, S. Puiseux Dao, and M. Edery, "Marked toxicity of Albizia bernieri extracts on embryo-larval development in the medaka fish (Oryzias latipes).," *Toxicon: official journal of the International Society on Toxinology*, vol. 64, pp. 29–35, Mar. 2013.

[10] M. L, I. M, P. E, and R. R, "Steroid and triterpenoid oligoglycosides of marine origin.," *Advances in experimental medicine and biology*, vol. 404, pp. 335–356, 1996.

[11] G. N and V. M. M, "Recent clinical experience with vaccines using MPL- and QS-21-containing adjuvant systems.," *Expert review of vaccines*, vol. 10, no. 4, pp. 471–486, 2011.

[12] S. Yao, L. Ma, J. Luo, J. Wang, and L. Kong, "New Triterpenoid Saponins from the Roots of Gypsophila paniculata L.," *Helvetica Chimica Acta*, vol. 93, pp. 361–374, 2010.

[13] A. Weng, M. Thakur, F. Beceren-Braun, D. Bachran, C. Bachran, S. B. Riese, K. Jenett-Siems, R. Gilabert-Oriol, M. F. Melzig, and H. Fuchs, "The toxin component of targeted anti-tumor toxins determines their efficacy increase by saponins.," *Molecular oncology*, vol. 6, no. 3, pp. 323–32, Jun. 2012.

[14] S. Bordbar, F. Anwar, and N. Saari, "High-value components and bioactives from sea cucumbers for functional foods--a review.," *Marine drugs*, vol. 9, no. 10, pp. 1761–805, Jan. 2011.

[15] G. Dong, T. Xu, B. Yang, X. Lin, X. Zhou, X. Yang, and Y. Liu, "Chemical constituents and bioactivities of starfish.," *Chemistry & biodiversity*, vol. 8, no. 5, pp. 740–91, May 2011.

[16] C. F. Franco, R. Santos, and A. V. Coelho, "Exploring the proteome of an echinoderm nervous system: 2-DE of the sea star radial nerve cord and the synaptosomal membranes subproteome.," *Proteomics*, vol. 11, no. 7, pp. 1359–64, Apr. 2011.

[17] C. Nielsen, *Animal evolution: Interrelationships of animal phyla.* Oxford: Oxford Univ. Press, 1995.

[18] L. C. Smith, J. Ghosh, K. M. Buckley, L. A. Clow, N. M. Dheilly, T. Haug, J. H. Henson, C. Li, C. M. Lun, A. J. Majeske, V. Matranga, S. V Nair, J. P. Rast, D. A. Raftos, M. Roth, S. Sacchi, C. S. Schrankel, and K. Stensvåg, *Invertebrate Immunity: Echinoderm Immunity.* Landes Bioscience and Springer Science+Business Media, 2010, pp. 260–301.

[19] M. S. Maier, R. Centurión, C. Muniain, and R. Haddad, "Identification of sulfated steroidal glycosides from the starfish Heliaster helianthus by electrospray ionization mass spectrometry," vol. 2007, no. vii, pp. 301–309, 2007.

[20] M. S. Maier, "Biological activities of sulfated glycosides from echinoderms," *Studies in Natural Products Chemistry*, vol. 35, pp. 311–354, 2008.

[21] H.-F. Tang, G. Cheng, J. Wu, X.-L. Chen, S.-Y. Zhang, A.-D. Wen, and H.-W. Lin, "Cytotoxic asterosaponins capable of promoting polymerization of tubulin from the starfish Culcita novaeguineae.," *Journal of natural products*, vol. 72, no. 2, pp. 284–9, Feb. 2009.

[22] F. Uckun, C. Mao, S. Jan, H. Huang, A. Vassilev, E. Sudbeck, C. Navara, and R. NArla, "SPIKET and COBRA compounds as novel tubulin modulators with potent anticancer activity," *Current opinion in investigational drugs*, vol. 1, no. 2, pp. 252–256, 2000.

[23] S. Fang, C. Hao, W. Sun, Z. Liu, and S. Liu, "Rapid analysis of steroidal saponin mixture using electrospray ionization mass spectrometry combined with sequential tandem mass spectrometry.," *Rapid communications in mass spectrometry: RCM*, vol. 12, no. 10, pp. 589–94, Jan. 1998.

[24] M. Sandvoss, a Weltring, a Preiss, K. Levsen, and G. Wuensch, "Combination of matrix solid-phase dispersion extraction and direct on-line liquid chromatography-nuclear magnetic resonance spectroscopy-tandem mass spectrometry as a new efficient approach for the rapid screening of natural products: application to the t," *Journal of chromatography. A*, vol. 917, no. 1–2, pp. 75–86, May 2001.

[25] A. a Kicha, A. I. Kalinovsky, N. V Ivanchina, T. V Malyarenko, P. S. Dmitrenok, S. P. Ermakova, and V. a Stonik, "Four new asterosaponins, hippasteriosides A - D, from

the Far Eastern starfish Hippasteria kurilensis.," *Chemistry & biodiversity*, vol. 8, no. 1, pp. 166–75, Jan. 2011.

[26] H.-F. Tang, Y.-H. Yi, L. Li, P. Sun, S.-Q. Zhang, and Y.-P. Zhao, "Asterosaponins from the starfish Culcita novaeguineae and their bioactivities.," *Fitoterapia*, vol. 77, no. 1, pp. 28–34, Jan. 2006.

[27] F. Song, M. Cui, Z. Liu, B. Yu, and S. Liu, "Multiple-stage tandem mass spectrometry for differentiation of isomeric saponins.," *Rapid communications in mass spectrometry: RCM*, vol. 18, no. 19, pp. 2241–8, Jan. 2004.

[28] Y. W. Ha, Y.-C. Na, J.-J. Seo, S.-N. Kim, R. J. Linhardt, and Y. S. Kim, "Qualitative and quantitative determination of ten major saponins in Platycodi Radix by high performance liquid chromatography with evaporative light scattering detection and mass spectrometry.," *Journal of chromatography. A*, vol. 1135, no. 1, pp. 27–35, Nov. 2006.

[29] R. Soares, C. Franco, E. Pires, M. Ventosa, R. Palhinhas, K. Koci, A. Martinho de Almeida, and A. Varela Coelho, "Mass spectrometry and animal science: Protein identification strategies and particularities of farm animal species.," *Journal of proteomics*, vol. 75, no. 14, pp. 4190–206, Jul. 2012.

[30] S. Liu, M. Cui, Z. Liu, F. Song, and W. Mo, "Structural analysis of saponins from medicinal herbs using electrospray ionization tandem mass spectrometry.," *Journal of the American Society for Mass Spectrometry*, vol. 15, no. 2, pp. 133–41, Feb. 2004.

[31] R. Li, Y. Zhou, Z. Wu, and L. Ding, "ESI-QqTOF-MS/MS and APCI-IT-MS/MS analysis of steroid saponins from the rhizomes of Dioscorea panthaica.," *Journal of mass spectrometry: JMS*, vol. 41, no. 1, pp. 1–22, Jan. 2006.

[32] V. U. Ahmad and A. Basha, Eds., "Marthasteroside A1," in *Spectroscopic Data of Steroid Glycosides: Cholestanes, Ergostanes, Withanolides, Stigmastane*, Springer New York, 2007, pp. 362–363.

[33] E. Breitmaier and W. Voelter, *Carbon-13 NMR Spectroscopy*. Weinheim: VCH Verlagsgesellschaft mbH, 1990.

[34] K. Bock and C. Pedersen, "A study of 13CH coupling constants in hexopyranoses," *Journal of the chemical society*, no. 3, pp. 293–297, 1974.

Chapter 6

Post-Translational Modification Profiling of Burn-Induced — Insulin Resistance and Muscle Wasting

Xiao-Ming Lu, Ronald G. Tompkins and
Alan J. Fischman

Additional information is available at the end of the chapter

http://dx.doi.org/10.5772/54849

1. Introduction

The maintenance of glucose levels represents one of the most tightly regulated systems in the body. All cells require glucose, however, it is only available from exogenous sources or hepatic production. Since glucose cannot be stored in significant amounts except as glycogen in the liver and muscle, glucose transport into the cell by specific transport proteins is critical for cell function. Insulin plays a major role in the maintenance of normal glucose levels. When blood glucose levels rise, insulin secretion is stimulated, resulting in increase in uptake of glucose by skeletal muscle via glucose transporter protein 4 (GLUT4), and decreased production by the liver. Binding of insulin to its receptor leads to activation of insulin receptor tyrosine kinase, which phosphorylates IRS proteins that function as docking platforms for the two main signalingpathways are responsible downstream regulation [1]; the phosphatidyl inositol 3-kinase (PI3K)-Akt/protein kinase B (PKB) pathway and the Ras-mitogen-activated protein kinase (MAPK) pathway. There appear to be several key proteins in the insulin/glucose and protein turnover regulatory cascade, including IRS-1 the predominent form of IRS in muscle. When levels of insulin and glucose are abnormally high in the fasting state, a condition called insulin resistance exists. Insulin resistance and muscle wasting during the persistent high grade inflammation induced by severe burn injury increases the patients risk for infection, sepsis, and death. Clinical data indicate that a resting metabolic rate switch occurs after burn injuries that involve ~40-60% total body surface area (TBSA). Based on studies of 189 pediatric burn patients [2,3,4], it was determined that burn size determines the inflammatory and hypermetabolic response to injury; serum glucose and insulin levels increased to 144 mg/dl and 32 ng/ml on day 8 after injury. Metabolic alterations such as abnormal cytokine release [5, 6], altered gene expression [7,8] and increased protein catabolism are common in patients with burn injuries [9,10,11]. Glucose intolerance and elevated insulin levels may contribute to hyperglycemia, even in non-diabetic patients [12,13,14,15,16,17]. Hyperglycemia and glucose intolerance are frequently associated with the metabolic response to major trauma. Following injury [18], burn shock [19,20] or systemic infection [21,22], oral and intravenous glucose tolerance tests have demonstrated delayed disposal of glucose from plasma into tissues. This "diabetes of injury" could be explained if there was an insulin deficiency, and several studies [23] have shown that early after trauma ("ebb phase") insulin concentrations are reduced even in the face of hyperglycemia. After resuscitation of trauma patients ("flow phase"), beta cell responsiveness to glucose administration and plasma insulin levels are appropriate or even higher than expected. However, despite this appropriate acute insulin response to glucose administration, glucose intolerance and hyperglycemia continue. This finding suggests that some of the tissues in trauma patients are relatively insensitive to the effects of insulin.

There are numerous reports that describe insulin resistance in burn patients and animal models [24,25,26,27,28,29,30,31,32,33,34,35,36,37,38,39]. Direct measurements show that liver and skeletal muscle are resistant tissues. In addition, lipolysis is not attenuated in trauma patients after glucose administration. The precise mechanism for insulin resistance after burns or other stressors is unknown. It is likely, however, that insulin binding to its membrane receptors is normal, and that there is a post receptor mechanism for the insulin resistance. Alterations in levels of cytokines, such as TNF, IL-1, and IL-6, have been reported in burn patients and animal models of burn injury by our laboratory and other investigators [38]. Infusion of endotoxin, TNF, and IL-1 can produce alterations in glucose metabolism and insulin resistance *in vivo* [40, 41]. In addition, it has also been shown that endotoxin [42] and IL-6 [43] can produce insulin resistance in isolated hepatocyte cultures and that IL-6 inhibits insulin mediated stimulation of glucokinase in isolated hepatocytes. Cortisol, glucagon and epinephrine, can produce insulin resistance [44]. These molecules oppose the actions of insulin and are termed counter-regulatory hormones. Since these counter-regulatory hormones are elevated, at least initially, after burn injury, it has been proposed that counter-regulatory hormones may play a role in burn induced insulin resistance. The levels of cytokines and counter-regulatory hormones are dramatically altered in burn patients and animal models [45,46]. It has been demonstrated that TNF suppresses insulin-induced tyrosine phosphorylation of insulin receptor, and inhibits downstream signaling from the insulin receptor [47,48]. Furthermore, the insulin resistance produced in spontaneously obese rats can be overcome by pretreatment of the animals with antibodies to TNF [49].

Although the number of investigations that address the mechanism(s) of insulin resistance in trauma patients has been limited, one important study [50] using the euglycemic insulin clamp technique demonstrated: (i) the maximal rate of glucose disposal is reduced in trauma patients; (ii) the metabolic clearance rate of insulin is almost twice normal in these patients; and (iii) post-trauma insulin resistance appears to occur in peripheral tissues, probably skeletal muscle, and is consistent with a post-receptor effect. Unfortunately, the procedures used in this study were not capable of independently accessing the contributions of glucose transport, phosphorylation, and subsequent intracellular metabolism of glucose. Ikezy*et al* [51] demonstrated that burn injury to rats resulted in impaired insulin-stimulated transport of [^{3}H]-2-deoxyglu-

http://dx.doi.org/10.5772/54849

cose into soleus muscle strips *in vitro*. These investigators also demonstrated that insulin stimulated phosphoinositide 3-kinase (PI3K) activity, that is pivotal for glucose transport in muscle by GLUT 4, was decreased by burn injury to rats as measured by its IRS-1 associated activity. These data are consistent with alterations in post-receptor signaling following burn injury, which results in burn induced insulin resistance and muscle wasting.

Dynamic and stress dependent multi-site phosphorylations of IRS-1 tyrosine, serine and threonine residues have been described to have both positive and negative insulin effects. IRS proteins contain a conversed pleckstrin homology (PH) domain located at their N termini and that anchors them to membrane phosphoinositides in close proximity to the insulin receptor. The PH domain is flanked by a phosphotyrosine-binding (PTB) domain. PhosporylatedSer/The residues in the PTB proximity are likely to dissociate IRS-IR binding and weaken insulin signaling. Tyrosine phosphorylations, in the N- or C-terminal regions of IRS-1 are generally considered to be positive PTM in the insulin signaling pathways. In other words, IRS-1 binds several Src homology 2 domain (SH2) proteins through its multiple tyrosine phosphorylation sites with YMXM or YXXM motifs to propagate the signal. In contrast, phosphorylations of serine and threonine residues at the C-terminal region are usually considered to be negative PTMs, however, some positive effects of serine phosphorylations have been reported. A number of phosphorylation sites have been identified with different approaches such as: radiolabeling with [γ- ^{32}p] ATP [52,53,54,55,56], immunoblotting with anti-phosphopeptide antibodies [57,58,59,60,61,62,63,64,65,66], studies with mutated IRS-1 [67,68,69] and HPLC online or offline interfaced with MALDI-TOF or ESI-TOF [70,71,72,73,74]. The large variation and poor reproducibility in the reported phosphorylation sites are explained by: method sensitivities, enzymatic and chemical stabilities of the phosphorylated sites and stimulus intensity /timing. Proposed mechanisms for impairment of the insulin signaling system by phosphorylations of serine and threonine residues include: feedback inhibition, cooperative interactions, uncoupling of the protein signaling network [75,76,77,78, 79] and ubiquitin-proteasome degradation [80,81,82,83,84,85,86]. It is fair to state that, to date, burn-induced phosphorylations patterns of IRS-1 are poorly understood. However, since these negative biological effects may provide some clues for exploring the mechanism of insulin resistance [87,88,89], after burn injury [90,91], evaluation of this issue has become a major focus of our laboratory.

Determination of the phosphorylation pattern of IRS-1 is essential for understanding the metabolic basis for many disease processes [92]. However, neither the causative factors nor the cellular mechanisms of the muscle wasting and insulin resistance associated with the massive acute inflammation induced by burn injury have been elucidated. Recent publications suggest that insulin resistance may be in part due to phosphorylation based negative-feedback in two different pathways: 1) Phosphorylated Ser/Thr residues in the IRS-1 phosphorylated tyrosine binding (PTB) domain may simply uncouple downstream processes from the insulin receptor β - subunit, terminating downstream signal transduction without changing IRS-1 protein integrity. 2) Phosphorylated Ser/Thr sites may become proteolytic targets for CUL7 E3 ubiquitin ligase in a manner that depends on the mammalian target of rapamycin (mTOR) and p70 S6 kinase activities. These Ser/Thr sites located in the proximal C-terminal region of IRS-1 may provide multiple cleavage sites. Other studies have shown a role for SOCS-1 and SOCS-3 with the elongin BC ubiquitin ligase complex in IRS protein degradation.

There are 50 to 70 potential phosphorylation sites in IRS-1, and some of these sites up- and/or down-regulate insulin signaling [93,94]. Sequencing of the human genome has allowed the identification of more than 500 kinases and 60 phosphatases which may be involved in the regulation of IRS-1 binding under physiological conditions [95]. To date, approximately 29 Ser/Thr phosphorylation sites in IRS1 have been reported from various *in vivo* and *in vitro* experiments [96,97,98]. Unfortunately, no systematic IRS-1 phosphorylation data associated with burn injury is currently available. Mapping of all the phosphorylation sites of IRS-1 remains a challenge issue. One of the major reasons for this is that intact IRS-1 is present at very low concentrations (~ 51.9 ng/gram muscle tissues as described below); even in tissues in which it is most abundant such as soleus muscle. However, it is possible to analyze these phosphor-Ser/Thr residues in response to burn injury with tandem mass spectrometry.

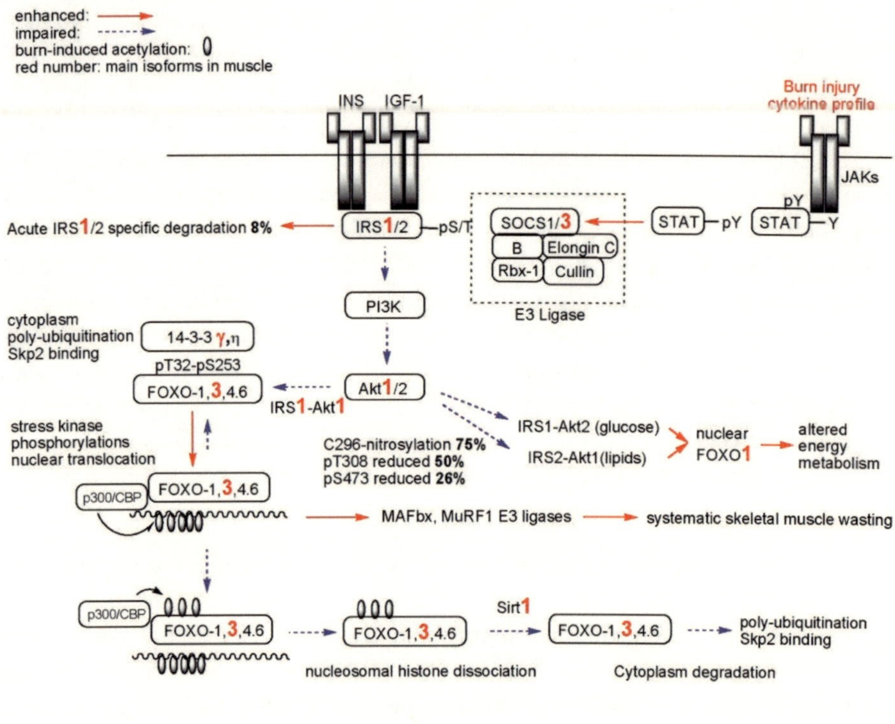

Figure 1. Insulin resistance and muscle wasting: unsymmetrical two tales in murine burn model. Insulin resistance and muscle wasting occurred at 10% and 70% likelihoods, respectively. IRS-1 integrity is reduced by 10% and thus is not a major caustic factor in downstream signaling. However, impaired Akt1/PKBα activity by 70% due to enhanced *S*-nitrosylation of Cys^{296} and reduction of phosphor-Thr^{308} and Ser^{473} has major impact on FOXO3 sub-cellular distribution and activities. Muscle wasting is significant in burned vs sham treated animals after day 3 post-burn injuries, but insulin resistance not significant under the same conditions.

We hypothesis that burn-induced PTMs that alter insulin sensitivity and muscle wasting occur not only at the IRS-1 level, but also at two critical downstream nodes: *S*-nitrosylated Cys^{296} in the Akt1 kinase loop and acetylated Lys residues in FOXO3. Specifically, (1) the docking platform integrity of IRS-1 may be partially disabled due to stress kinase mediated Ser/Thrphosphorylations which become E3 ligase targets. In other words, the reduction in glucose transport in skeletal muscle following burn injury may secondarily affect abundance and/or phosphorylation of IRS-1. (2) *S*-nitrosylated Cys^{296} interacts with phosphor-Thr^{308} in regulation of Akt1/PKBα kinase loop conformational changes which consequently inhibit kinase activity. (3) In addition of FOXO3 phosphorylation and reversible acetylation play major roles in transcriptional activities which trigger apoptosis and muscle wasting under the conditions of impaired Akt1/PKBα and IGF1 signaling as in the above two hypothesis. In contract to other biochemical approaches that are currently in use, all these PTM effects, such as E3 ligases cleaved IRS-1 fragments as well as site specific PTMs, can only be unambiguously analyzed with sensitive NanoLC-Q-TOF tandem mass spectrometry techniques. However, a major limitation of this approach is the low abundance of the signaling proteins for *in vivo* studies. Figure 1 illustrates the genesis of insulin resistance and muscle wasting at several crucial nodes: insulin resistance has been observed at 10% likelihood, while muscle wasting occurs at 70% likelihood in our murine models described below.

2. Materials

Methanol, acetonitrile (LC-MS Chromasolv, ACN), formic acid (FA), glacial acetic acid, LC-MS grade water, dithiotheretol (DTT) and iodoacetic acid, iodoacetamide, [Glu^1]-Fibrinopeptide B, methyl methanethiolsulfonate (MMTS), *S*-nitrosoglutathione (GSNO), sodium L-ascorbate, neocuproine, *N,N*-dimethylformamide (DMF), dithiothreitol (DTT), dimethyl sulfoxide (DMSO), Trypsin digestion kits (#PP0100), Phenylmethanesulfonyl fluoride (PMSF, cat# P-7626) and goat IgG were obtained from Sigma Chemical Co. (St. Louis, MO). SDS-PAGE ready gels (7.5%, #161-1100), SDS-PAGE ready gels (12 % Tris-HCl, #161-1102),SDS-PAGE ready gels (4-15% Tris-HCl, #161-1122), Laemmli sample buffer (#161-0737) and Coomassie brilliant blue R250 (#161-0436) were obtained from BIO-RAD (Hercules, CA, USA). Streptavidin agarose CL-4B was a product of Fluka (Cat#: 85881, Milwakee, WI). HPDP-Biotin (Cat#: 21341) and iodoacetyl-LC-Biotin (Cat#: 21333), immobilized monomeric avidin beads (Cat#: 20228), Iodoacetyl-LC-Biotin (Cat#: 21333) were purchased from Pierce (Rockford, IL).

Recombinant rat IRS-1 (#12-335, lot# 23015A purchased in 2005), assay buffer 5X (#20-145) and Mg^{++}/ATP 5X (#20-113), Anti-Akt1/PKBα monoclonal antibody (Cat# 05-798, Lot: 26860) and inactive Akt1/PKBα (Cat#: 14-279) were obtained from Upstate Technology (Lake Placid, NY, USA). Anti-ubiquitin (rabbit polyclonal, Ab19247) and anti-C-terminal IRS-1 (rabbit polyclonal, Ab653) antibodies were purchased from Abcam (Cambridge, MA, USA). Anti-N-terminal IRS-1 (rabbit polyclonal, SC560) was obtained from Santa Cruz Biotechnology (Santa Cruz, CA, USA). Protein G agarose (cat# 16-266) was obtained from Millipore (Billerica, MA, USA). Cell lysis buffer (cat# 9803), anti-FOXO3 rabbit antibodies (Cat#2497) were purchased from

Cell Signaling (Beverly, MA, USA). IRS-1 (total) ELISA kit (KHO0511), Akt pThr308 ElISA kit (KHO0201) and pSer473 kit (KHO0111) were purchased from Invitrogen (Carlsbad, CA, USA).

TRI reagent solution (cat# AM9738) was a product of Applied Biosystem (Framingham, MA, USA). 1-bromo-3-chloropropane (cat# BP 151) was purchased from Molecular Research Center, Inc. (Cincinnati, OH, USA). Qproteome cell compartment kit (Cat#: 37502) was obtained from Qiagen(Valencia, CA, USA).

The diet with depletion of L-Leu was obtained from Dyets, Inc., Bethlehem, Pennsylvania, DYET #510133, meets 1995 NRC nutrient requirements. [isopropyl-$^2H_7$]-L-Leu was product of Cambridge Isotope Lab (Andover, MA, USA).

Protein molecular weight markers (Cat#928-40000), secondary antibody (Cat# 926-3221, anti-Rabbit IgG) were purchased from LI-COR Biosciences (Lincoln, NE, USA). All PCR primers were obtained from the Massachusetts General Hospital primer bank.

3. Methods

3.1. Degradation of recombinant human IRS-1 stimulated with high insulin dose

Mammalian 293 cells were transfected with a recombinant IRS-1 FLAG tagged plasmid using a liposome reagent and Opti-MEM medium to deliver the plasmid DNA into the cells. Transfected cells were grown to confluence and placed in serum-free Dulbecco's modified Eagle's medium. The cells were then treated with insulin (1 μM) for 10 min. The medium was aspirated, and the cells were lysed in Reporter lysis buffer with phosphatase cocktail inhibitors containing 50 nM Potassium Bisperoxo(bipyridine)oxovanadate and 5 nMCalyculin A (Discodermia calyx) at 4°C. Fragments of Flag-IRS-1 C-terminal were immunoprecipitated with mAb to the first C-terminal 14 amino acid residues of IRS-1. The reaction mixtures were gently stirring in PBS (200 ml) at 4°C for 1 hr and excess mAb was removed with PBS (1 ml x 3). Flag-IRS-1 was released and cysteine residues were alkylated with Laemmli sample buffer (with 3% 2-mercaptoethanol, 100 mM DTT, 50 ml) for 5 min at 95°C and then 1 hr at room temperature under stirring. The reaction mixtures were separated by SDS-PAGE (7.5% Tris-HCl); IRS-1 bands stained with Coomassie brilliant blue R-250 were excised. In-gel trypsin digestion was performed (0.4 μg trypsin in 70 ml reaction buffer, 37°C, and overnight).

3.2. Mouse burn model

The protocol for the studies was approved by the Massachusetts General Hospital and Shriners Hospital for Children Animal Care Committees. Our animal care facility is accredited by the Association for Assessment and Accreditation of Laboratory Animal Care. Male CD-1 mice (Charles River Breeding Laboratories, Wilmington, MA, USA) weighing about 22-25 g were used. Sixteen animals were used for full thickness third degree burn injury produced under anesthesia (ketamine xylazine). After clipping of back hair, animals were placed in a template designed to expose 25% of their dorsum, and immersed into a water bath at 90?C for 9 second. After burn, the animals were immediately resuscitated with saline (2ml / mouse) by intraperitoneal injection. Buprenorphin (0.1 mg/kg, I.P.) was administered every 6-12 hours after injury. The sham group (n=5, matched for weight) was treated in the same manner as the burn group (n=14) with the exception that they were exposed to warm water (~36°C). The mice were sacrificed by cervical dislocation and skeletal and liver were dissected and quickly placed in liquid nitrogen. All biological studies were performed with skeletal muscle excised from the animals at day 7 after burn injury or sham treatment.

3.3. Skeletal muscle preparation

Due to sequence analysis using NanoLC-Q-TOF tandem mass spectrometry for very low abundant IRS-1 in muscle, total whole body skeletal muscle (~2.5-3.0 g/animal) was evaluated; fast and slow twitch muscles could not be studied independently. The muscle groups studied included: trapezius, gluteus superficialis, rectus femorus, latissimusdorsi, shoulder deltoid, serratus anterior, vastusmedialis, semitendinosus, biceps femoris, adductor longus, gracilis, triceptsbrachi, soleus and rectus abdominus. The muscle was harvested by careful dissection which excluded skin, bone and other non muscular tissues. Immediately after dissection, tissue samples were immersed in liquid nitrogen. Frozen tissue samples were cut into pieces smaller than ~50 mg, and homogenized by 5 strokes over 30 seconds (full speed, model CTH-115, Cole Parmer). For tandem mass spectrometry, muscle tissue samples were processed in freshly prepared Cell Signaling lysate buffer (5 ml per gram tissue) containing fresh PMSF (1mM) on ice. Homogenates were sonicated briefly in ice cold water, and centrifuged at 14,000 g for 10 minutes at 4°C. Supernatants were collected and stored at -80°C for further studies.

3.4. IRS-1 in-gel digestion

skeletal muscle were processed in freshly prepared Cell Signaling lysate buffer (5 ml per 1 gram tissues) containing fresh PMSF (1 mM) on ice. The homogenates were sonicated briefly in ice-cold water, and centrifuged at 14,000 g for 10 minutes. The supernatants were collected and mixed with protein G agarose beads (100 ml, 50% slurry) for 2 hours to remove IgG and non-specific proteins. The protein G beads were removed by centrifugation at 14,000 g for 30 seconds. Anti-C-terminal IRS-1 antibody (Ab653, 2 ml) was added to the supernatants to immunoprecipite IRS-1 (overnight at 4°C). The immune complexes were recovered by adding protein G agarose slurry (50%, 100 ml) with rotating for two hours at room temperature. The recovered beads (~ 50 ml) were washed (six times) with PBS (1 ml) and treated with Laemmli sample buffer (2X, 50 ml) containing 2-mercaptoethanol (3%, v/v, 100 mM DTT) at 95°C for 5 min. SDS-PAGE separation and in-gel trypsin digestion were described as above.

3.5. Skeletal muscle IRS-1 ELISA

Mouse skeletal muscle tissue (20 mg) was homogenized with a TissueRuptor using a Qproteome cell compartment kit according to the manufacture's protocol. IRS-1 C-terminal fragments in cytosolic, membrane, nuclear and cytoskeletal fractions were measured using IRS-1 (total) ELISA kit. Homogenate aliquots (100 μl) from muscle tissue harvested from 16 burned and 8 sham treated muscle tissues were diluted with Standard Diluent Buffer (400 μl) provided from the ELISA kits. IRS-1 standard calibration curves were prepared according to the manufacturer's protocol. Diluted tissue lysates (100 μl) were pipetted into the 96-well plates. The ELISA plates were gently shaken to capture IRS-1 at 4°C overnight. Rabbit anti-ubiquitin antibody, rabbit anti-N-terminal IRS-1 antibody and rabbit anti-C-terminal IRS-1 antibody were diluted by 500 fold using horseradish peroxidase (HR) diluents at room temperature. After six washings (0.4 ml Wash Buffer, gentle shaking for 30 seconds) at room temperature, rabbit anti-IRS-1 antibody provided with the IRS-1 ELISA kit together with the three detection antibodies (100 μl) were pipetted into each well. Detection was performed by gentle shaking with the detection antibodies at room temperature for 1 hour. After removal of excess detection antibodies, anti-rabbit IgG-HRP antibody was added and analyzed according to the manufacturer's directions.

3.6. RT-PCR analysis of degradation pathways

To understand the roles of FOXO3 in skeletal muscle wasting as well as to evaluate FOXO3 degradation, we need to first distinguish FOXO3 and 14-3-3γ mediated proteasomal proteolysis (MuRF1, MAFbx/atrogin1) and lysosomal autophagy (Bnip3, Atg4a, Atg12, Gabarapl1) degradation pathways at the mRNA level. These studies will be performed in both thermally injured (n=16) and sham treated animals (n=6). Skeletal muscle excised from the animals on day 3,7 and 14 after burn injury or sham treatment is frozen, tissue samples (~50 mg) are cut into small pieces in RNase-free tubes, and homogenized with 5 strokes (5 seconds each) of an Omni TH-tissue homogenizer in sterilized Eppendorf tubes (2 ml) containing TRI reagent solution. RNA extraction is performed according to the TRI standard protocol. With this procedure the average 260nm/280nm ratio is ~ 1.95, and the RNA yield is ~1.2 μg/mg skeletal muscle. The quality of the isolated RNA is assessed with agarose gel electrophoresis. Samples are analyzed in triplicate using the comparative threshold cycle SYBR green method. Expression levels of target genes are corrected by normalization to the expression level of GAPDH, and relative expression levels are calculated: $\Delta C_t = C_t$(target gene)- C_t(GAPDH), $\Delta\Delta C_t = \Delta C_t$(burn) - ΔC_t(sham), targeted gene normalized to the endogenous reference is given by: $2^{-\Delta\Delta Ct}$. The primers that will be used for RT-PCR are tabulated below (F= forward, R=reverse):

FOXO3	F: CCTACTTCAAGGATAAGGGCGAC,	R: GCCTTCATTCTGAACGCGCATG
14-3-3γ	F: GGACTATTACCGTTACCTGGCAG,	R: CTGCATGTGCTCCTTGCTGATC
MuRF1	F: TACCAAGCCTGTGGTCATCCTG,	R: TCTTTTGGGCGATGCCACTCAG
Bnip3	F: GCTCCAAGAGTTCTCACTGTGAC,	R: GTTTTTCTCGCCAAAGCTGTGGC
Atg4a	F: CAGTCTCCACAGCGGATGAGTA,	R: GTGTGATGGGTGCTTCTGAACC
Atg12	F: GAAGGCTGTAGGAGACACTCCT,	R: GGAAGGGGCAAAGGACTGATTC
Gabarapl1	F: GTGGAGAAGGCTCCTAAAGCCA,	R: AGGTCTCAGGTGGATCCTCTTC
GAPDH	F: GTCTCCTCTGACTTCAACAGCG,	R: ACCACCCTGTTGCTGTAGCCAA

Table 1. PCR primers for proteasomal proteolysis and lysosomal autophagy analysis

http://dx.doi.org/10.5772/54849

Using these primers, GAPDH mRNA levels were not significantly different between burned and sham treated mice 16.12 ±0.93 vs 15.62±2.98 (p=0.162, unpaired t-test).

3.7. Mapping of Akt1/PKBα cysteine residues

Inactive Akt1/PKBα (10 μg, 0.18 nmol, in 10 μl stock solution) was transferred into a siliconizedEppendorf tube (0.6 ml) containing Laemmli sample buffer (2X,10 μl, pH adjusted to 8.0) and DDT (2 μl, 20 nmol, PBS, pH = 8.0) and the solution was kept at 95°C for 5 min. Freshly prepared iodoacetyl-LC-Biotin (15 μl, 55 nmol, in DMF) was added to the denatured protein solution followed by stirring for additional 15 min at room temperature. The resulting biotinylated Akt1/PKBαwas purified by SDS-PAGE (4-15% Tris-HCl) and stained with Coomassie brilliant blue R-250. The protein bands were excised (~ 1 mm size) and digested (Akt1/PKBα: trypsin = 25, over night at 37°C) with a trypsin profile IGD kit. The biotinylated peptide mixture was captured by gentle stirring with streptavidin agarose CL-4B (30 μl packed) at room temperature for 1 hr (final vol. 100 μl). The streptavidin beads were washed with PBS (0.5 ml x 3), followed by water/acetonitrile (ACN 10%, 0.5 ml x 3). Biotinylated peptides were released from the streptavidin beads with formic acid (FA, 70%, 100 μl) at room temperature for 15 min with brief vortexing. The supernatant containing biotinylated peptides was transferred into a new vial and the formic acid was evaporated with a SpeedVac. The biotinylated peptide mixture was resuspended in water/acetonitrile (ACN, 2%, with 0.1% FA, 70 μl) and aliquots (10 μl) were analyzed.

3.8. Identification of disulfide bonds in inactive Akt1/PKBα

Inactive Akt1/PKBα (10 μg, 0.18 nmol, in 10 μl stock solution) was transferred into a siliconizedEppendorf tube (0.6 ml) containing Laemmli sample buffer (2X, 10 μl, pH = 8.0) and iodoacetamide (2 μl, 20 nmol, PBS, pH = 8.0). The mixture solution was kept at 95°C for 5 min and stirred at room temperature for additional15 minutes. The Akt1/PKBαderivative was purified by SDS-PAGE (4-15% Tris-HCl) and stained with Coomassie brilliant blue R-250. The protein bands were excised (~ 1 mm size) and digested (Akt1/PKBα: trypsin = 25, overnight) with a trypsin profile IGD kit. Supernatant (~ 70 μl) was neutralized with formic acid (5 μl) and aliquots of the final solution (10 μl) were analyzed.

3.9. Analysis of NO acceptor sites in inactive Akt1/PKBα

Three samples of inactive Akt1/PKBα (10 μg, 0.18 nmol, in 10 μl stock solution) were treated with GSNO (250 nmol, 50 μl PBS, pH = 8.0) for 5 min at room temperature in the dark in siliconizedEppendorf tubes (0.6 ml). Separation of Akt1/PKBα and GSNO was achieved by two successive acetone/water precipitations (0.3 ml, 70% ACN) at – 40°C for 10 min. The supernatants (containing GSNO) were removed by centrifugation at 14,000 X g for 2 minutes. The kinase pellets were resuspended in blocking buffer (100 μl, 20 mMTris-HCl, pH 7.7, 2.5% SDS, 20 mM MMTS, 1 mM EDTA, 0.1 mMneocuproine) at room temperature for 1 hr with gently stirring (I mm ID X 5 mm bar). Excess MMTS was removed by acetone (100%, 0.3 ml) precipitation (as above) and the protein pellets were resuspended in PBS (50 μl, pH = 8.0). Freshly prepared iodoacetic acid (5 μl, 2 mM in PBS, pH = 8.0), Biotin-HPDH (5 μl, 2 mM in

DMSO), iodoacetyl-LC-Biotin (5 μl, 2 mM in DMF) and sodium ascorbate (20 μl, 5 mM, PBS) were added to the three vials containing nitrosylated Akt1/PKBα. The reaction mixtures were stirred at room temperature for 5 min (iodoacetic acid and iodoacetyl-LC-Biotin) or 1 hr for the thiol-disulfide exchange reaction. Aliquots of SDS sample buffer (2x, with 3% 2-mercaptoethanol, 100 mM DTT, 50 μl) were added to the protein solutions and the mixtures were incubated at 95°C for 5 min. The derivatized proteins were separated with SDS-PAGE Ready gels. The gels were stained with Coomassie brilliant blue R-250 and the Akt1/PKBα bands were excised as 1 X 1 mm pierces. The proteins were digested with the trypsin profile IGD kit. Carboxylmethylcysteine (CMC) containing peptides were neutralized with FA (5 μl) and sequenced via parent ion discovery trigged by the CMC immonium ion (134.02 ± 0.05 mDa). Biotinylated peptides were sequenced with data dependent acquisition after capture with streptavidin agarose beads. Ten μl aliquots of each final solution were analyzed.

3.10. Analysis of the Cys^{296}-Cys^{310} disulfide bond formation in Akt1/PKBα after treatment with *S*-nitrosoglutathione

Inactive Akt1/PKBα (10 μg, 10 μl, 0.18 nmol) and freshly prepared GSNO (5 μl, 250 nmol, PBS, pH = 8.0) were stirred in an Eppendorf tube (0.6 ml) in the dark at room temperature for 1 hr. Separation of Akt1/PKBα and GSNO was performed with acetone/water (70%) as above. The kinase pellet was resuspended in PBS (10 μl) and SDS sample buffer (with 100 mM of iodoacetamide, 10 μl, 1 mmol) was added. The cysteine alkylation was performed at room temperature for 15 min. The protein samples were separated with SDS-PAGE Ready gels and digested as above. Aliquots of the final solution (10 μl) were analyzed.

3.11. Measurement of the free and disulfide bonded Cys^{296} in Akt1/PKBα from soleus muscle of burned rats

The lysates (~10 mg/ml total soleus proteins) were diluted to about 3-5 mg protein / ml protein with PBS, and filtered through 0.22 μm membranes. Immunoprecipitation was performed as following: anti-Akt1/PKBαmAb (Upstate, clone AW24, 5 μg) and prewashed protein G agarose beads (50 μl, packed) were kept at 4°C for 1 hrs under gently stirring, without washing the beads, the soleus lysates (5 ml) were added and maintained under stirring for another 90 minutes. The non-specific proteins were washed with PBS three times, then treated with Laemmli sample buffer (pH adjusted to 8) containing acetyl-LC-Biotin (400 μM) at 95°C for 5 min. The procedures for SDS-PAGE separation and in-gel trypsin digestion were the same as described above.

3.12. Metabolic labeling with [isopropyl-$^2H_7$]-L-Leu and natural L-Leu Diets

The diet with depletion of L-Leu was obtained as L-amino acids defined diet for rats and mice. For producing the light diet, natural L-Leu was added to the diet powder (1% by weight) and producing the heavy diet, the same amount of [isopropyl-$^2H_7$]-L-Leu was added to the diet powder. For both diets, a minimal amount of water was added to make biscuits of adequate size. The biscuits were dried at room temperature for 1 week as suggested by Dyets in order to maintain the original nutrients. Burned and sham treated mice were caged separately and

http://dx.doi.org/10.5772/54849

maintained in a temperature controlled facility with a 12-h light/dark cycle. Burned mice were fed with the diet containing [isopropyl-$^2H_7$]-L-Leu and sham treated mice fed with the diet containing natural L-Leu. Five grams of light and heavy diets were provided daily to each mouse for 7 days. The animals had ad libitum access to water.

3.13. Biotinylation of Cys^{296} in Akt1/PKBα kinase loop

Following immunoprecipitation of metabolically labeled Akt1/PKBα, Laemmil sample buffer (50 μl, X2) was added to the washed immunocomplex beads (packed 50 μl, washed with PBS, 1 ml X three 5 min cycles). This was followed by addition of freshly prepared Iodoacetyl-LC-Biotin solution (10 μl, stock solution: 2 mg in 1ml of DMF). Cysteine acylation was performed at room temperature for 15 min with stirring. The reaction was quenched by addition of 2-mercaptoethanol (5 μl). The beads were then heated at 95°C for 5 min and kept at room temperature for 30 min prior to loading on SDS-PAGE gels.

3.14. Avidin purification

Immobilized monomeric avidin beads (30 μl, 50 % aqueous slurry) were placed in siliconized polypropylene Eppendorf tubes (0.6 ml), and washed with PBS. The digested peptides (70 μl) were added to the packed avidin beads (15 μl) and the mixture was placed on a rocking platform for 30 min to capture the biotinylated peptides. Supernatant was collected, dried via Speed-Vac, and resuspended in mobile phase A (as described below, 15 μl) for control peptide ^{252}FYGAEIVSALDYLHSEK^{268} analysis. The beads were then washed with PBS (200 μl X 3), followed by ACN/water (10/90 = v/v, 200 μl X 3). The biotinylated peptides were recovered by addition of formic acid (30 μl, 70%) and gently rocking for 5 min at room temperature. This recovery step was repeated three time and the supernatants were combined, dried via Speed-Vac, and resuspended in mobile phase A (15 μl) for biotinylated loop peptide ^{290}ITDFGLCK^{297} analysis.

3.15. Measurements of skeletal muscle Akt1 $pThr^{308}$ and $pSer^{473}$

According to the manufacture's protocols of the $pThr^{308}$ and $pSer^{473}$ ELISA kits, one unit of phosphorylation standard is defined as the amount of Akt $pThr^{308}$ or $pSer^{473}$ derived from 500 pg or 100 pg of Akt protein, which is phosphorylated by MAPKAP 2 and PDK 1. Muscle tissues lysates obtained with the Cell Signaling buffer described as above were used for measurement of Akt $pThr^{308}$ and $pSer^{473}$. The phosphorylation levels were normalized to tissue weight.

3.16. Western blot and acetylation characterization of muscle FOXO3 post burn injury

Immunoprecipitations of muscle lysates from burned and sham treated mice were performed using anti-C-terminal antibody (sc-34895, 2 μg). SDS-PAGE was performed with 12% Ready Gels and protein molecular weight markers. Western blot analysis was performed with primary rabbit antibodies (Cell Signaling, Cat#2497, 20 μl + Tween-20, 20 μl + Odyssey blocking buffer, 20 ml) at 4°C overnight, and secondary antibody (Odyssey, Cat# 926-3221, anti-Rabbit IgG 2 μl + Tween-20 20 μl + Odyssey blocking buffer, 20 ml) at room temperature for 1 hour.

The membrane was scanned over near-infrared range. Recombinant human FOXO3 was loaded onto the 12% Ready Gels with intact and reduced goat IgG. Two FOXO3 bands were also found with molecular weights of above 87 and 80 kDa as compared with intact IgG (150 kDa) and reduced IgG heavy chains (50 kDa). The FOXO3 bands were digested and analyzed for acetylation using DDA approach.

3.17. NanoLC-Q-TOF^{micro}

All experiments were performed using a Waters CapLC-Q-TOF^{micro} system (Waters Corporation, Milford, MA, USA). An analytical column (75 μm I.D. X 150 mm, Vydac C18, 5 μm, 300 A, LC Packings, Dionex Company, San Francisco, CA) was used to connect the stream select module of the CapLC and the voltage supply adapter for ESI. After washing with mobile phase C (auxiliary pump, 0.1% formic acid in water/acetonitrile, 2% acetonitrile) for 2 minutes, the trapped peptides were back washed from the precolumn onto the analytical column using the 10-position stream switching valve. A linear gradient was used to elute the peptide mixture from mobile phase A (0.1% FA in water/ACN, 2% ACN) to mobile phase B (0.1% FA in ACN). The gradient was segmented as follow: isocratic elution with 2% solvent B for 3 min, 2-80 % solvent B from 3 to 45 min and 80 to 2% B from 45-50 min. The gradient flow rate was adjusted to ~70 nl/min. The electrospray voltage was set to ~ 3000 V to obtain an even ESI plume. Sample cone and extraction cone voltages were set at 45 and 3 V, respectively. The instrument was operated in positive ion mode with the electrospray source maintained at 90°C. The instrument was calibrated with synthetic human [Glu^1]-Fibrinopeptide B (100 fmol/μl in acetonitrile/water = 10:90, 0.1% formic acid, v/v) at an infusion rate of 1 μl/min in TOF MS/MS mode. The collision energy was set at 35 V. Instrument resolution for the [Glu^1]-Fibrinopeptide B parent ion, m/z = 785.84, was found to be ~5000 FWHM. Neutral loss for p-Ser and p-Thr parent ion discovery was set at 97.977 ± 0.03 Da with CE 35 and 5 V, respectively. All data were acquired and processed using MassLynx 4.1 software.

4. Results and discussion

4.1. Phosphorylated Ser/Thr triggers skeletal muscle IRS-1 C-terminal degradation

A total of 260 tryptic IRS-1 peptides, both doubly and triply charged under ESI, were located within the Q-TOF mass survey window setting (from m/z 400 to 1200). The chromatographic elution time window was ~30 min under our NanoLC gradient conditions and it was impossible to chromatographically separate the digested IRS-1 peptide mixture at the single peptide level; since many of the tryptic peptides overlapped. To overcome this problem, up to eight precursor ions were set for MS survey which provided secondary mass resolution in addition to the chromatographic separation. False positive precursor ions attributable to contaminations were eliminated by IRS-1 MS/MS sequence analysis. The NanoLC interfaced with Q-TOF settings that we used also had some false negative discoveries. These missed precursor ions may be due to their week hydrophobic properties (escaping from the trapping C18 column for desalting), week ionization, miss-digestion of large peptides and chemical alternations in predictable peptide structures. However, the confidently identified precursor ions represent desirable candidate peptides for *in vivo* phosphorylation studies. Thus, unambiguously discovered peptides were selected as relative MS fingerprints for IRS-1 protein expression as well as PTM analysis in insulin treatment studies. Confirmation of the phosphorylation of Ser/Thr sites was performed by the following three step procedure: (1) Phosphorylated parent ion discoveries by MS survey via neutral loss (H_3PO_4) or phosphor-Tyr immonium ion approaches; the peptide mass tolerance was set at 0.2 Da; (2) Analysis of candidate parent ions with PepSeq of MassLynx V4.1 software to verify IRS-1 tryptic peptide sequences. Mercaptocysteine was searched as a fixed modification, whereas oxidation of methionine and phosphorylations were searched as variable modifications. (3) Confirmations of phosphorylated Ser/Thr sites with the diagnostic mass difference of 80.00 ± 0.15 Da (HPO_3 moiety) between phosphorylated and non-phosphorylated y or b ions, as well as phosphor-Tyr containing ions with S/N > 2. Figure 2, 3, 4 demonstrate the neutral approach to identify phosphor-Ser/Thr sites, while tryptic peptides containing phosphor-Tyr sites are as shown in Figure 5, 6, 7.

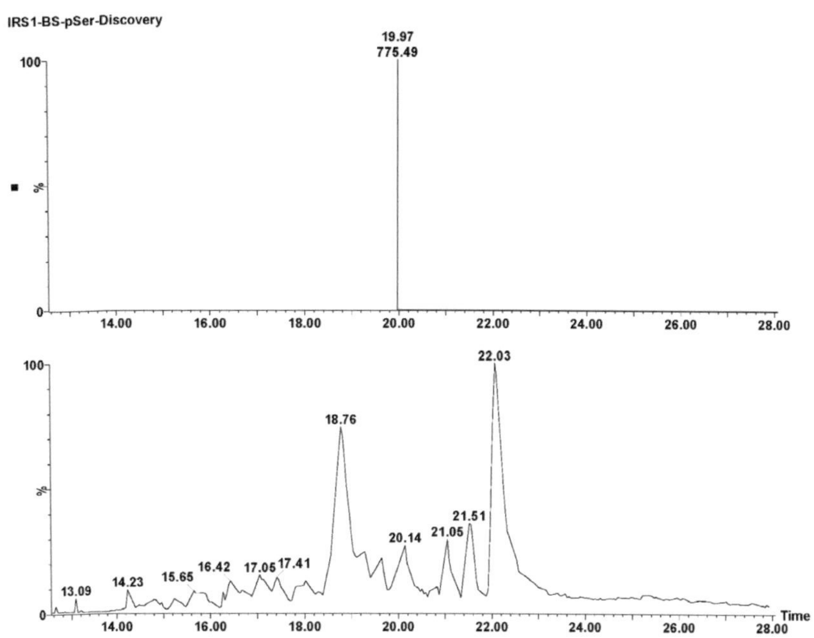

Figure 2. NanoLC base peak ion chromatogram of tryptic IRS-1 parent ion discovery with the neutral loss approach. Top panel: TOF MS/MS BPI chromatogram of IRS-1 doubly charged tryptic peptide [298]SRTESITATSPASMVGGKPGSFR[320] (m/z 776.43), eluted at retention time 19.97 min, discovered with neutral loss of H_3PO_4. Bottom panel: TOF MS BPI neutral loss survey chromatogram obtained with collision energy 5 V.

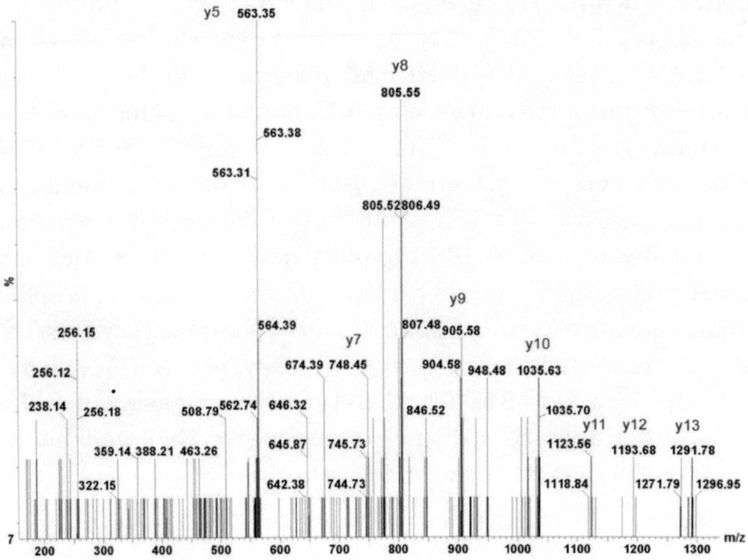

Figure 3. Sequence profile of IRS-1 phospho-Ser/Thr peptide acquisition triggered with the neutral loss approach. Doubly charged tryptic ^{298}SRTESITATSPASMVGGKPGSFR^{320} (m/z 770.43) parent ion eluted at 19.97 min as shown in the top panel Figure 2. The y ion series ranging from y5 to y13 confirm the correct sequence.

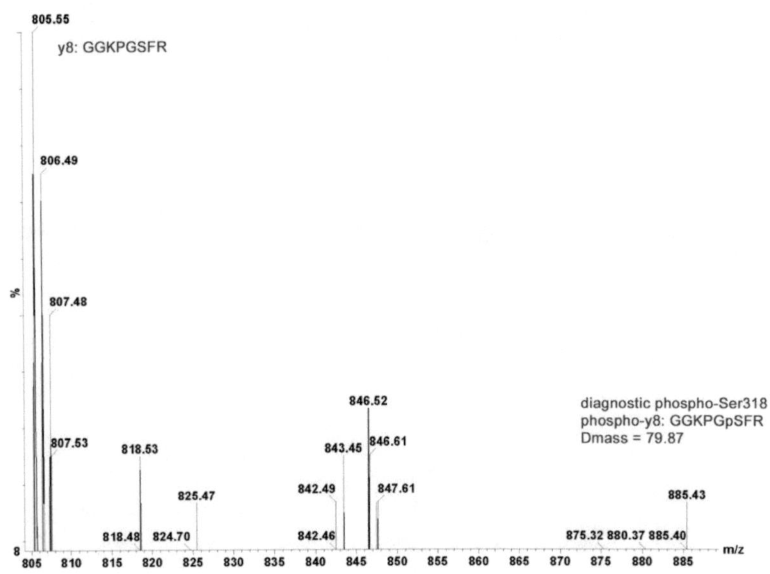

Figure 4. The zoom spectrum of Figure 3 shows diagnostic phosphor-Ser^{318} in the ^{298}SRTESITATSPASMVGGKPGpSFR^{320} peptide. Non-phospho-y8 ion (GGKPGSFR, m/z 805.56) and phosho-y8 ion (GGKPGpSFR, m/z = 885.43) indicates Δmass shift of 79.87 Da for HPO_3 modification.

http://dx.doi.org/10.5772/54849

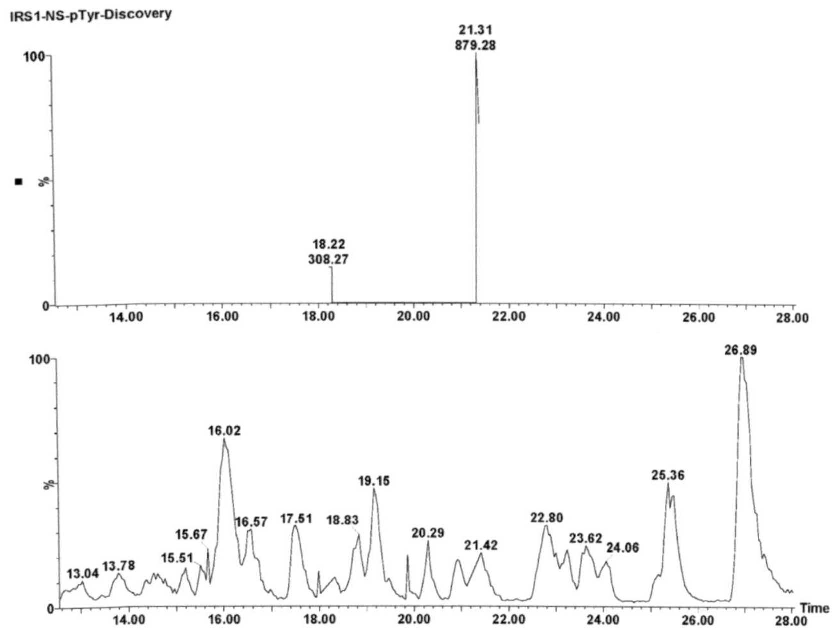

Figure 5. NanoLC base peak ion chromatogram of tryptic IRS-1 parent ion discovery with phospho-Tyr immonium ion approach. Top panel: phospho-Tyr parent ion eluted at retention time 21.31 min with triply charged m/z 879.28. Singly charged contaminant eluted at retention time 18.22 min with m/z 308.27. Immonium ion survey collision energy was kept between 5 and 100 V. Bottom panel: TOF MS BPI p-Tyr immonium ion survey chromatogram obtained with collision energy 5 V.

Having validated the site specific phosphorylation methods as described above, an *invitro* transfected IRS-1 model system was developed in order to analyze those stress induced phosphorylation sites and its degradation Typical MS/MS sequence data of insulin dependent phosphorylation sites $pSer^{641}$ are shown in Figure 8.

The striking insulin dependent phosphorylation pattern indicates that $pThr^{475}$, $pThr^{477}$ and $pSer^{641}$ were induced by high dose insulin stress. These phosphorylated sites at high dose insulin stimulation provided the first clue for understanding possible mechanism(s) for insulin resistance up stream of the insulin/IRS-PI3K-Akt-FOXO and growth factors-PI3K-Akt-FOXO pathways. In order to evaluate IRS-1 degradation at these phosphorylation sites, SILAC was used for relative quantification of IRS-1 at the insulin dosage. Tryptic peptide T23 (^{162}EVWQ-VILKPK^{171}) labeled with heavy isotope (under insulin stress) and light isotopes (without insulin) was used as a mass marker to evaluate IRS-1 protein level. Relative peak areas of precursor peptides indicated that at least 50% of IRS-1 was degraded rapidly. The critical question is whether IRS-1 degradation is trigged at the three phosphorylated sites? The predicated C-terminal fragment cleaved at sites $pThr^{475}$ /$pThr^{477}$ is expected at 80,673 Da and the second fragment cleaved at site $pSer^{641}$ expected at 64,441 Da. When C-terminal specific

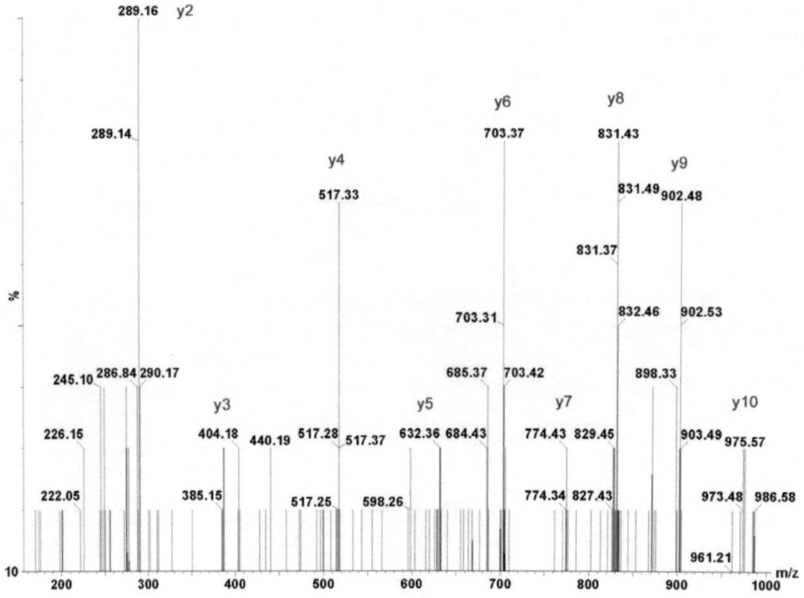

Figure 6. Sequence profile of phopspho-Tyr^{489} peptide acquisition triggered with the immonium ion approach. Triply charged Parent ion ^{489}YIPGATMGTSPALTGDEAAGAADLDNR^{515} (m/z 879.28)elutedat 23.31 min as shown in the top panel of Figure 5, MS/MS acquisition was obtained with collision energy of 35 V. The y ion series ranging from y5 to y13 confirmed the correct sequence.

mAb was used to repeat the insulin stimulation studies, SDS-PAGE showed that the IRS-1 band was reduced by ~50% with insulin stress as compared with the control; which is in agreement with the SILAC result. The multiple bands located between 50 kDa (IgG heavy chain) and 100 kDa (dimmer of heavy chain, 2-mercaptoethanol and DTT are not sufficient to achieve complete reduction of all disulfide bonds) were excised, digested and subjected to NanoLC-Q-TOF sequence analysis. The 65% sequence coverage confirmed that the FLAG tagged human IRS-1 bands were slightly lower in MW than the standard rat IRS-1 band. One fragment band (~ 80 kDa estimated from SDS-PAGE) was confirmed with two human IRS-1 sequences: ^{639}SVSAPQQIINPIR^{651} and ^{1017}TGIAAEEVSLPR^{1028}. At the same time the cleavage site precursor ion (^{472}GPS$_{P}$TL$_{P}$TAPNGHYILSR^{487}) was no longer detected. Another fragment band (~ 65 kDa from SDS-PAGE) was confirmed with ^{1017}TGIAAEEVSLPR^{1028} only. For the same reason, the precursor ion (^{639}SV$_{p}$SAPQQIINPIR^{651}) corresponding to this cleavage was missed from our MS survey list. These three facts confirm a negative regulated mechanism: stressed cells at the high insulin dose activate unknown kinases to phosphorylate threonine and serine residues located in the middle of the C-terminus of IRS-1 (for human IRS-1, C-terminus refers from the PTB domain residue aspartic acid 262 to the last glutamine 1242) and the multiple phosphorylated sites may trigger the ubiquitin-proteosome pathway to yield these major fragments. The C-terminus of IRS-1 cleaved around pThr^{475} /pThr^{477} afforded the fragment with MW ~ 80 kDa, while the fragment with MW ~65 kDa was related to pSer^{641}. The

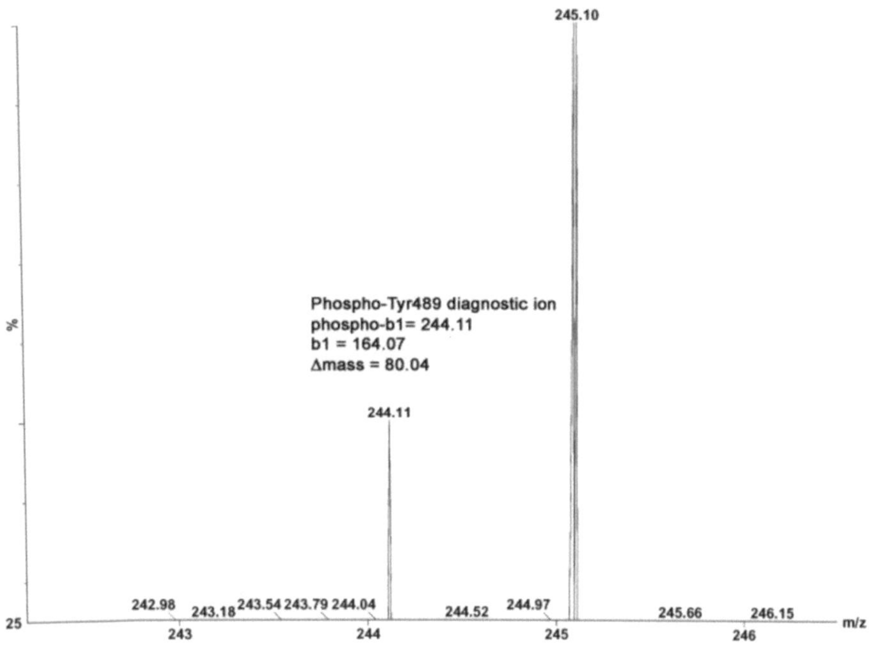

Figure 7. The zoom spectrum of Figure 6 shows Diagnostic phospho-Tyr[489] in the IRS1 triply charged parent ion [489]YIPGATMGTSPALTGDEAAGAADLDNR[515]. Non-phospho-b1 ion (Tyr, m/z 164.07) and phosho-b1 ion (pTyr, m/z = 244.11) indicates Δmass shift 80.04 for the HPO_3 modification.

observation that serine phosphorylation decreases insulin-stimulated tyrosine phosphorylation of IRS-1 and the observation of proteolytic turnover of the protein suggest the IRS-1 functions in both positive (N-terminal) and negative (C-terminal) feedback loops, The negative feedback is related to serine phosphorylation at the N-terminal half of the protein, with the C-terminal boundary at approximately amino acid residue 574 [99]. Positive signaling effects at low insulin dosages were associated with $pSer^{308}$, $pThr^{305}$ and $pTyr^{1012}$. Phosphorylated Tyr^{1012} may be the one of the downstream SH2 domain binding sites since it possesses the characteristic sequence YADM. Thus the sequence specific Ser/Thr kinase list might present pharmaceutical targets for modulating insulin resistance.

In vitro phosphorylation sites of rat IRS-1 C-terminal region provided "similarity" degradation references for further *in vivo* studies. The IRS-1 fragment sizes estimated from SDS-PAGE and their sequences are listed in Table 2.

For quantitative measurement of IRS-1 degradation in muscle of burned mice, additional studies were performed to explore sub-cellular distributions, C-terminal fragments and ubiquitinated IRS-1. An antibody specific to the 14 C-terminal amino acid residues of IRS-1 was used to capture IRS-1 irrespective of its post-translational modifications and integrity. Subsequently anti-ubiquitin, anti-C-terminal and anti-N-terminal polyclonal antibodies were used as the primary antibodies for ELISA analysis. The sub-cellular distribution of skeletal

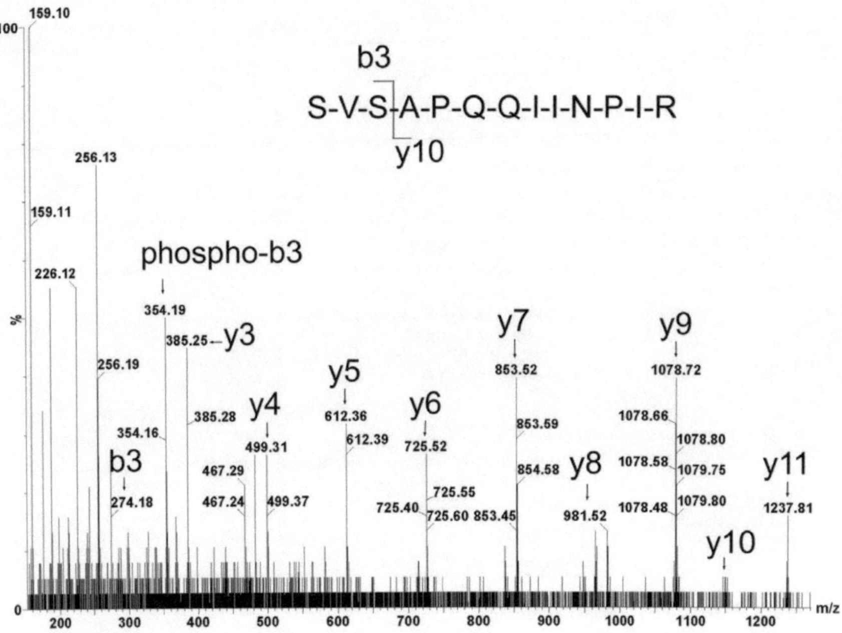

Figure 8. Analysis of $pSer^{641}$ peptide of recombinant human IRS-1 stimulated with high insulin dose. Doubly charged parent ion was discovered with the neutral loss approach: $[M+2H]^{2+}$ = 711.91, ^{639}SVpSAPQQIINPIR^{651}. ^{639}Ser-Val, b2 ion = 187.12. No corresponding phosphorylated ^{639}Ser b2 ion was observed, however, ^{639}Ser-Val-Ser^{641}, b3 ion at m/z = 274.14 and phosphorylated b3 ion at m/z = 354.17 (Δmass = 80.03 Da), indicated phosphorylation of Ser^{641} rather than Ser^{639}.

position	$M+H^+$	Sequence	Sequenced in SDS-PAGE bands (kDa)
1170-1180	1263.67	SLNYIDLDLAK	95, 44, 42
1156-1169	1363.61	ESAPVCGAAGGLEK	95, 44, 42
993-1010	1984.92	QSYVDTSPVAPVSYADMR	44
1135-1155	2242.11	HSSASFNVWLRPGDLGGVSK	95

Table 2. Tandem mass spectrometry (MS/MS) characterization of mouse skeletal muscle IRS-1 C-terminal fragments after burn injury

muscle IRS-1 post-burn injury is illustrated in Figure 9. The physiological distribution pattern in sham treated mice demonstrates nearly equal amounts of membrane bound IRS-1 (102.7 ng/g) and the IRS-1 in the cytosolic and nuclear compartments (49.1 and 44.9 ng/g). No detectable IRS-1 was observed in the cytoskeletal compartment.

The total cellular IRS-1 from the three compartments was found to be 196.7 ng/g. Results with the anti-N-terminal antibody data indicated that about 26.3% of the IRS-1 pool remained as intact protein. Thus, the majority of IRS-1 was present as C-terminal fragments. Ubiquitinated

http://dx.doi.org/10.5772/54849

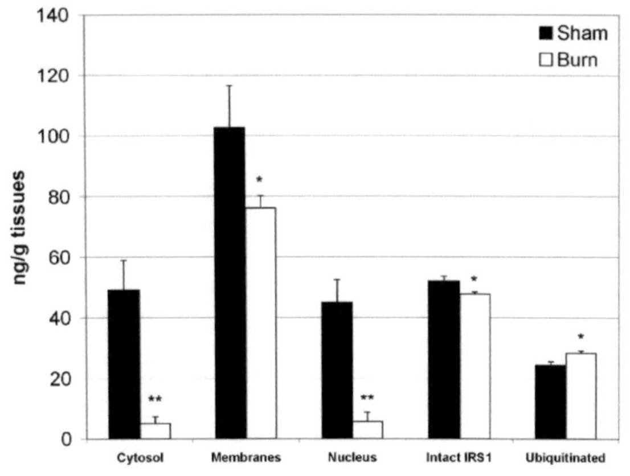

Figure 9. Quantitative measurement of IRS-1 integrity and sub-cellular distribution. IRS-1 was captured with anti-C-terminal mAb, and detected with anti-ubiquitin, anti-N-terminal, and anti-C-terminal rabbit polyclonal antibodies. For total intact and ubiquitinated IRS-1, sub-cellular components were isolated using a Qproteome cell compartment kit according to the Qiagen protocol. Values represent mean ± sem for 14 burned and 5 sham treated mice. *: $p<0.05$, **: $p<0.005$.

IRS-1 was found to represent 12.4% of total IRS-1. Burn-induced changes in the sub-cellular distribution of IRS-1 were clearly driven by the 15.9 % increase in ubiquitination. Consequently, total IRS-1 in the three sub-cellular compartments was reduced by 55.8%, while intact cellular IRS-1 was decreased by 7.7%. A striking feature revealed from the sub-cellular distribution pattern of IRS-1 is that equilibrium between the cytosolic and nuclear compartments occurs by day 7 after burn injury.

The level of intact IRS-1 protein was found to be only ~51.9 ng/g in the skeletal muscle, which is too low to map phosphorylation sites with tandem mass spectrometry. However, those burn-induced phosphor-Ser/Thr sites provide one to get into the insight of the mechanism of insulin resistance and muscle wasting at the initial Ins/Ir/IRS-1 signaling transduction level. On the other hand, with the mixed-muscle preparations that were evaluated, it was not possible to determine the percentage of slow and fast twitch fibers. These issues in conjunction with the small amount of skeletal muscle harvestable from mice, the low level of IRS-1 in muscle and the low sensitivity of the site specific MS/MS sequencing for low abundant phosphorylated residues are an unavoidable limitation of current studies. The *in vitro* and *in vivo* IRS-1 data suggest that in 8-10 week old mice with burn injury insulin resistance occurs in only ~10% of the animals. The observations that significant muscle wasting occurs both clinically and in animal models (~70% of animals) suggest a pivotal role for downstreamAkt1/PKBα.

4.2. *S*-nitrosylated Cys[296] catalyzes disulfide bond formation with Cys[310] in Akt1/PKBα | | active loop

Akt1/PKBα is a central mediator of the IR/IRS/ PI3K/FOXO pathway. In addition, to the role of reversible phosphorylation/ dephosphorylation at Thr[473] and Ser[308] in its regulation, reversible inactivation can also be mediated by *S*-nitrosylation at cysteine residues. We performed *in vitro* and *in vivo* studies to verify this hypothesis. Here, for the first time, tandem mass spectrometry data revealed that *S*-nitrosylated Cys[296] mediates kinase loop conformational changes mediated via *S*-nitrosylation and phosphorylation.

For the *in vitro* studies, Akt1/PKBα was *S*-nitrosylated with the NO donor *S*-nitrosoglutathione (GSNO) and derivatized by 3 methods. The derivatives were isolated by SDS-PAGE, trypsinized and analyzed by tandem MS. For the *in vivo* studies, Akt1/PKBα in muscle lysates from burned rats was immunoprecipitated, derivatized with HPDP-Biotin and analyzed. The *in vitro* studies provided unambiguous MS fingerprints for the *in vivo* studies. The *invivo* studies demonstrated that NO free radical reacts with the free thiol of Cys[296] to produce a Cys[296]-SNO intermediate which accelerates interaction with vicinal Cys[310] to form a Cys[296]-Cys[310] disulfide linkage, at the same time, dephosphorylation at Thr[308] was observed. The disulfide bond between Cys[296] and Cys[310] was not detected in lysates from sham animals. As a result of this dual effect produced by burn injury, the loose conformation that is slightly stabilized by the kinase loop Lys[297]-Thr[308] salt bridge may be replaced by a more rigid structure which may block substrate access and down-regulate activity. *S*-nitrosylated C[296], located inside the Akt1 activity loop, was observed in tryptic peptide ITDFGLCK. Also, significant reductions in phosphorylation of Ser[473] and Thr[308] of Akt1 were measured as 26.2% ($p<0.05$) and 49.8% ($p<0.005$), respectively.

Akt1/PKBα consists of three structural features: the N-terminal pleckstrin homology (PH) domain, a large central kinase domain and a short C-terminal hydrophobic motif. High specific binding of the PH domain with membrane lipid products of PI3-kinase recruits Akt1/PKBα to the plasma membrane where phosphorylations of Thr[308] in the kinase domain and Ser[473] located in the C-terminal hydrophobic motif occur. Phosphorylation of Thr[308] partially stimulates kinase activity; however, additional phosphorylation of Ser[473] is required for full activity. Activation is associated with a disordered to ordered transition of a specific αC helix of Akt1/PKBα via an allosteric mechanism. A salt bridge between the side-chain of Lys[297] and the phosphate group of pThr[308] in this αC helix contributes to an ordered activation segment from [292]DFG to APE[319] [99,100,101,102]. Reversible dephosphorylations of Thr[308] and Ser[473] by protein phosphatase 2A (PP2A) and PH domain leucine-rich repeat protein phosphatase (PHLPPα) also occur in the Akt1/PKBα activation/deactivation cycle [103,104,105,106]. In addition to the role of reversible phosphorylation/dephosphorylation in the regulation of Akt1/PKBα activity, this kinase is also reversibly inactivated by *S*-nitrosylation under conditions that result in persistently increased production of nitric oxide; such as after burn injury [107,108,109,110]. Thiol titration and NMR data indicate that a disulfide bond (Cys[60]-Cys[77]) exists in the kinase PH domain [111]. A second disulfide bond in the critical kinase activation loop (Cys[297]-Cys[311]) has been reported to be associated with dephosphorylation under oxidative stress *in vitro*[112]. In addition, it has been shown that when Cys[224] of Akt1/PKBα is mutated to a Ser residue, the kinase becomes resistant to NO donor-induced *S*-nitrosylation and inactivation; suggesting that this residue is a major *S*-nitrosylation acceptor site [109]. *In vivoS*-nitrosylations of the insulin receptor (β) and Akt1/PKB*α* result in reductions in their kinase activities [108]. These data suggest that the redox status of Akt1/PKB*α*, regulated by NO, is a second factor in the post translational modifications that modulate kinase activity (via dynamic conformational changes) and thus GLUT-4 trafficking and cellular FOXO translocation. Nevertheless, up to now, published data on the reversible phosphorylation(s) and *S*-nitrosylation(s) relevant to Akt1/PKB*α* activation, conformation and regulation have not provided conclusive information about their interrelationships nor critical *S*-nitrosylation sites involved in the kinase activation/ deactivation cycle.

Recent technical developments have made it feasible to study the molecular details of these important processes. These techniques include: 1. sensitive and site-specific procedures for the detection of *S*-nitrosylation based upon NanoLC interfaced with tandem MS/MS; 2. the Biotin-Switch method for qualitative discrimination of thiol state between free, disulfide bonded and *S*-nitroylated cysteine residues under carefully defined conditions [113,114,115,116,117,118]; and 3. highly specific anti-Akt1/PKB*α*mAb's that can be used to immunoprecipitate quantities of the protein that are sufficient to yield SDS-PAGE bands with Coomassie brilliant blue R-250 staining which are compatable with tandem MS analysis.

The following issues need to be taken in considerations: 1. the ability of Cys^{296} to chemically quench elevated levels of free radicals, specifically nitric oxide; 2. loop conformational changes associated with two types of PTM; 3. quantitative proteomics of Akt1/PKB*α* by stable isotope labeling in mice. We obtained MS/MS sequence data to characterize the thiol states of Cys^{296} in the kinase activity loop of Akt1/PKB. These measurements were possible despite the extremely low level of nitrosylated protein (at the 10^{-15}pmol level, the chance of positive hits is ~25% with lysates prepared from 25 mg of soleus muscle). The biochemical role of *S*-nitrosylation at Cys^{296} was characterized as an intermediate state which reduces the kinetic barrier to form the disulfide bond with Cys^{310} within the activity loop. This occurs simultaneously with dephosphorylation of $pThr^{308}$ after burn injury. The facts that no other disulfide bonds associated with Cys^{296} were detected suggest that they may be thermodynamically forbidden; due to geometry and/or dihedral angle strain. The data obtained with soleus muscle from burned and sham treated rats indicates that NO mediated formation of the Cys^{296}-Cys^{310} disulfide bond (which likely down-regulates kinase activity) plays a reciprocal role with formation of a Lys^{297}-$pThr^{308}$ salt bridge (which up-regulates kinase activity) during disease associated reversible activation/deactivation processes.

To further the proof-of-concept about formation of a Cys^{296}-Cys^{310} disulfide bridge after burn injury, metabolically labeled Akt1/PKB*α* was characterized with NanoLC-Q-TOF tandem mass spectrometry based on the classic isotope dilution principle. Akt1/PKB*α* in liver extracts from mice with burn injury that were fed with [$^2H_7$]-L-Leu was immunoprecipitated and isolated with SDS-PAGE. Two tryptic peptides, one in the kinase loop and a control peptide just outside of the loop were sequenced. Their relative isotopologue abundances were determined by stable isotope labeling by amino acids in mammalians (SILAM)[119]. Relative quantifications based on paired heavy/light peptides were obtained in 3 steps. 1. Homogenization of mixtures of equal amounts of tissue from burned and sham treated animals (i.e., isotope dilution) and acquisition of uncorrected data based on parent monoisotopic MS ion ratios; 2. Determination of isotopic enrichment of the kinase from burned mice on Day 7; and 3. Enrichment correction of partially labeled heavy and light monoisotopic MS ion ratios for relative quantification of bioactivity (loop peptide) and expression level (control peptide). Our data demonstrate that protein synthesis and enrichment after injury were dependent on tissue and turnover of individual proteins. Three heavy and light monoisotopic ion ratios for albumin peptides from burned mice indicated ~55% enrichment and ~16.7 fold down regulation. In contract, serum amyloid P had ~66% enrichment and was significantly up regulated. Akt1/PKBα had ~56% enrichment and the kinase level in response to burn injury was up regulated compared with the control peptide. However, kinase bioactivity, represented by the Cys^{296} peptide, was significantly reduced. Overall, we demonstrate that 1. Quantitative proteomics can be performed without completely labeled mice; 2. Measurement of enrichment of acyl-tRNAs is unnecessary and 3. Cys^{296} plays an important role in kinase activity after burn injury.

Stable isotope labeling by amino acids in cell culture (SILAC) provides relative quantification of *in vitro* protein synthesis and functional proteomics under conditions that mimic disease states [120,121,122,123,124]. Typically, two cell populations are cultured for six doublings times; control cell medium contains the natural amino acid (e.g., $^{12}C_6$-Lys and/or $^{12}C_6$-Arg, 99% natural abundance), and the second medium contains the same levels of amino acids with heavy isotopes (e.g., $^{13}C_6$-Lys and/or $^{13}C_6$-Arg, 98% abundance) and disease related stimuli. The two cell populations are mixed with equal amounts of total proteinand digested peptides are accurately measured by mass spectrometry with a mass difference of 6 Da for singly charged parent ions. Six doubling times allows isotopic enrichment of the precursor acyl-tRNA pool to reach ~98% in cancer cell lines. Labeling above 95% is generally required for comparative and quantitative proteomics by MS. Thus, the relative abundance of any paired peptide's monoisotopic MS ion chromatogram with SILAC can be used to measure protein synthesis in comparison with the controls under *in vitro* conditions. The SILAC approach has been used with *C. elegans*fed with >98% ^{15}N labeled *E. coli* [125], skeletal muscle from chickens fed with a synthetic diet containing 50% of [$^2H_8$]-Val [126,127], partially labeled rat diet with >99% ape ^{15}N algal cells for 44 days [128] and F1-F4 offspring of mice fed with lysine-free diet containing 1% of L-$^{13}C_6$-Lys [129]. Complete labeling has been reported to be achieved by the F2 generation. Metabolic labeling with ^{15}N can be performed efficiently and economically, however, data interpretation can be challenging since the monoisotopic peak can shift, due to the distribution of positional isotopomers as a function of labeling time [130,131]. Global labeling with ^{15}N has been used as a tool for characterization of enrichment under partially labeling conditions [132,133,134]. Stable isotope labeled amino acids, such as L-$^{13}C_6$-Lys and L-$^{13}C_6$-Arg, provide ideal residues at C-terminal labeling positions for trypsin digestion. Protein synthesis depends on 2 factors: acyl-tRNA levels and protein turnover rate. These factors are tissue, cell type, time and treatment dependent. To minimize individual variability, full incorporation of L-$^{13}C_6$-Lys can be achieved in mice; however, it is very costly.

Analysis of the hypermetabolic/inflammatory response under acute phase conditions is very challenging for several reasons: 1. Significant changes in protein expression are associated with high levels of reactive oxygen species (ROS) and post translational protein modifications; i.e. not only protein levels but also biological activities have to be quantified; 2. Individual protein enrichments and incorporated isotope distributions may vary with the partially isotope enriched precursor t-RNA pool (>50%) and corresponding protein turnover rates during the acute phase response.

To address these considerations and explore the feasibility of the basic SILAC approach in animals under acute phase and partial isotope labeling conditions, a mouse model with full-thickness 40% TBSA burn was used to proteomically characterize liver Akt1/PKBα | | from the perspectives of both protein expression and biological activity. [Isopropyl-$^2H_7$]-L-Leu was selected for labeling based on 4 considerations: 1. L-Leu is an essential amino acid with high abundance in proteins. 2. Compared with other amino acids, [isopropyl-$^2H_7$]-L-Leu is relatively inexpensive; 3. None of the 7 deuterium atoms of [isopropyl-$^2H_7$]-L-Leu are attached at the α-carbon which may be exchangeable with hydrogen atoms; thus in contrast to studies with [$^2H_{10}$]-Leu, MS offset can be eliminated as a confounding variable; 4. The hydrophobicity of L-Leu reduces false negative discovery during C18 reversed phase trapping and desalting.

It has been reported that NO production is elevated by stressors such as burn injury and in patients with type 2 diabetes [110,135,136]. It has also been shown that the Cys^{297}–Cys^{311} disulfide bond in the critical kinase activation loop of Akt1/PKBα may be formed in association with dephosphorylation under oxidative stress *in vitro* [112]. Thus, we hypothesized that reversible *S*-nitrosylation at either Cys^{296} or Cys^{310} in the kinase active loop may be a PTM factor which complements reversible phosphorylation at Thr^{308} in the regulation of kinase activity and sought to determine how *S*-nitrosylation interacts with phosphorylation during the Akt1/PKBα activation cycle [103]. To address these issues, GSNO was used as the only NO donor in a model *S*-nitrosylation system to randomly target the seven cysteine residues of the kinase at pH = 8. The nucleophilic role of sulfhydryl groups is well documented and it is clear that cysteine residues located in the enzyme hydrophobic loop are important catalytic entities in both transfer and addition reactions. Vicinal Cys^{296} and Cys^{310} take advantage of the pK_a for dissociation of the thiol to thiolate and these electron-rich thiolate groups can lead to formation of an intradomain disulfide bond [137].Therefore, Cys^{296} and Cys^{310} are potential *S*-nitrosylation sites as predicted from the 3D structure of the kinase. NO donors, such as thioredoxin and thiol/disulfide oxidoreductases were excluded from the system to prevent possible interferences [138,139], however, a small amount of 2-mercaptoethanol (~0.05% v/v) was necessary to prevent oxygen effects.

The simple, but well-defined, *S*-nitrosylation reaction model was used to probe for particular NO acceptor sites in human Akt1/PKBα (inactive, 89% pure containing 2-mercaptoethanol and EGTA, Upstate) in three steps: A. Mapping of all cysteine residues with DTT reduction, iodoacetyl-LC-Biotin alkylation and affinity capture provided relative MS ionization efficacies and charge states; B. Detection of disulfide bonds with and without GSNO, provided an understanding of NO-mediated disulfide bond formation. C. MS/MS pinpointed the *S*-nitrosylated sites with three different thiol-specific derivatives. False negatives may occur with the Biotin-Switch method, whereas false positives are more common with the other methods, however, thiolether derivatives can be identified with MS/MS data. The findings of these

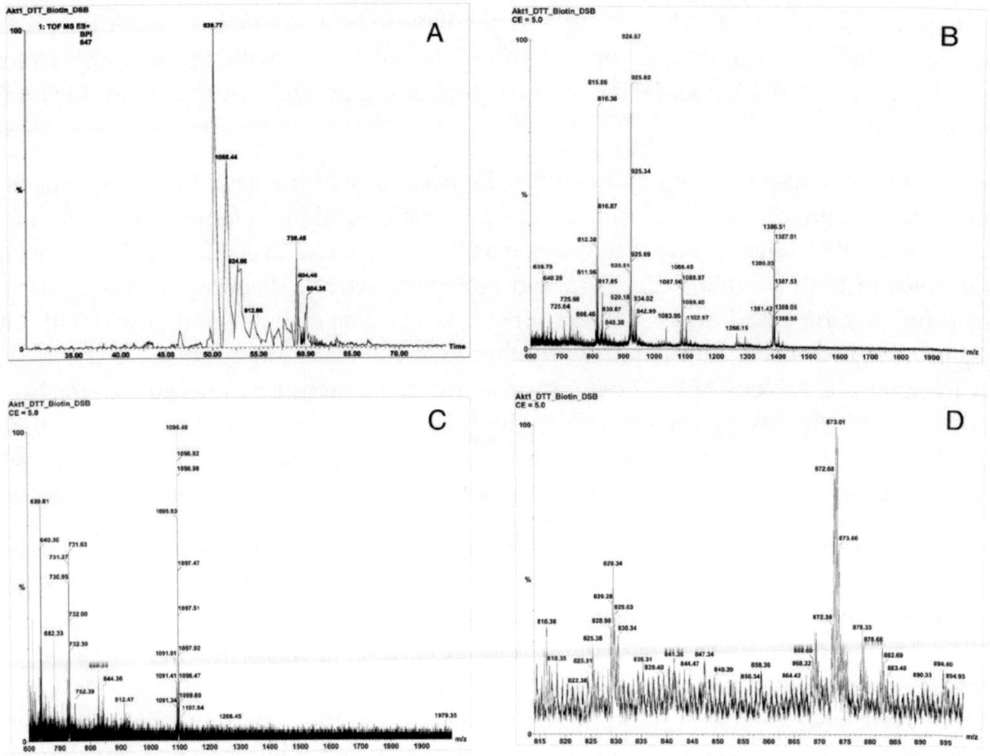

Figure 10. Mapping of cysteine residues in inactive Akt1/PKBα (a) Base peak intensity (BPI) NanoLC chromatogram of affinity capture of all seven cysteine residues that were biotinylated with iodoacetyl-LC-Biotin (b) TOF MS analysis of parent ions co-eluted at retention time of ~53 min. Parent ions m/z 924.67 and m/z 1386.51 are triply and doubly charged ions from the same tryptic peptide ^{308}TFCGTPEYLAPEVLEDNDYGR^{328} which contains Cys^{310}. Parent ion m/z 1266.09 is a triply charged ion from the tryptic peptide, ^{437}YFDEEFTAQMTITPPDQDDSMECVDSER^{465}, which contains Cys^{460}. Parent ion m/z 815.87 is a doubly charged ion derived from the tryptic peptide, ^{77}CLQWTTVIER^{86}, which contains Cys^{77}. The parent ion at m/z 1088.49 results from CH_4 neutral loss from m/z 1096.46 as shown in Figure 10C. (c) TOF MS analysis of parent ions co-elutting at retention time of ~50.8 min. Parent ions m/z 731.33 and m/z 1096.46 are triply and doubly charged ions from the same tryptic peptide, ^{49}ESPLNNFSVAQCQLMK^{64}, which contains Cys^{60}. Parent ion m/z 639.79 is doubly charged and is derived from tryptic peptide, ^{290}ITDFGLCK^{297}, which contains Cys^{296}. (d) TOF MS analysis of parent ions co-eluting at retention time of ~53.5 min. Parent ion m/z 829.00 is triply charged and derived from tryptic peptide, ^{329}AVDWWGLGVVMYEMMCGR^{346}, which contains Cys^{344}. Parent ion m/z 872.70 is triply charged and derived from tryptic peptide, ^{223}LCFVMEYANGGELFFHLSR^{241}, which contains Cys^{224}.

studies were used to study the biological consequences of *S*-nitrosylation of Akt1/PKBα in soleus muscle from burned rats. This *in vivo* system was used because soleus muscle is an insulin sensitive tissue with relatively high levels of IRS-1.

A base peak intensity (BPI) Nano-LC chromatogram of all seven affinity captured cysteine residues that were biotinylated with iodoacetyl-LC-Biotin is shown in Figure 10A. Cysteine residue monoisotopic mass of $C_3H_5NOS = 103.01$ Da was replaced with derivatizedCys residue monoisotopic mass of $C_{21}H_{35}N_5O_4S_2$ = 485.21 Da. The relative simplicity of the NanoLC chromatogram indicates the high purification efficacy for removing non-biotinylatedtryptic peptides from streptavidin agarose beads. Three predominate TOF MS tryptic parent ions were identified; m/z 639.81 (T41, M+2H$^+$ = 639.83) eluting at 50.5 min, m/z 1088.49 (T9, M-CH_4+2H$^+$ = 1088.03) at eluting at 51.5 min and m/z 924.67 (T44, M+3H$^+$ = 924.43) eluting at 53 min are doubly and triply charged tryptic peptides containing Cys^{296}, Cys^{310} and Cys^{60}, respectively. Figure 10B shows the parent ions co-eluting at ~ 53 min as well as the charge state assignments. Parent ions m/z 924.67 (T44, M+3H$^+$ = 924.43) and m/z 1386.51 (T44, M+2H$^+$ = 1386.14) are triply and doubly charged ions from the same tryptic peptide, ^{308}TFCGTPEYLAPEVLEDNDYGR^{328}, which contains Cys^{310}. Parent ion m/z 1266.09 (T58, M+3H$^+$ =1266.41) is triply charged and derived from the peptide, ^{437}YFDEEFTAQMTITPPDQDDSMECVDSER^{465}, which contains Cys^{460}. Parent ion m/z 815.87 (T11, M+2H$^+$ = 815.93) is doubly charged from the peptide, ^{77}CLQWTTVIER^{86}, which contains Cys^{77}. Parent ion m/z 1088.49 resulted from CH_4 neutral loss from m/z 1096.48. Figure 10C shows TOF MS parent ions that co-eluted at ~50.8 min; chromatographic peak tailing the most intense peak at 50.5 min. Parent ions m/z 731.33 (T9, M+3H$^+$ = 731.03) and m/z 1096.46 (T9, M+2H$^+$ = 1096.04) are triply and doubly charged ions from the same tryptic peptide, ^{49}ESPLNNFSVAQCQLMK^{64}, which contains Cys^{60}. Parent ion m/z 639.81 (T41, M+2H$^+$ =639.83) is a doubly charged ion from the tryptic peptide, ^{290}ITDFGLCK^{297}, which contains Cys^{296}. Figure 10D shows the TOF MS parent ions that co-eluted at ~53.5 min. Parent ion m/z 829.00 (T45, M+3H$^+$ = 829.05) is triply charged and derived from the tryptic peptide, ^{329}AVDWWGLGVVMYEMMCGR^{346}, which contains Cys^{344}. Parent ion m/z 872.70 (T32, M+3H$^+$ = 872.43) is triply charged and derived from the tryptic peptide, ^{223}LCFVMEYANGGELFFHLSR^{241}, which contains Cys^{224}. No doubly charged T58, T45 or T32 ions were observed. It is clear that the ionization efficacies for the peptides containing Cys^{296} (M+2H$^+$), Cys^{310} (M+2H$^+$ and M+3H$^+$), Cys^{60} (M+2H$^+$ and M+3H$^+$) and Cys^{77} (M+2H$^+$) are much higher than for the triply charged peptides containing Cys^{460} (M+3H$^+$), Cys^{334} (M+3H$^+$) and Cys^{224} (M+3H$^+$) under the same conditions.

When Akt1/PKBα was treated with GSNO without cleavage of disulfide bonds and the free cysteine residues were alkylated with iodoacetamide, two intradomain disulfide bonds were identified: Cys^{60}-Cys^{77} in the PH domain and Cys^{296}-Cys^{310} in the kinase active loop.

The monoisotopic parent ion with m/z = 821.35, shown in Figure 11A, represents two tryptic peptides containing the Cys^{296}-Cys^{310} disulfide bond in the kinase loop. The isotopic peaks at m/z 821.61 and m/z 821.35 are attributed to the M + 1 and M + 0 ions. A mass difference of 0.26 Da (expected 0.25 Da) indicated 4 positive charges: two at n-terminals and two at side chains of the c-terminals of the dipeptides. The expected quadruply charged disulfide bond linked Cys^{296} and Cys^{310} containing peptides (T41-SS-T44, M + 4H$^+$) were calculated to be m/z 821.38 [(894.45 + 2387.06 + 4)/4]. The monoisotopic parent ion with m/z = 764.41, shown in Figure 11B, represents the two tryptic peptides containing the Cys^{60}-Cys^{77} disulfide bond in the PH domain. The quadruply charged state is calculated as m/z 764.66 (M + 1) – 764.41 (M + 0) = 0.25 which indicates 4 positive proton charges. The quadruply charged disulfide bond linked Cys^{60} and Cys^{77} containing peptides (T9-SS-T11, M + 4H$^+$) are calculated as m/z 764.37 [(1806.86 + 1246.63 + 4)/4]. Without GSNO treatment, only the Cys^{60}-Cys^{77} disulfide bond was detected. The mass accuracies for the two measurements were found to be 36 ppm (Cys^{296}-Cys^{310}

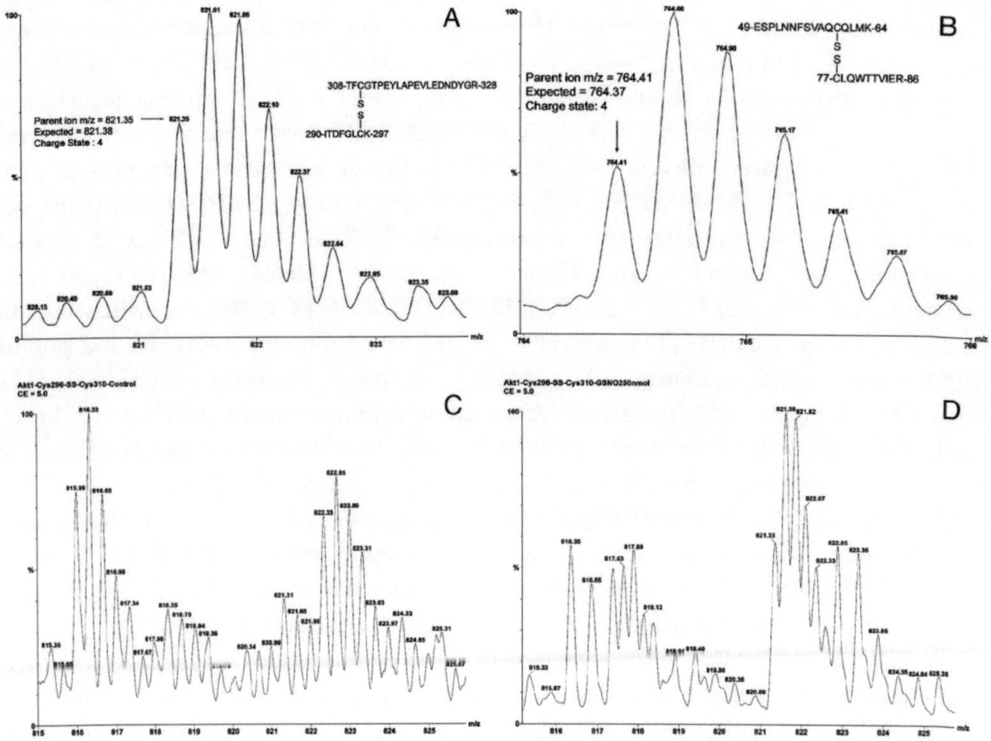

Figure 11. Detections of two intradomain disulfide bonds in Akt1/PKBα (a) Detection of intradomain Cys^{296}-Cys^{310} disulfide bond in the kinase loop. Inactive Akt1/PKBα (10 μg) was treated with GSNO and iodoacetamide (50 μM) in Laemmli sample buffer. In-gel trypsin digestion was performed after SDS-PAGE separation (BIO-RAD, 4-15% Tris-HCl). Monoisotopic parent ion at m/z 821.35, charge state: 4. Expected quadruply charged disulfide linked Cys^{296} and Cys^{310} containing the peptide at m/z 821.38. (b) Detection of the intradomain Cys^{60}-Cys^{77} disulfide bond in the PH domain. Monoisotopic parent ion at m/z 764.41, charge state: 4. Expected quadruply charged disulfide bond linked Cys^{60} and Cys^{77} containing peptide at m/z 764.37. (c) Free thiol state of Cys^{310} in the kinase loop without NO donor. The triply charged parent ion m/z 815.99: ^{308}TFCGTPEYLAPEVLEDNDYGR^{328} (expected: m/z 816.03, carboxyamidomethylcysteine, CAM derivative) represents the completely free thiol state of Cys^{310}, while the triply charged m/z 821.31 is not from disulfide linked Cys^{296}-Cys^{310} dipeptides (expected charge state: 4). The Cys^{296}-Cys^{310} disulfide bond was not detected in the absence of NO donor. (d) Nitric oxide promotes the formation of the Cys^{296}-Cys^{310} disulfide bond in the kinase loop. Inactive Akt1/PKBα (10 μg) was treated with GSNO (250 nmol, 50 μl PBS, pH = 8.0, 1 hr at room temperature in the dark) prior to alkylation with iodoacetamide and SDS-PAGE. The doubly charged m/z 816.35 ion is not from a Cys^{310} containing tryptic peptide (expected charge state: 3), and quadruply charged m/z 821.33 occurs at the expense of diminished triply charged Cys^{310} peptide. The free thiol of Cys^{310} is completely converted into the disulfide bond with Cys^{296}.

disulfide bond linked dipeptides) and 78 ppm (Cys^{60}-Cys^{77} disulfide bond linked dipeptides). The impact of GSNO on Cys^{296}-Cys^{310} disulfide bond formation is demonstrated in Figure 11C and D. The *S*-nitrosylation reaction without GSNO (Figure 11C) shows the triply charged tryptic peptide, ^{308}TFCGTPEYLAPEVLEDNDYGR^{328}, (CAM derivative) containing Cys^{310} at m/z 815.99 (expected monoisotopic parent ion: 816.03). The observed M+1 isotopic peak was at m/z 816.33. The difference between the isotopic M+1 and M+0 peak of 0.34 Da indicates 3

http://dx.doi.org/10.5772/54849

proton charges. In contrast, the triply charged ions at m/z 821.31 and m/z 821.65 (difference = 0.31 Da) do not represent the quadruply charged Cys^{296}-Cys^{310} dipeptides in Figure 11C. The triply charged Cys^{310} containing peptide was found to be totally absentwith GSNO treatment as shown in Figure 11D. The doubly charged ions at m/z 816.35 and m/z 816.85 (difference = 0.50 Da) are not related to the triply charged tryptic peptide ^{308}TFCGTPEYLAPEVLEDN-DYGR^{328} (CAM derivative) containing Cys^{310} at m/z 815.99 as shown in Figure 11C. In contrast, the ions at m/z 821.33 and m/z 821.58 (difference = 0.25 Da) are indeed from quadruply charged Cys^{296}-Cys^{310} linked dipeptides. Since quadruply charged Cys^{296}-Cys^{310} linked dipeptides are formed at the expense of triply charged Cys^{310} containing peptide after GSNO treatment, it is obvious that *S*-nitrosylation and disulfide bond formation occur simultaneously in the kinase loop.

We next sought to determine which cysteine residue is the NO acceptor that initializes Cys^{296}-Cys^{310} disulfide bond formation. There are three possibilities for the two cysteine residue thiol states: single *S*-nitrosothiol, double *S*-nitrosothiols and nitroxyl disulfide. The last case (nitroxyl disulfide) can be ruled out from the list, since expected net mass increases of 28 Da (NO - 2H = 30 - 2 Da) were not observed for the corresponding dipeptides. The second case, double *S*-nitrosothiols of Cys^{296} and Cys^{310}, may occur if both pKa's are acidic inside the kinase loop. The Biotin-Switch method was used to identify the *S*-nitrosothiol within the loop under gentle reaction conditions (GSNO 250 nmol, 1 hour). In addition, two other thiol-specific reagents, iodoacetic acid and iodoacetyl-LC-Biotin (leaving molecule: HI, fast and quantitative), were evaluated.

Chem derivatives	Parent calc.	Parent found	y2 ion calc.	y2 ion found
CMC	953.45	953.42	308.13	308.17
HPDP-Biotin	1323.64	1323.68	678.32	678.29
Acetyl-LC-Biotin	1277.65	1277.58	632.33	632.38

Table 3. Characterization of the thiol-specifically modified Akt1/PKBαpeptide ^{290}ITDFGLCK^{297}

Confirmations of the *S*-nitrosylation sites were performed by the following 3 step procedure: A. Parent ion discoveries with automated data dependent acquisition (DDA); the peptide mass tolerance was 0.2 Da for the carboxymethyl cysteine (CMC) immonium ion. Under these conditions, only a few false positive ions were observed and these were eliminated manually from the expected CMC parent ion list. B. Confidently discovered parent ions were analyzed with PepSeq of MassLynx V4.1 software; oxidation of methionine was searched as a variable modification. C. For peptides, with MS/MS scores < 35, manual interpretations of candidate parent ions were performed with the following procedure: continuum MS/MS spectra were smoothed, the upper 80% was centroided and cysteine residues were confirmed with three different thiol-specifically derivatized y ions. Cysteine residue monoisotopic mass C_3H_5NOS = 103.01 Da was replaced with CMC residue monoisotopic mass $C_5H_7NO_3S$ = 161.01 Da, HPDP-Biotin derivatized adduct residue monoisotopic mass $C_{22}H_{37}N_5O_4S_3$ = 531.20 Da and iodoacetyl-

LC-Biotin derivatized adduct residue monoisotopic mass $C_{21}H_{35}N_5O_4S_2$ = 485.21 Da, respectively.

Table 3 shows the expected results of Cys^{296}*S*-nitrosylation in the kinase loop with the three different chemical modifications. The resulting *S*-nitrosylatedCys was reduced with ascorbate and then derivatized with iodoacetic acid to afford the CMC derivative (the Cys residue with a monoisotopic mass C_3H_5NOS = 103.01 Da was replaced by the CMC residue with a monoisotopic mass $C_5H_7NO_3S$ = 161.01 Da) for sequence analysis. The CMC derivative of the y2 ion of the doubly charged tryptic peptide, ^{290}ITDFGLCK^{297}, was confirmed at m/z 308.17 (expected 308.13 = 161.01 + 145.10 +2.02). The Cys HPDP-Biotin adduct (Cys residue monoisotopic mass C_3H_5NOS = 103.01 Da was replaced with the adduct residue monoisotopic mass $C_{22}H_{37}N_5O_4S_3$ = 531.20 Da) was used for sequence analysis. The corresponding y2 ion of the Biotin-HPDP derivatized, ^{290}ITDFGLCK^{297}, was confirmed at m/z 678.29 (expected 678.32 = 531.20 + 145.10 +2.02). The CysIodoacetyl-LC-Biotin adduct (Cys residue monoisotopic mass C_3H_5NOS = 103.01 Da was replaced with adduct residue monoisotopic mass $C_{21}H_{35}N_5O_4S_2$ = 485.21 Da) was used for peptide sequence analysis. The corresponding y2 ion of iodoacetyl-LC-Biotin derivatized, ^{290}ITDFGLCK^{297} was confirmed at m/z 632.38 (expected 632.33 = 485.21 + 145.10 +2.02). Since the y2 ions of ^{296}Cys-Lys^{297} produced with the three different derivatization procedures were unambiguously observed it is likely that Cys^{296} is a favorable *S*-nitrosylation site under the conditions used. Although studies with mutated Akt1/PKBα| | (C^{224}S) indicated that Cys^{224} is a major S-nitrosylation acceptor site *in vitro*, the biological role of *S*-nitrosylated Cys^{224} in kinase regulation needs to be further explored. In the current study it was determined that significant *S*-nitrosylation of Cys^{224} is improbable, since using the three alkylation approaches and trypsin digestion, the levels of positive ionization of Cys^{224} containing peptides were below the level of detection. This failure in detection of *S*-nitrosylated Cys^{224} might be a false negative under our experimental conditions and clearly warrants further investigation. Nevertheless, our findings clearly demonstrate that *S*-nitrosylated Cys^{296} is directly relevant to the kinase activation regulation cycle.

One possible explanation for the kinetics of Cys^{296}-Cys^{310} disulfide bond formation in the kinase loop may be that there is a high kinetic barrier without GSNO. Due to its highly labile nature [140], *S*-nitrosylated Cys^{296}, which forms rapidly in the presence GSNO, may function as an intermediate state. Since this intermediate is likely to have a lower kinetic barrier for Cys^{296}-Cys^{310} disulfide bond formation, the overall speed of the reaction should increase greatly. It has been reported that trans-nitrosylation reactions between vicinal thiols can occur and accelerate disulfide bond formation [141]. The well characterized Cys^{296}-Cys^{310} disulfide bond can be used as a signature peptide for detection of *S*-nitrosylation of Cys^{296} after immunoprecipitation. The separation of tryptic peptide mixtures with our NanoLC interfaced Q-TOF is demonstrated in Figure 12 (bottom panel). The extracted mass ion peak m/z 821.62, as shown in Figure 12 (top panel), is the M+1 isotopic peak of the quadruply charged dipeptides (the most intense isotopic peak due to high number of carbon atoms).

The *in vitro* system allowed us to determine conditions that are favorable for evaluation of *S*-nitrosylation of Cys^{296} by MS/MS and was useful for studying the mechanism of intradomain disulfide bond formation. The reason for using inactive Akt1/PKBα (unphosphorylated) in these studies was to find possible *S*-nitrosylation sites in relationship with the following

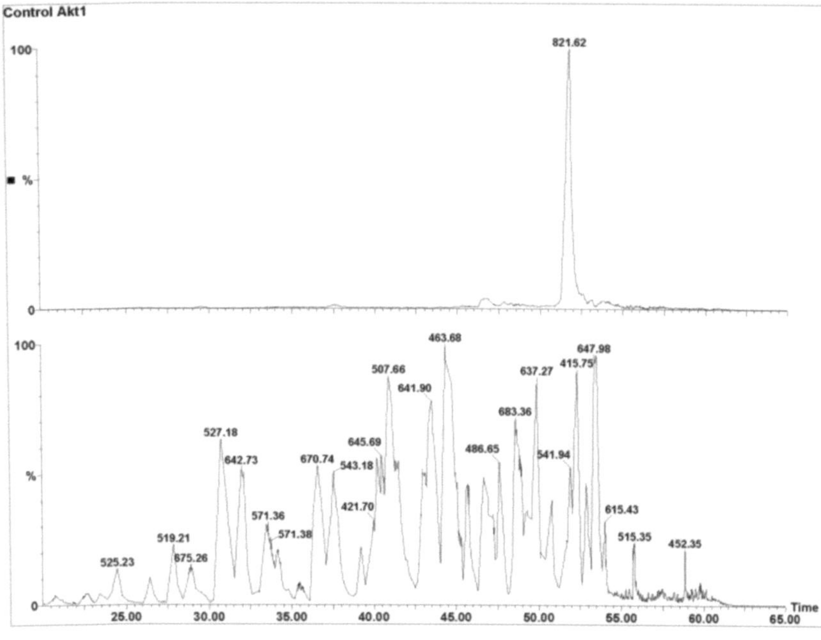

Figure 12. NanoLC chromatogram of tryptic peptides of Akt1/PKBα in soleus muscle Top panel: Mass ion chromatogram of the dipeptides m/z 821.62: M+1 isotopic peak of the quadruply charged dipeptides (intensity of M+0 monoisotopic peak is lower than M+1 due to isotope abundant as shown in Figure 11A). Bottom panel: BPI chromatogram of the Akt1/PKBαtryptic peptides after immunoprecipitations and in-gel digestion from NanoLC interfaced with Q-TOF tandem mass spectrometry.

published data: 1. Akt1/PKBα undergoes transient phosphorylation/ dephosphorylation which regulates the kinase activity conformation cycle; 2. Kinase disulfide bond formation, Cys^{297}-Cys^{311}, and dephosphorylation at pThr^{308} are induced simultaneously by H_2O_2 oxidative stress *in vitro*; 3. High levels of nitric oxide production occur both after burn injury and in diabetic patients. Previous results from our laboratory have indicated that there is *S*-nitrosylation at Cys^{296} in rat soleus muscle. A parention at m/z 690.83 containing Cys^{296} (T41-T42: ^{290}ITCFGLCKEGIK^{301}) was observed with CAM immonium trigged parent ion discovery, however, MS/MS sequencing data was not obtained. As a continuation of these studies to explore *S*-nitrosylation in the kinase active loop, large amounts of rat soleus muscle lysate (~ 3-5 mg/ml total proteins, 3 ml for each experiment, day 4 after 40% TBSA, 3rd degree burn) were used. In the present study, detailed MS/MS analysis of HPDP-biotinated free Cys^{296} peptide and Cys^{296}-Cys^{310} disulfide bound dipeptides of Akt1/PKBα were performed with lysates of rat soleus muscle after burn injury. The tryptic parent ion derivatized from free Cys^{296} after burn injury was observed at m/z 662.84 (M+2H$^+$, expected 662.82) and the MS/MS sequence data is shown in Figure 13. A low sequence score of 18 was obtained from the parent ion with S/N = 3. However, the critical diagnostic y2, y4 and y5 ions at m/z 678.29, m/z 849.34 and m/z 995.51 confirmed that trace amounts of free Cys^{296} are indeed present after intrado-

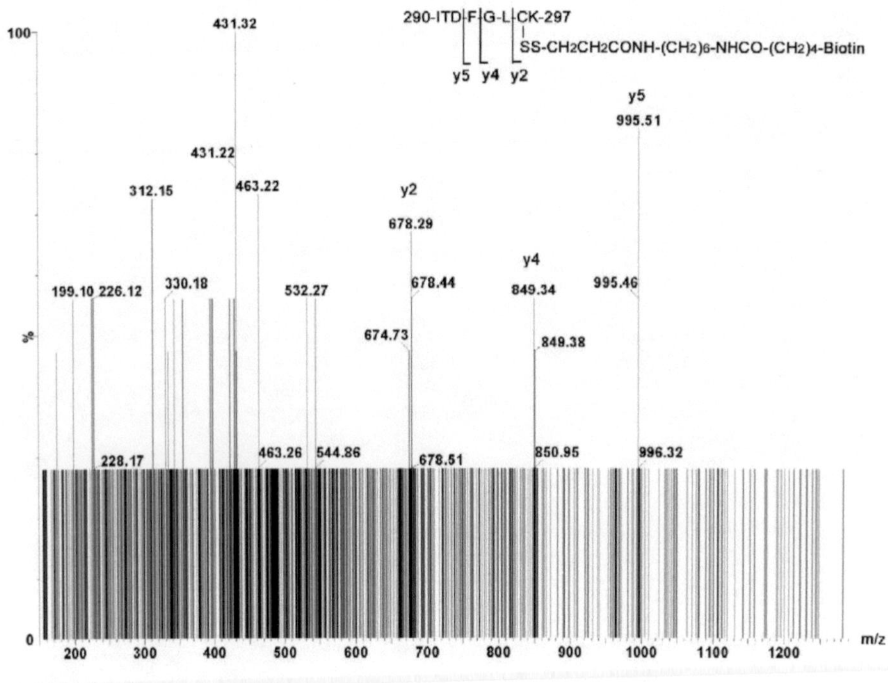

Figure 13. Sequence analysis of biotinated free Cys^{296} peptide of Akt1/PKBα after burn injury Rat soleus muscle lysates (30 mg total protein) were treated with anti-Akt1/PKBαmAb and in-gel biotination was performed with HPDP-Biotin. Parent ion m/z 662.84 (M+2H$^+$, expected 662.82) was sequenced. Cys residue monoisotopic mass C_3H_5NOS = 103.01 Da is replaced with the adduct residue monoisotopic mass $C_{22}H_{37}N_5O_4S_3$ = 531.20 Da. A low sequence score of 18 was obtained from the parent ion with S/N = 3, however the critical diagnostic y2, y4 and y5 ions at m/z 678.29, 849.34 and 995.51 confirmed that trace amounts of free Cys^{296} are presentafterburn injury.

main disulfide bond formation induced by burn injury. In addition, partial sequencing data for Cys^{296}-Cys^{310} disulfide linked dipeptides is shown in Figure 14.

The phosphorylation status of Akt1 Thr^{308} and Ser^{473} were evaluated by ELISA and the results were expressed as units per gram tissues. Figure 15 shows that phosphorylations of Akt1 at Thr^{308} and Ser^{473} in skeletal muscle of burned mice were reduced by 49.8% ($p<0.005$) and 26.2% ($p<0.05$) compared with sham treated control animals.

The C-terminal y ion series of Cys^{310} containing peptide, ^{308}TFCGTPEYLAPEVLEDNDYGR^{328}, was observed for the quadruply charged parent ion (T41-SS-T44, M + 4H$^+$). Cys^{296}-Cys^{310} disulfide linked dipeptides were not observed in muscle lysates from sham treated animals. The chance of obtaining the MS/MS sequence using our *in vivo* experimental conditions is only about 20-25%. This indicates that one interpretable MS/MS outcome (score > 25) is expected in 4 or 5 independent experiments in which 3 successive injections are performed. Nevertheless, these MS/MS data for peptides containing free Cys^{296} and Cys^{296}-Cys^{310} linked dipeptides are sufficient to verify our hypothesis that *S*-nitrosylation promotes intradomain disulfide bond formation and dephosphorylation at pThr^{308} after burn injury as illustrated in Figure 16. Due to the high lability of Cys^{296}-SNO,direct identification of this species *in vivo* was not possible.

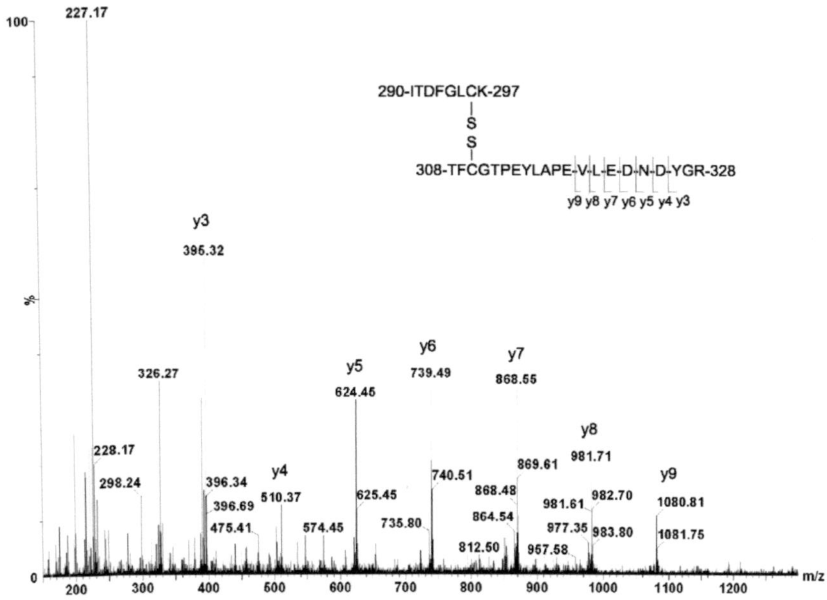

Figure 14. Identification of the Cys^{296}-Cys^{310} disulfide linked peptide with dephosphoryated Thr^{308} in soleus muscle from burned rats MS/MS sequence of Cys^{296}-Cys^{310} disulfide linked dipeptides: C-terminal y ion series (y3 to y9) of Cys^{310} containing peptide, ^{308}TFCGTPEYLAPEVLEDNDYGR^{328}, were observed from the quadruply charged parent ion (T41-SS-T44, M + $4H^{+}$).

Proposed mechanism for burn-induced Akt1/PKBα kinase loop conformational changes via phosphorylation and *S*-nitrosylation cross-taking in skeletal muscle. Phosphorylation of Thr^{308} stabilizes the disordered loop structure between ^{292}DFG and APE^{319} via a salt bridge with Lys^{297} as illustrated in the loop peptide 1, which up-regulates Akt1/PKBα kinase activity. NO free radical production is increased after burn injury, consequently, a large portion of Cys^{296} undergoes *S*-nitrosylation at Cys^{296} (peptide 2), however, some free Cys^{296} remains, which can be biotinylated for MS/MS confirmation (peptide 3). *S*-nitrosylation activates Cys^{296}-Cys^{310}intradomain disulfide bond formation (peptide 4). *S*-nitrosylation at Cys^{296} is associated with dephosphorylation of Thr^{308} and inaccessibility to the kinase site as shown in Akt1 crystal structure [142]; which down-regulates kinase activity.

S-nitrosylation of Akt1/PKBα is a key factor for understanding the regulation of glucose transport and downstream protein synthesis. A recent report demonstrated that blockade of iNOS prevents the *S*-nitrosylations of Akt and IRS-1 and results in insulin resistance *in vivo* [143]. Although it is clear that two PTMs of Akt1/PKBα, phosphorylation at Thr^{308} and *S*-nitrosylation at Cys^{296}, are critical for the regulation of Akt1/PKBα activity under stress conditions, there are still many unanswered questions concerning how reversible phosphorylation/ dephosphorylation and *S*-nitrosylation/denitrosylation modulate Akt1/PKBα activity.

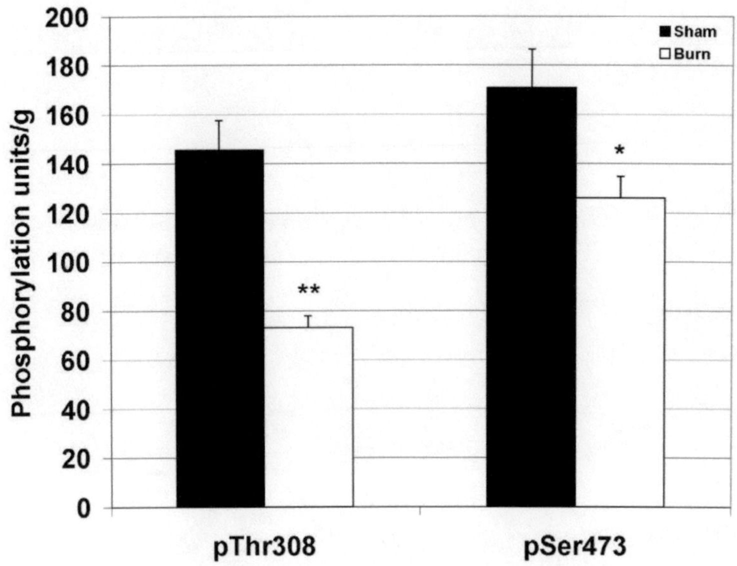

Figure 15. Impaired phosphorylation of Thr^{308} and Ser^{473} of Akt1 in skeletal muscle of burned mice. Skeletal muscle tissues from burned mice were homogenized with Cell Signaling buffer and phosphorylation levels of Thr^{308} and Ser^{473} in Akt1 were measured by ELISA. Akt $pThr^{308}$ ELISA kit (KHO0201) and $pSer^{473}$ kit (KHO0111) were purchased from Invitrogen. The phosphorylation units were normalized to tissue weight. Values represent mean ± sem for 15 burned and 8 sham treated mice. *: $p<0.05$, **: $p<0.005$.

For example, it has been reported that the Cys^{296}-Cys^{310} disulfide bond is present only when there is binding of substrate to the active kinase loop and phosphorylation at Thr^{308}; indicating that both disulfide bond formation as well as phosphorylation of Thr^{308} are important for kinase activity. In contrast, this disulfide bond was not observed under similar conditions in two studies of the ternary structure of the kinase; even though, oxidative stress was shown to induce dephosphorylation of $pThr^{308}$ and disulfide bond formation in the kinase loop in an *in vitro* study [112].

In summary, our data establishes that Cys^{296} is an important *S*-nitrosylation site in the kinase loop of Akt1/PKBα under gentle reaction conditions: (a) iodoacetic acid as previously described; (b) the HPDP-Biotin switch method and (c) the iodoacetyl-LC-Biotin method to ensure indirect capture of Cys^{296}-SNO which may be undetectable with HPDP-Biotin. The corresponding derivatized y2 ions (^{296}Cys-Lys^{297}) in the tryptic peptide (Ile-Thr-Asp-Phe-Gly-Leu-Cys-Lys) were obtained with mass sequences to eliminate false positive discovery. Although no other *S*-nitrosylated cysteine residues were detected, it is possible that *S*-nitrosylations at Cys^{224}, Cys^{344} and Cys^{460} were missed due to very low ionizations (i.e., false negative discoveries). As a consequence of *S*-nitrosylation at Cys^{296}, there is rapid disulfide bond formation with vicinal Cys^{310} in the kinase loop. This affords a stable disulfide bond linked quadruply charged parent ion at m/z 821.35 ($M + 4H^+$). Partial sequencing data for Cys^{296}-Cys^{310} linked dipeptides from soleus muscle lysates indicated that burn injury is associated with bothdephorsphorylation of $pThr^{308}$ and disulfidebond formation. Current qualitative results have

http://dx.doi.org/10.5772/54849

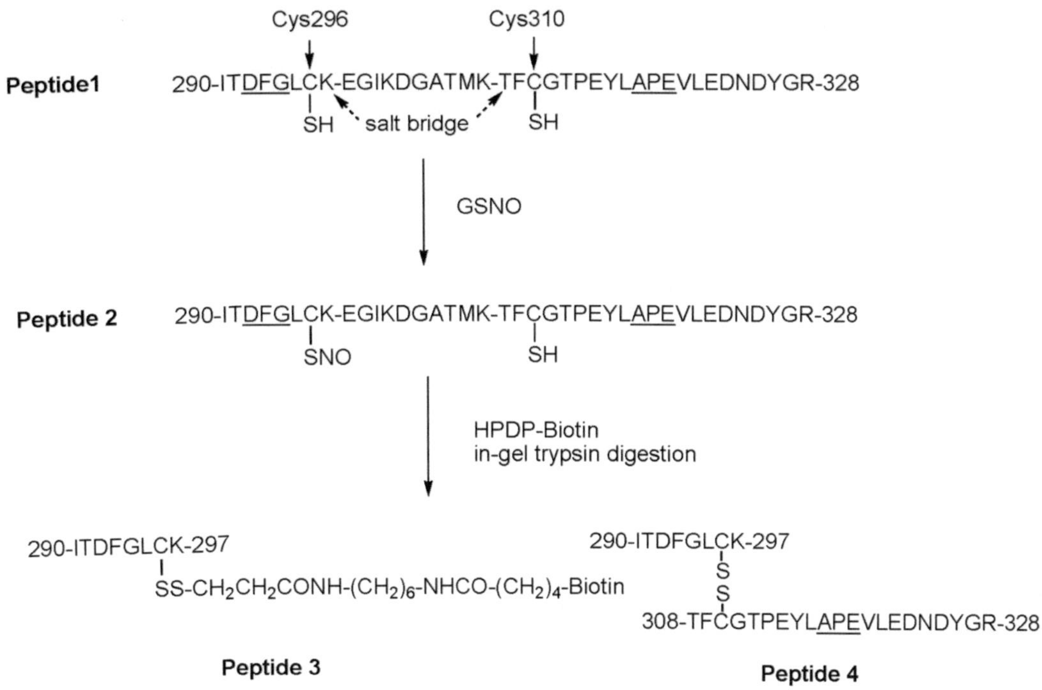

Figure 16.

provided important mechanistic information; however, quantitative measurements of Cys^{296}thiol states post-burn injury remain very challenging.

The essential issue for any isotope dilution method is to precisely characterize the heavy isotope labeled internal standard in terms of atomic and chemical purities. To determine the relative quantification of liver Akt1/PKBα after burn injury, two typical serum acute phase proteins, negative regulated albumin and positive regulated amyloid P component, as well as liver Akt1/PKBα were characterized in a preliminary study with tissue and blood samples from 3 mice with burn injury (40% TBSA). To eliminate possible mathematical and biological complexities associated with of multiple isotopomer population distributions for individual tryptic peptides produced with partial labeling conditions, peptides with only one instance of [isopropyl-$^2H_7$]-L-Leu were selected for measurement of relative labeling efficiencies. A tryptic peptide may be positively charged at its N-terminal α-amine group and the side-chain amine group of a Lys residue or the guanido group of an Arg residue; thus, a doubly charged parent ion, $[M+2H^+]$, may be observed with ESI mass spectrometry. In addition, triply charged tryptic parent ions, $[M+3H^+]$, may be obtained for peptides containing proline or histidine residues or with larger size peptides. Peptides with one instance of [isopropyl-$^2H_7$]-L-Leuincorporation yield paired light and heavy parent ions with monoisotopic mass ion differences of 3.5 Da (doubly charged) or 2.3 Da (triply charged) under ESI conditions. Charge state dependent DDA allows these multiply charged peptides to be focused in the CID chamber with charged argon cleavages. The singly charged and predominated light and heavy MS/MS y ion series from the light and heavy parent ions are produced with mass difference of 7 Da. This allows unambiguous relative quantification of parent ion enrichments from possible false positive discoveries. Characteristics of three proteins with enrichments of greater than 50% are shown in Table 4.

	Sequence, (charge state observed)	Enrichments %, (SD)
albumin	^{243}**L**SQTFPNADFAEITK^{257}, (2)	53 (3.2)
	^{559}HKPKATAEQ**L**K^{669}, (2)	57 (3.8)
	^{439}APQVSTPT**L**VEAAR^{452}, (2)	54 (4.1)
amyloid P component	^{66}SQS**L**FSYSVK^{75}, (2)	66 (4.9)
	^{88}VGEYS**L**YIGQSK^{99}, (2)	65 (4.6)
	^{147}APPSIV**L**GQEQDNYGGGFQR^{166}, (3)	69 (5.2)
liver Akt1/PKBα	^{9}EGW**L**HKR^{15}, (2)	59 (4.0)
	^{184}EVIVAKDEVAHT**L**TENR^{200}, (3)	56 (2.7)
	^{290}ITDFG**L**B*KEGIKDGATMK^{307}, (3)	55 (3.3)

Table 4. Protein enrichment levels on day 7 after 3rd degree burn of 40% TBSA

The negative acute phase protein albumin and the positive acute phase protein amyloid P component had enrichments of ~55% and ~66%, respectively. The enrichment level (56%) of liver Akt1/PKBα was found to very similar to that of albumin. These enrichment values represent ultimate [isopropyl-$^2H_7$]-L-Leuincorporation in each individual protein which can be used as the isotopic correction factor for the light and heavy parent ion MS ratio obtained by mixing exact the same weight of labeled and non-labeled liver tissues.

Akt1/PKBα was immunoprecipitated from the mixture of [isopropyl-$^2H_7$]-L-leucine labeled liver from burned mice an equal amount tissue from sham treated animals and processed further by the methods described above. The relative expression of Akt1/PKBα at the protein level from livers of burned and sham treated mice is shown in Figure 17.

The triply charged monoisotopic parent ion at m/z 647.99 was detected for the control peptide ^{252}FYGAEIVSALDYLHSEK^{268}; calculated [M+3H$^+$] = 647.99. Two heavy monoisotopic parent ions at m/z 650.34 and m/z 652.36 indicates one and two instances of [isopropyl-$^2H_7$]-L-Leu incorporation into the control peptide. Triply charged MS differences were found to be 2.3 Da (calculated MS difference for one heavy Leu incorporation: 7/3 = 2.3 Da) and 4.3 Da (calculated MS difference for two heavy Leu incorporation: 14/3 = 4.6 Da), respectively. MS/MS y ion series from y3 to y12 of the m/z 647.98 confirms the control peptide for studying protein expression. The intensities of the m/z 650.34 and m/z 652.36 ions represent the heavy Akt1/PKBα populations from burn injured mice, whereas the m/z 647.99 ion is derived from the sham treated animals. Estimated total ion intensity was ~9.5 after burn injury and ~6.5 after sham treatment. Due to the low S/N of ~2 for the heavy ions and the enrichment of 56% in Table 1, Akt1/PKBα protein expression, was observed to be up-regulated in response to burn injury the

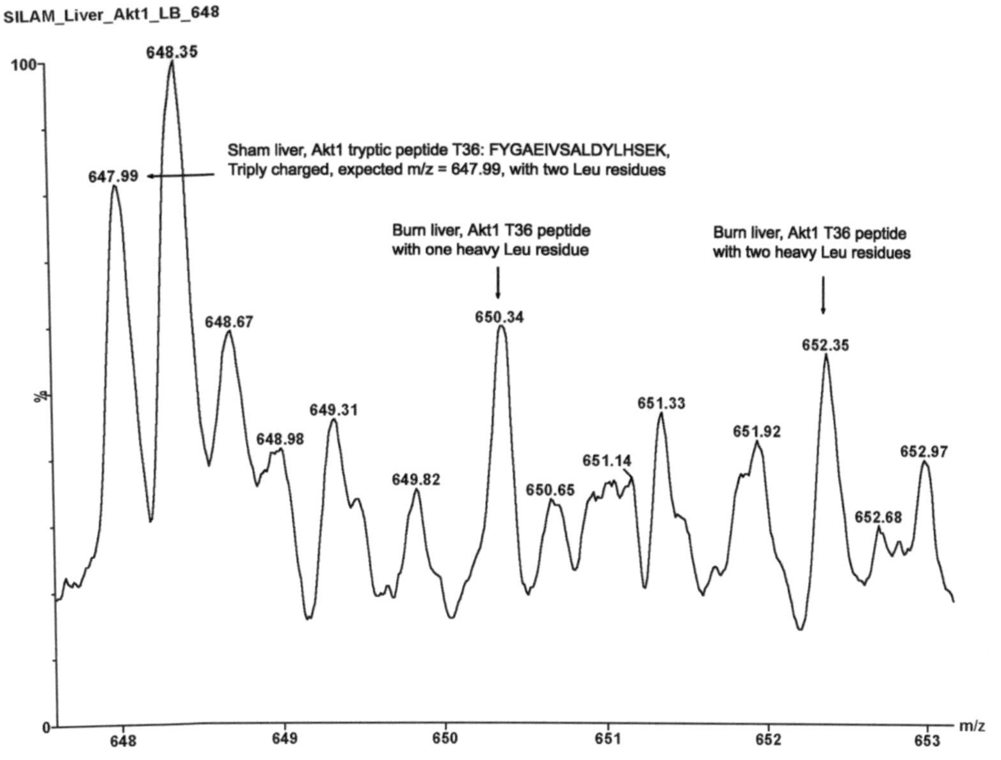

Figure 17. Changes in liver Akt1/PKBα expression at protein level after burn injury A triply charged monoisotopic parent ion at m/z 647.99 was found for the control peptide [252]FYGAEIVSALDYLHSEK[268]; calculated [M+3H$^+$] = 647.99. Two heavy monoisotopic parent ions at m/z 650.34 and m/z 652.36 indicate one and two instances of [isopropyl-2H7]-L-Leu incorporation into the control peptide. Akt1/PKBα protein expression, estimated from both heavy ions, was found to be up regulated after correction for both enrichment and background.

mice.However, the heavy ion for the biotinylated peptide, [290]ITDFGLCK[297], which was used as a marker for kinase activity, was significantly reduced (almost to background) after injury as illustrated in Figure 18.

Biotinylated light peptides [290]ITDFGLCK[297] of Akt1/PKBα from sham treated mice was detected at m/z 639.88 and was doubly charged as indicated by the natural abundance carbon isotope peak at m/z 640.33. Three biotinylated y2, y4 and y6 ions at m/z 632.44, 802.51 and 1064.59 confirmed the loop peptide sequence with biotin modification as shown in Figure 19. The corresponding y2 ion of iodoacetyl-LC-Biotin derivatized, [296]CK[297], was confirmed at m/z 632.44 (expected 632.33 = 485.21 + 145.10 +2.02). DDA with low S/N occurred *in vivo* studies was performed with continuum mode to enhance the parent ion discovery. On the other hand, centroided spectra are found to be necessary to obtain accurately the diagnostic modifications in the y ions. Biotinylated heavy peptide [290]ITDFGLCK[297] in Akt1/PKBα from burn injured mice (n = 3) was identified at m/z 643.38 with its natural carbon isotopic peak at m/z 643.88. A MS

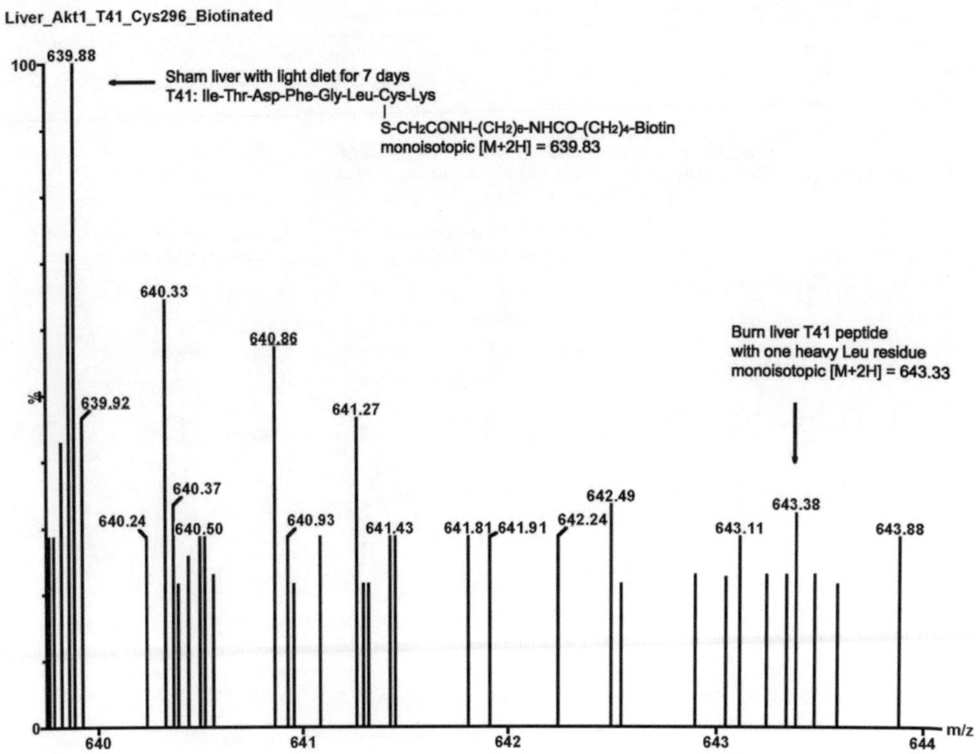

Figure 18. Liver Akt1/PKBα activity measurement via the loop peptide Light peptide, [290]ITDFGLCK[297], of Akt1/PKBα from sham treated mice was detected at m/z 639.88; doubly charged as indicated by the natural abundance carbon isotope peak at m/z 640.33. Biotinylated heavy peptides [290]ITDFGLCK[297] of Akt1/PKBα from the burn injured mice were detected at m/z 643.38; doubly charged as indicated by the natural abundance carbon isotope peak at m/z 643.88. The MS difference of 3.5 Da between the paired light and heavy parent ions indicates one instance of [isopropyl-$^2H_7$]-L-Leu incorporation into the heavy ion at m/z 643.38 after burn injury. The intensity of the m/z 643.38 ion indicates that the loop peptide containing Cys[296] was markedly reduced (almost to baseline) in response to burn injury (n = 3).

difference of 3.5 Da between the paired light and heavy parent ions clearly indicated that one instance of [isopropyl-$^2H_7$]-L-Leu was incorporation into the doubly charged parent ion at m/z 643.38 with doubly charged state (n = 3). MS ion intensity at m/z 643.38 indicated that loop peptide containing Cys[296] was almost undetectable after burn injury. These observations were evaluated with MS/MS sequencing; peptide charge status and MS shift of the isotope labeled paired peptides *in vivo*.

The incorporation efficiencies of isotopically labeled peptides in Table 3 demonstrates that amyloid P component was 10% higher than albumin; suggesting a faster turnover rate during up regulation. Serum albumin and liver Akt1/PKBα appear to have similar enrichments ~55%. Classically, individual protein fractional synthesis rate (FRS) is calculated by the relative isotope enrichment ratio of the labeled protein vs. precursor acyl-tRNA over the labeling time period

http://dx.doi.org/10.5772/54849

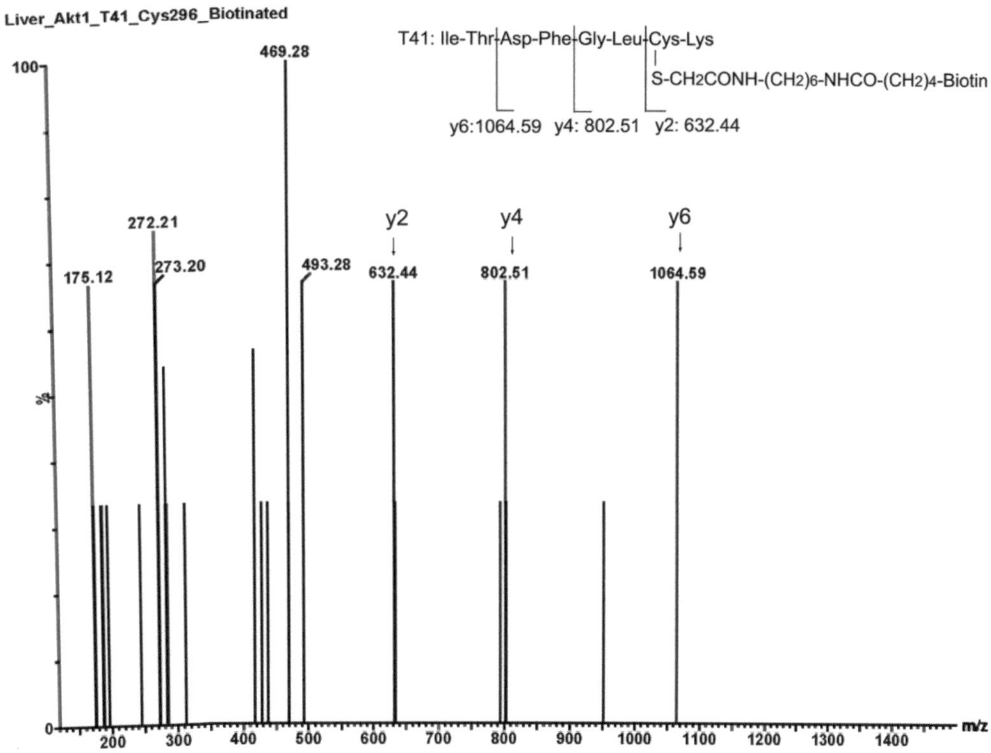

Figure 19. Identification of the kinase loop peptide derivatized with the iodoacetyl-LC-Biotin Cysteine residue monoisotopic mass C_3H_5NOS = 103.01 Da was replaced with the iodoacetyl-LC-Biotin derivatized adduct monoisotopic mass $C_{21}H_{35}N_5O_4S_2$ = 485.21 Da. Three biotinylated y2, y4 and y6 ions at m/z 632.44, 802.51 and 1064.59 unambiguously confirmed the loop peptide sequence with biotinylated mass shifts for kinase bioactivity measurements.

for a given isotope tracer [144,145]. FSR is a very important parameter for assessing effects of clinical interventions by comparisons between patients and healthy controls. In general, information about protein synthesis obtained with FRS and partially labeled SILAM are very similar and either can be used to optimize therapeutic strategies.

Our previous studies with thermally injured rats have demonstrated that there is no apparent alteration in binding of insulin to its receptors in liver, skeletal muscle or adipose tissue. Thus, acute and chronic insulin resistances induced by surgical trauma, burn injury, hemorrhage and sepsis are primarily post-receptor effects in the insulin-like growth factor-phosphatidylinositol-3 kinase-Akt pathway. Phosphorylations of specific Ser and Thr residues in the C-terminus of IRS-1 induce its degradation via the ubiquitin-proteosome pathway; which may early biological effect after receptor binding. Impaired Akt1/PKBα kinase activity after injury may be a later downstream event. Deficiency of Akt1/PKBα causes decreased somatic cell and body size [146], while knockout of Akt2/PKBα leads to insulin resistance [147]. Akt1/PKBα is involved in cellular survival pathways, by inhibiting apoptotic processes and stimulating protein synthesis pathways. It is also a key signaling protein in cellular pathways of skeletal muscle differentiation [148,149]. Currently, assays of Akt1/PKBα | | activity in vitro and in vivo are performed with antibodies specific for the phosphorylated Ser^{473} and Thr^{308} residues which are critical for stabilizing the global and loop active conformations of the kinase. Difficulties with using anti-phospho-serine, but not anti-phospho-tyrosine antibodies, have been occurred in our phosphoproteomic research. NO production is elevated after burn injury and in patients with type 2 diabetic and it has been shown that the Cys^{297}-Cys^{311} disulfide bond in the kinase loop may be formed in association with dephosphorylation under oxidative stress in vitro. Reversible S-nitrosylation at Cys^{296} in the kinase loop is another PTM which complements reversible phosphorylation at Thr^{308}in the regulation of kinase activity. It has been shown that Akt1/PKBα undergoes transient phosphorylation/dephosphorylation which regulates the kinase active conformation cycle; kinase disulfide bond formation, Cys^{297}-Cys^{311}, and dephosphorylation at pThr^{308} are induced simultaneously by H_2O_2 oxidative stress *in vitro* [46];and high levels of nitric oxide production occurs in both burn injured rats and diabetic patients. Freethiol group of Cys^{296} undergoes loop conformational changes by capture of nitric oxide, or chemical modifications with other reactive oxygen species produced under the burn injury; thus blocking substrate recognition. Intact loop peptide with a trace amount of free cysteine in the peptide population, ^{290}ITDFGLCK^{297}, after burn injury was developed as an unambiguous index for bioactivity. However, this peptide is not related to kinase protein expression in responses to the burn, since varying degrees of different thiol modifications in the loop may occur at the same time. In contrast, the control peptide, ^{252}FYGAEIVSALDYLHSEK^{268}, locatedjust outside of kinase loop, was a useful index of protein level. Kinase bioactivity measured with tandem mass spectrometry was comparable with previously reported data measured with immune complex kinase assay and anti-pThr^{308} as well as anti-Ser^{437}mAbs, whereas protein levels were slightly increased in responses to injury. MS/MS sequence analysis and [isopropyl-$^2H_7$]-L-Leu incorporation in the paired peptides indicated that after thermal injury kinase activity is significantly reduced, despite increased protein expression. These findings indicate that neither complete labeling of nor measurement of acyl-tRNA enrichment are necessary or critical for quantitative proteomics with SILAM. Cys^{296}thiol state is considered as one of the important factors for the kinase activity. The limitations of partially labeled SILAM for clinical studies are: 1. Specific protein enrichment must be measured in tissues labeled with heavy isotopes under stress conditions; unfortunately, many proteins of clinical interest occur at low abundance and thus there is a high rate of false negative discovery. 2. Sequence confirmation of individual proteins requires that SDS-PAGE bands be visible by Coomassie brilliant blue R-250 staining (at least 0.1 μg). Despite these limitations our observations may provide new insights into the treatment of muscle wasting and other aspects of insulin resistance after critical injury.

As the central mediator of the IR/IRS/ PI3K/FOXO pathway, Akt1/PKBα kinase loop conformational changes are induced via a transition from the physiological salt bridge Lys^{297}-Ser^{308} and the pathphsiological disulfide bond Cys^{296}-Cys^{310}, which inhibits kinase substrate recognition. Impaired Akt1/PKBα kinase activity and enhancement of the activities of other stress kinases leads to FOXO3 translocation from the cytosolic compartment into the nuclear compartment, where FOXO3 transcriptional activity is further regulated by reversible acetylation.

4.3. Acetylation of transcription factor FOXO3 in muscle wasting post-burn injury

Skeletal muscle serves as the major protein reservoir from which amino acids can be mobilized for gluconeogenesis, new protein synthesis or as an energy source. With starvation and in many systemic disease states, including sepsis, cancer, burn injury, diabetes, cardiac and renal failure, there is generalized muscle wasting, which results primarily from increased breakdown of muscle proteins combined with reduced protein synthesis in most of these conditions [150,151]. In all these catabolic states, the loss of muscle mass involves a common pattern of transcriptional responses, including induction of genes for protein degradation and decreased expression of genes for growth-related and energy-yielding processes [152]. In atrophying muscles, two independent degradation pathways, lysosomal autophagy and proteasomal proteolysis are activated to catalyze the degradation of muscle proteins, including myofibrillar components and organelles [153,154,155,156,157,158]. Recent findings suggest that FOXO1 is a major regulator of energy metabolism in general (159) while FOXO3 may play significant roles in skeletal muscle wasting in responses to stresses [160,161,162,163,164].

FOXO3 activity is highly regulated by post-translational modifications, including phosphorylation, acetylation and ubiquitination in response to oxidative stress [165,166,167,168,169,170]. Under physiological conditions, insulin induces FOXO3 phosphorylation in muscle via IGF-1/insulin-IRS-PI3K-Akt, leading to the exclusion of FOXO3 from the nucleus and binding with 14-3-3γ protein. Consequently poly-ubiquitination and degradation occur in the cytoplasm (171,172,173,174,175). Therefore, the finely tuned equilibrium between FOXO3 transcription activities in the nuclear compartment and degradation in the cytosolic compartment is maintained. However, pathophysiologic changes not only impair Akt/PKB activity (reduced levels of pSer^{308} and pThr^{473} and enhanced Cys^{296}S-nitrosylation as discussed above), but also increase the activities of a number of stress kinases which phosphorylate FOXO3 at sites different from those acted upon by IGF-1/insulin-IRS-PI3K-Akt. This results in nuclear translocation and transactivation with modulation of FOXO3 activities by p300/CB-mediated acteylation and Sirt1- mediated deacetylation [176,177,178,179,180].

Within thenucleus, FOXO3 binds to the target gene promoter; p300/CBP is recruited to the DNA-FOXO3 complex and transcription of target proteins is stimulated; initially by acetylating nucleosomal histones. Subsequently, there is p300/CBP mediated acetylation of FOXO3 which leads to dissociation from the promotor.At the same time, Sirt1 may stimulate or maintain the binding of FOXO3 to DNA which stimulates deacetylation of acetylated FOXO3 under conditions of oxidative stress.FOXO3 may also be monoubiquitinated, which enhances its transcriptional activity. Recent data has shown that nuclear Sirt1 deacetylation may render the acetylated FOXO3 lysine residues (Lys^{242}, Lys^{259}, Lys^{290}, Lys^{569} and possible Lys^{270}, Lys^{271}) susceptible to polyubiquitination. Degradation of deacetylated FOXO3 appears to be mediated by Skp2, a subunit of E3 ubiquitin ligase, which also binds to the Ser^{256} residue that is phosphorylated by Akt/PKB. These regulatory pathways are illustrated in Figure 1. Therefore, the hypothesis is that, burn injury stimulates muscle FOXO3 activities by altering an intricate combination of phosphorylation, acetylation and ubiquitination,named "the FOXO3 code" [181]. These PTMs are likely to occur concurrently and to affect each other, leading to burn induced muscle wasting. Investigations of the complicated interlocking processes mediating post translational modulations of regulatory proteins with a focus on nuclear protein FOXO3,

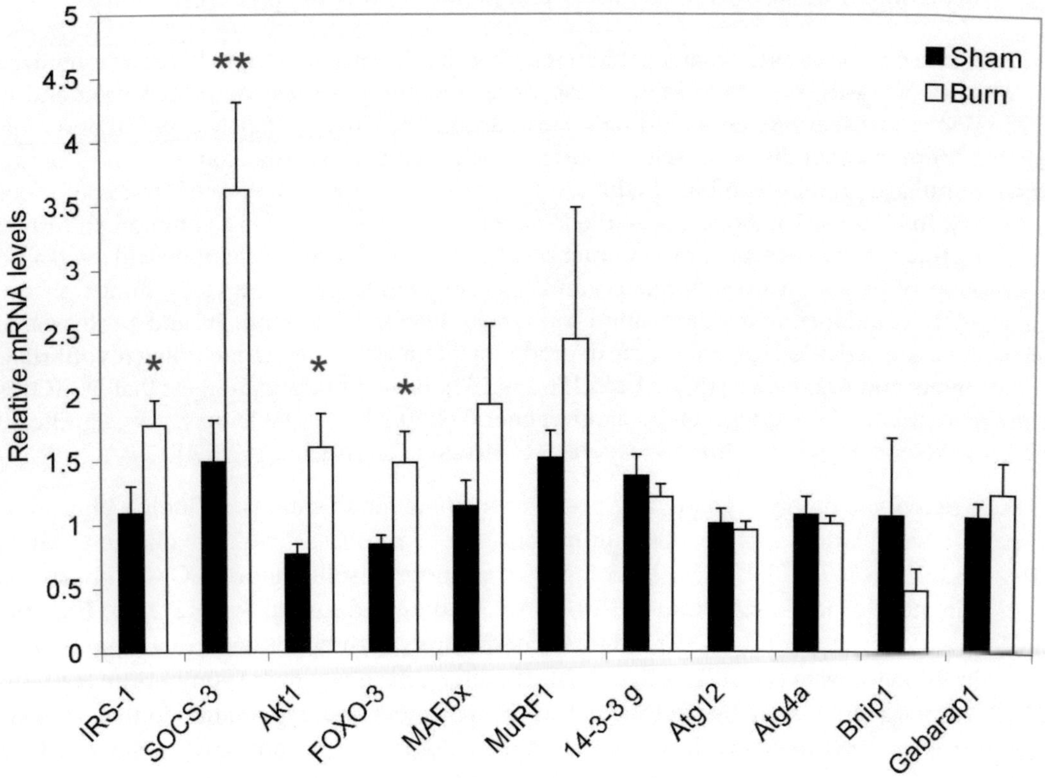

Figure 20. Burn-induced proteasomal and lysosomal proteolysis gene expression in mouse skeletal muscle. Gene profiles in sham treated (n=8) and burned mice; 3rd degree of 30% TBSA on day 7 after injury (n=15) indicate reduced cytosolic FOXO3 degradation and enhancement in the proteasomal proteolysis pathway.

in relation will lead to new knowledge about the mechanism(s) of muscle wasting after burn injury. The effects of FOXO3 PTMs on its function have been studied extensively, but discrepant results have been reported by many investigators under different conditions. Unfortunately, little information about FOXO3 PTM in muscle after burn injury is currently available.

Determination of acetylation state of lysine residues in FOXO3 protein is dependent on NanoLC-Q-TOF tandem mass spectrometry technology. Unlike labile phosphorylated or O-GlcNac modified Ser residues, acetylated lysine residues are stable during tissue extraction processes. The likelihood of false negative findings is minimal. Therefore, NanoLC-Q-TOF tandem mass spectrometry provides accurate site-specific identification of acetylation on lysine residue by detecting a mass shift (Δmass) of 42.01 Da [182]. In this project, we propose to explore the relationship between FOXO3 acetylation and muscle wasting after burn injury.

Initially, quantitative real-time RT-PCR was performed to evaluate factors related to muscle wasting at the mRNA level. IRS-1, SOCS3, Akt1, FOXO3, MAFbx, MuRF1, 14-3-3γ, Atg12, Atg4a, Bnip3, and Gabarapl1 mRNA levels were measured as shown in Figure 20. In contrast to the decrease in cellular IRS-1 protein levels, its mRNA expression was increased by 35%

($p<0.05$). SOCS-3 and Akt1 mRNA expressions were also increased by 140% ($p<0.005$) and 110% ($p<0.05$), respectively. Increased Akt1 mRNA expression was observed even though there were decreased phosphorylations of Akt1 Ser473 and Thr308, and increased S-nitrosylation of Cys296 in the kinase loop. These data suggest that impairment of the Akt mediated anabolic pathway show an early tendency for transcriptional recovery on day 7 after injury. In contrast, significant up-regulation of FOXO3 and no change in 14-3-3γ mRNA indicates that cytosolic FOXO3 degradation via the 14-3-3γ complex continues to be reduced in responses to the burn injury on day 7. Atg proteins, Binlp1, Gabarapl1 and many other proteins act together to generate double-membrane autophagosomes, which transfer their contents to lysosomers. However, all of these autophagy-related mRNAs were not significantly changed. In contrast, increased atrogin-1/MAFbx and MuRF-1 mRNAs, although not significant on Day 7, suggest that E3 ligase promoted proteasomal proteolysis is mainly responsible for muscle wasting after burn injury, challenging the lysosome hypothesis [183,184].

The activity of FOXO3 is dependent on sub-cellular location which is regulated by a broad range of PTMs: phosphorylation, acetylation and ubiquitination. Specifically, FOXO3 regulation mechanisms in association with nucleosomal histones are primarily controlled by reversible acetylations as illustrated in Figure 1. Nineteen phosphorylated residues are listed in the UniProtKB/Swiss-Prot and five acetylated sites in FOXO3 and seven sites in FOXO1 are observed [185]. However, these data are not consistent between laboratories. For the first time, two PTM isomers of muscle FOXO3 induced by burn injury were unambiguously confirmed at the amino acid sequence level with the NanoLC-Q-TOF approach. As illustrated in Figure 22 (left panel) Western blot analysis confirmed the SDS-PAGE FOXO3 band splitting in skeletal muscle of burned mice. The apparent SDS-PAGE MW of FOXO3 in skeletal muscle of sham treated mice was ~87 kDa (672 AA, calc MW: 71,064) from varying amounts of FOXO3 in lanes S30, S15 and S5. One extra band, located at apparent molwt of ~80 kDa as seen in lanes B30, B15 and B5, was detected in skeletal muscle from burned mice. These two FOXO3 isomers were clearly verified with recombinant human FOXO3 as shown in the right panel of Figure 21.

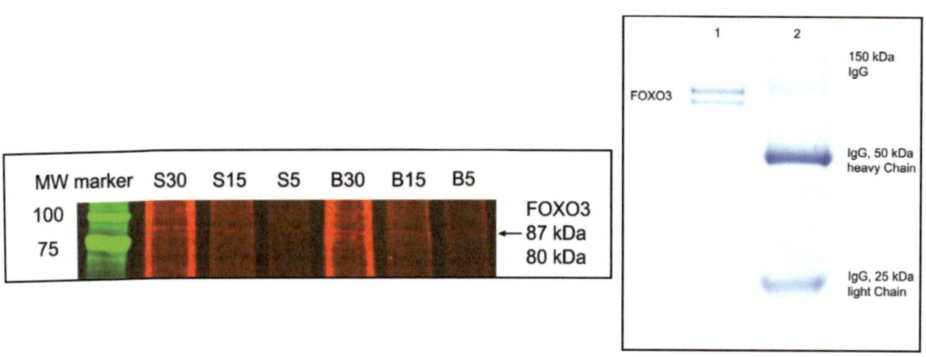

Figure 21. SDS-PAGE band splitting of FOXO3 Left panel:Immunoprecipitations of muscle lysates from burned and sham treated mice were performed using anti-C-terminal antibody (sc-34895, 2 μg). The membrane was scanned over near-infrared range. Right panel:Recombinant human FOXO3 was loaded onto the 12% Ready Gels with intact and reduced goat IgG. Two FOXO3 bands were also found with molecular weights of above 87 and 80 kDa as compared with intact IgG (150 kDa) and reduced IgG heavy chains (50 kDa).

NanoLC-Q-TOF tandem mass spectrometry data revealed that burn-induced skeletal muscle FOXO3 undergoing multiple phosphorylations and acetylations. These PTMs increase overall FOXO3 negative charge which changes electrophoretic mobility during SDS-PAGE. Both FOXO3 SDS-PAGE bands, obtained *in vitro* and *in vivo*, were unambiguously confirmed with MS/MS sequencing. Criteria for positive skeletal muscle FOXO3 PTM identification were defined as follows: 1. Tryptic peptides in digests must be unambiguously confirmed with MS/MS sequencing with reference to protein data banks; 2. Both SDS-PAGE bands are verified as FOXO3 isomers with at least two peptide sequence matches; 3. Mass accuracy of phosphorylated and acetylated MS/MS ion shifts are: 79.97 ± 0.10 and 42.01 ± 0.10 Da; 4. S/N of phosphorylated and acetylated MS/MS ions are >2. FOXO3 acetylated at the 241-Lys residue (~80 kDa) in mouse muscle after burn injury was sequenced as shown in Figure 22.

Our MS/MS data confirmed phosphorylation and acetylation in two domains of FOXO3, the FOXO3 DNA binding domain and the FOXO3 transactivation/chromatin remodeling domain as shown below:

FOXO3 DNA binding domain

Human FOXO3 tryptic peptide T4, triply charged

VLAPGGQDPGSGPATAAGGLSGGTQALLQPQQPLPPPQPGAAGGpS144GQPR

Burned mouse skeletal muscle FOXO3 tryptic peptide T18, doubly charged

SSWWIINPDGG**ACK241**

FOXO3 transactivation/Chromatin remodeling domain

Human FOXO3 tryptic peptide T30-31, doubly charged

ACK271AALQTAPEpS280ADDpS284PSQLSACK290

In summary. Under physiological conditions, insulin induces FOXO3 phosphorylation in muscle via IGF-1/insulin-IRS-PI3K-Akt, leading to the exclusion of FOXO3 from the nucleus and binding to 14-3-3γ protein with subsequent poly-ubiquitination and degradation in the cytoplasm. Similarly, acetylation of FOXO3 results in neutralization of the positive charges on lysine residues and facilitates entry into the nuclear compartment. In the nucleus FOXO3 up-regulates genes mediating skeletal muscle protein degradation and down-regulates genes mediating skeletal muscle protein synthesis. The net result of the processes is muscle wasting. In primitive man (i.e. "cave-man") this was a highly adaptive process. For example when a cave-man suffered from major trauma such as being "mauled by a saber tooth tiger" and survived the insult to return to his cave, skeletal muscle wasting was critical for survival. Since primitive man probably did not have significant amounts of adipose tissue and glycogen stores provide limited substrates for energy production and anabolic function survival depended on mobilization of skeletal muscle (in addition to some nutritional supplementation by friends and relatives).

In modern society, after major trauma, the victim is usually confined to an intensive care unit and nutritional metabolic requirements after injury are met by carefully controlled enteral and

http://dx.doi.org/10.5772/54849

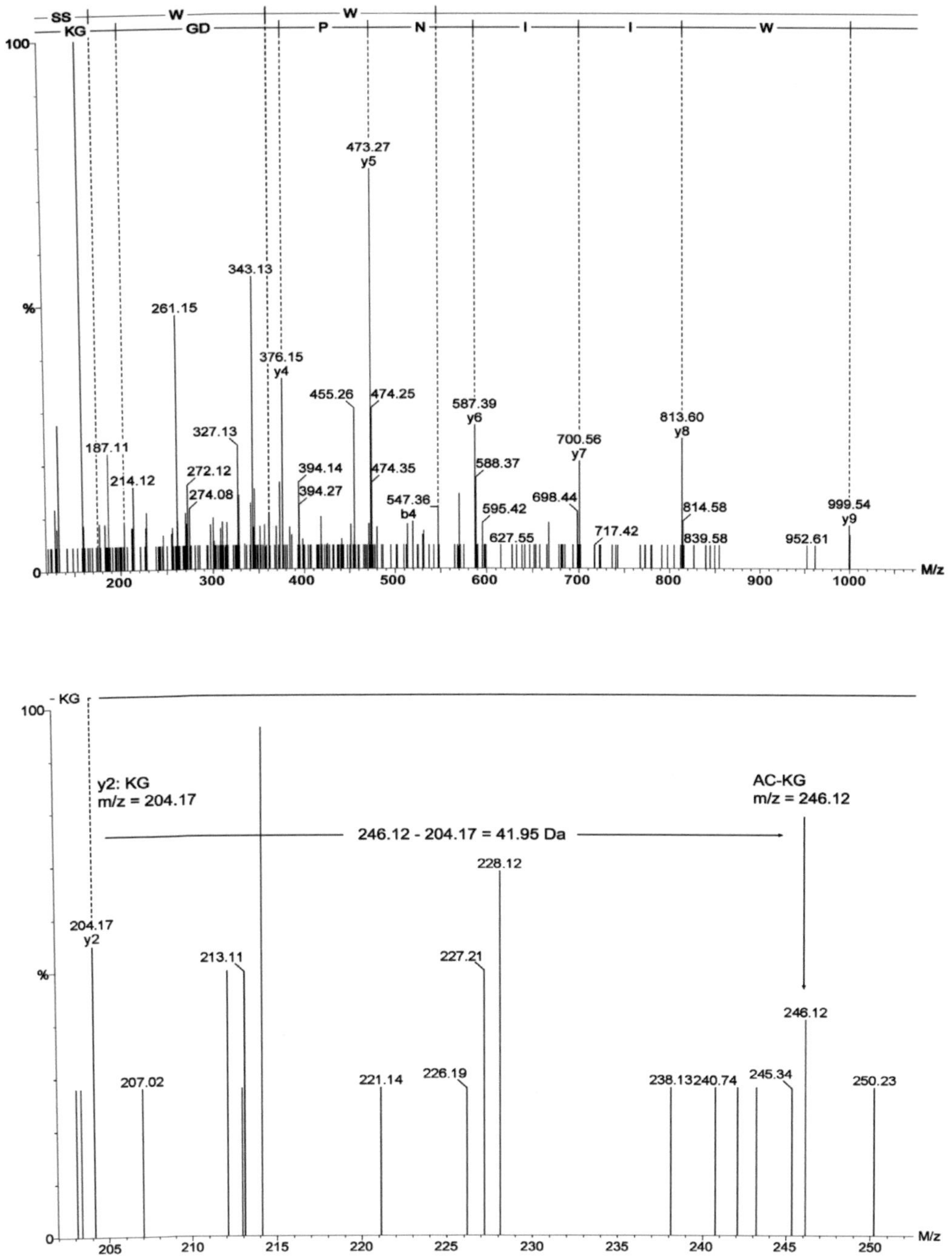

Figure 22. Site-specific pinpointing of acetylated Lys241 of FOXO3 in burned mouse muscle. Upper panel: Identification of mouse FOXO3 peptide T18 $[M+2H]^{+2}$ = m/z 680.34, found: m/z 680.52. Lower panel: Zoom of the T18 peptide y2 ion m/z 204.17 (241-Lys-Gly) and corresponding acetylated y2 ion m/z 246.12 (AC-241-Lys-Gly) indicates a mass shift of 41.95 Da.

parenteral nutrition. However the processes mediating FOXO3 entry in to the nucleus continue to be manifest and muscle wasting persists leading to weakness and in severe cases respiratory failure. Thus, a critical survival mechanism in primative man has transitioned to a major factor in morbidity and mortality for victims of severe trauma and burns in today's society.

5. Conclusion

PTM profiling of burn-induced IRS-1 C-terminal phosphorylation, S-nitrosylation of Akt1/ PKBα I I Cys^{296} and acetylation of FOXO3 Lys^{241}, Lys^{271} and Lys^{290} expands our understanding of insulin resistance and muscle wasting after burn injury. These findings reveal that Cys^{296}-Cys^{310} disulfide bond formation together with dephosphorylation of Thr^{308} in the kinase Akt1/ PKBα I I loop regulates FOXO3 sub-cellular distribution and transcriptional activity. The PTM profiling enables new recognition patterns for partner's molecules turn "on" and "off" of enzyme activity and control the lifetime and location of the mediators in insulin signal transduction [137,186]. IRS-1 integrity is reduced by 10% which is not a major factor in downstreamsignaling. However, impaired Akt1/PKBa activity by 70% due to enhanced S-nitrosylation of Cys^{296} and reduction of phosphor-Thr^{308} and Ser^{473} has major impact on FOXO3 sub-cellular distribution and activities. Muscle wasting but not insulin resistance is significant in burned vs sham treated groups between days 3 and 7 post-burn injury. Our studies provide a deep insight into the interrelationships between burn-induced oxidative and metabolic stresses and muscle wasting in human patients [187].

Author details

Xiao-Ming Lu[1,2], Ronald G. Tompkins[1,2] and Alan J. Fischman[1,2]

1 Surgical Service, Massachusetts General Hospital and Harvard Medical School, Boston, MA, USA

2 The Shriners Hospitals for Children, Boston, MA, USA

References

[1] Taniguchi CM, Emanuelli B, Ronald KC. Critical nodes in signaling pathways: insights into insulin action. Nature Reviews Molecular Cell Biology 2006; 7:85-96.

[2] Jeschke MG, Mlcak RP, Finnerty CC, Norbury WB, Gauglitz GG, Kulp GA, Herdon DN. Burn size determines the inflammatory and hypermetabolic response. Critical Care 2007; 11:R90.

[3] Gauglitz GG, Halder S, Boehning DF, Kulp GA, Herdon DN, Barral JM, Jeschke MG. Post-burn hepatic insulin resistance is associated with endoplasmic reticulum (ER) stress. Shock 2010; 33(3):299-305.

[4] Evers LH, Bhavsar G, Mailander P. The biology of burn injury. Experimental Dermatology 2010; 19:777-783.

[5] Przkora R, Herdon DN, Finnerty CC, Jeschke MG. Insulin attenuates the cytokine response in a burn wound infection model. Shock 2007; 27(2):205-208.

[6] Jeschke MG, Boehning DF, Finnerty CC, Herndon DN. Effect of insulin on the inflammatory and acute phase response after burn injury. Critical Care Medicine 2007; 35(9 Suppl): S519-S523.

[7] Barrow RE, Dasu MRK, Ferrando AA, Spies M, Thomas ST, Perez-Polo JP, Herndon DN. Gene expression patterns in skeletal muscle of thermally injured children treated with oxandrolone. Annual Surgery 2003; 237(3):422-428.

[8] Dasu MR, Barrow RE, Herndon DN. Gene profiling in muscle of severely burned children: Age-and Sex-dependent changes. The Journal of Surgical Research 2005; 123:144-152.

[9] Pidcoke HF, Wade CF, Wolf SE. Insulin and burned patient. Critical Care Medicine 2007; 35(9): suppl. S524-S530.

[10] Gauglitz GG, Herndon DN, Kulp GA, Meyer III WJ, Jeschke MG. Abnormal insulin sensitivity persists up to three years in pediatric patient post-burn. The Journal of Clinical Endocrinology & Metabolism. 2009; 94(5):1656-1664.

[11] Gauglitz GG, Herndon DN, Jeschke MG. Insulin resistance postburn: Underlying mechanisms and current therapeutic strategies. Journal of Burn Care & Research 2008; 29:683-694.

[12] Khoury W, Klausner JM, Benabraham R, Szold O. Glucose control by insulin for critically ill surgical patients. The Journal of Trauma 2004; 57(5):1132-1138.

[13] Carter EA, Burks D, Fischman AJ, White MF, Tompkins RG. Insulin resistance in thermally-injured rats is associated with post-receptor alterations in skeletal muscle, liver and adipose tissue. International Journal of Molecular Medicine 2004; 14:653-658.

[14] Johan Groeneveld AB, Beishuizen A, Visser FC. Insulin: a wonder drug in the critically ill? Critical Care 2002; 6(2):102-105.

[15] Ikezu T, Okamato T, Yonezawa K, Tompkins RG, Martyn JAJ. Analysis of thermal injury-induced insulin resistance in rodents. Journal of Biological Chemistry 1997; 272 (40):25289-25295.

[16] White MF. Insulin signaling in health and disease. Science 2003; 302:1710-1711.

[17] Zhang Q, Cater EA, Ma B-Y, White MF, Fischman AJ, Tompkins RG. Molecular mechanism(s) of burn-induced insulin resistance in murine skeletal muscle: role of IRS phosphorylation. Life Science 2005; 77:3068-3077.

[18] Carey LC, Lowery BD, Cloutier CT. Blood sugar and insulin response of humans in shock. Annual Surgery 1970; 172:342-350.

[19] Allison SP, Hinton P, Chamberlain MJ. Intravenous glucose-tolerance, insulin, and free-fatty-acid levels in burned patients. Lancet 1968; 2:1113-1116.

[20] Taylor FHL, Levenson SM, Adams MA. Abnormal carbohydrate metabolism in human thermal burns. The New England Journal of Medicine 1944; 231:437-445.

[21] Rayfield EJ, Curnow RT, George DT, Beisel WR. Impaired carbohydrate metabolism during a mild viral illness. The New England Journal of Medicine 1973; 289:618-621.

[22] Williams JL, Dick GF. Decreased dextrose tolerance in acute infectious disease. Archives of Internal Medicine 1932; 50:801-818.

[23] Wilmore DW, Mason AD Jr, Pruitt BA Jr. Insulin response to glucose in hypermetabolic burn patients. Annual Surgery 1976; 183:314-320.

[24] Mizock BA. Alterations in carbohydrate metabolism during stress: a review of the literature. The American Journal of Medicine 1995; 98:75-84.

[25] Grecos GP, Abbott WC, Schiller WR, Long CL, Birkhahn RH, Blakemore WS. The effect of major thermal injury and carbohydrate-free intake on serum triglycerides, insulin and 3-methylhistidine excretion. Annual Surgery 1984; 200:632-637.

[26] Thomas R, Aikawa N, Burke JF. Insulin resistance in peripheral tissues after a burn injury. Surgery 1979; 86:742-747.

[27] Turinsky J, Patterson SA. Proximity of a burn wound as a new factor in considerations of postburn insulin resistance. The Journal of Surgical Research 1979; 26:171-174.

[28] Woolfson AMJ, Heatley RV, Allison SP. Insulin to inhibit protein catabolism after injury. The New England Journal of Medicine 1979; 300:14-17.

[29] Wolfe RR, Drukot MJ, Wolfe MH. Effect of thermal injury on energy metabolism, substrate kinetics and hormonal concentrations. Circulatory Shock 1982; 9:383-394.

[30] Wolfe RR, Durkot MJ, Allsop JR, Burke JF. Glucose metabolism in severely burned patients. Metabolism 1979; 28(10):1031-1039.

[31] Jahoor F, Herndon DN, Wolfe RR. Role of insulin and glucagon in the response of glucose and alanine kinetics in burn-injured patients. The Journal of Clinical Investigation 1986; 78:807-814.

[32] Jahoor F, Shangraw RE, Miyoshi H, Wallfish H, Herndon DN, Wolfe RR. Role of insulin and glucose oxidation in mediation the protein catabolism of burns and sepsis. American Journal of Physiology 1989; 257:E323-E331.

[33] Black PR, Brooks DC, Bessey PQ, Wolfe RR, Wilmore DW. Mechanism of insulin resistance following injury. Annual Surgery196:420-435.

[34] Frayn KN. Effects of burn injury on insulin secretion and sensitivity to insulin in the rat in vivo. European Journal of Clinical Investigation 1975; 5(4):331-337.

[35] Allsop JR, Wolfe RR, Burke JF. Glucose kinetics and responsiveness to insulin in the rat injured by burn. Surgery Gynecology and Obstetrics. 1978; 147:565-573.

[36] Frayn KN, Le Marchand-Brustel Y, Freychet P. Studies on the mechanism of insulin resistance after injury in the mouse. Diabetologia 1978; 14:337-341.

[37] Turinsky J, Saba TM, Scovil WA, Chesnut T. Dynamics of insulin secretion and resistance after burns. The Journal of Trauma 1977; 17:344-350.

[38] Turinsky J. Glucose metabolism in the region recovering from burn injury: effect of insulin on 2-deoxyglucose uptake in vivo. Endocrinology 1983; 113:1370-1376.

[39] Wogensen L, Jensen M, Svensson P, Worsaae H, Welinder B, Nerup J. Pancreatic beta-cell function and interleukin-1 beta in plasma during the acute phase response in patients with major burn injuries. European Journal of Clinical Investigation 1993; 23:311-319.

[40] Lang CH, Dobrescu C, Burke JF. Tumor necrosis factor impairs insulin action on peripheral glucose disposal and hepatic glucose output. Endocrinology 1992; 130:43-52.

[41] Ling PR, Bristrian BR, Mendez B, Igtfan NW. Effects of systemic infusion of endotoxin, tumor necrosis factor, and interleukin-1 on glucose metabolism in the rat: relationship to endogenous glucose production and peripheral tissue glucose uptake. Metabolism 1994; 43:279-284.

[42] Portoles MT, Pagan R, Ainaga MJ, Diaz-Laviada I, Municio AM. Lipopolysaccharide-induced insulin resistance in monolayers of cultured hepatocytes. British Journal of Experimental Pathology 1989; 70:199-205.

[43] Christ B, Nath A, Heinrich PC, Jungermann K. Inhibition by recombinant human interleukin-6 of the glucagon-dependent induction of phosphopyruvate carboxykinase gene expression in cultured rat hepatocytes: regulation of gene transcription and messenger RNA degradation. Hepatology 1994; 20(6):1577-1583.

[44] Cryer PE. Hypoglycemia: the limiting factor in the management of IDDM. Diabetes 1994; 43:1378-1389.

[45] de Bandt JP, Chollet-Martin S, Hernvann A, Lioret N, du Roure LD, Lim SK, Vaubaudole M, Guiechot J, Saizy R, Giboudeau J. Cytokine response to burn injury: relationship with protein metabolism. The Journal of Trauma 1994; 36(5):624-628.

[46] Burke JF, Wolfe RR, Mullanye CJ, Matthews DE, Bier DM. Glucose requirements following burn injury. Parameters of optimal glucose infusion and possible hepatic and respiratory abnormalities following excessive glucose intake. Annual Surgery 1979; 190(3):274-283.

[47] Feinstein R, Kanetyh H, Papa MZ, Lunenfield B, Karazik A. Tumor necrosis factor alpha suppresses insulin-induced tyrosine phosphorylation of insulin receptor and its substrates. Journal of Biological Chemistry 1993; 268:26055-26058.

[48] Hotamisligil GS, ?rray DL, Choy ?, Spiegelman BM. Tumor necrosis factor inhibits signaling from the insulin receptor. Proceeding of the National Academy of Sciences of United States of America 1994; 91:4854-4858.

[49] Hotamisligil GS. Reduced tyrosine kinase activity of the insulin receptor in obesity-diabetes: central role of tumor necrosis factor. The Journal of Clinical Investigation 1994; 94:1543-1549.

[50] Wilmore DW, Aulick HL, Goodwin CW. Glucose metabolism following severe injury. Acta Chirurgica Scandinavica Supplementum 1980; 498:43-47.

[51] Ikezu T, Okamoto T, Yonezawa K, Tompkins RG, Martyn JA. Analysis of thermal injury-induced insulin resistance in rodents. Implication of postreceptor mechanisms. Journal Biological Chemistry 1997; 272:25289-95.

[52] Sun XJ, Crimmins DL, Myers MG Jr., Miralpeix M, and White MF. Pleiotropic insulin signals are engaged by multisite phosphorylation of IRS-1. Molecular and Cellular Biology 1993; 13(12):7418-7428.

[53] Liberman Z, and Eldar-Finkelman H. Serine 332 phosphorylation of insulin receptor substrate-1 by glycogen synthase kinase-3 attenuates insulin signaling. Journal of Biological Chemistry 2005; 280(6):4422-4428.

[54] De Fea K, Roth RA. Protein kinase C modulation of insulin receptor substrate-1 tyrosine phosphorylation requires serine 612. Biochemistry. 1997; 36(42):12939-12947.

[55] Goodyear LJ, Giorgino F, Sherman LA, Carey J, Smith RJ, and Dohm GL. Insulin receptor phosphorylation, insulin receptor substrate-1 phosphorylation, and phosphatidylinositol 3-kinase activity are decreased in intact skeletal muscle strips from obese subjects. The Journal of Clinical Investigation 1995; 95:2195-2204.

[56] Tanasijevic MJ, Myers MG Jr, Thoma RS, Crimmins DL, White MF, and Sacks DB. Phosphorylation of the insulin receptor substrate IRS-1 by casein kinase II. Journal of Biological Chemistry 1993; 268(24):18157-18166.

[57] Giraud J, Hass M, Feener EP, Copps KD, Dong X, Dunn SL, and White MF. Phosphorylation of IRS1 at Ser-522 inhibits insulin signaling. Molecular Endocrinology 2007; 21(9):2294-2302.

[58] Luo M, Langlais P, Yi Z, Lefort N, Filippis EAD, Hwang H. Christ-Roberts CY, and Mandarino LJ. Phosphorylation of human insulin receptor substrate-1 at serine 629 plays a positive role in insulin signaling. Endocrinology 2007; 148(10): 4895-4905.

[59] Scioscia M, Gumaa K, Kunjara S, Paine MA, Selvaggi LE, Rodeck CH, and Rademacher TW. Insulin resistance in human preeclamptic placenta is mediated by serine phosphorylation of insulin receptor substrate-1 and -2. Journal of Clinical Endocrinology 2006; 91(2):709-717.

[60] Nawaratne R, Gray A, Jogensen CH, Downes CP, Siddle K, and Sethi JK. Regulation of insulin receptor substrate 1 pleckstrin homology domain by protein kinase C: role of serine 24 phosphorylation. Molecular Endocrinology 2006; 20(8):1838-1852.

[61] Danielsson A, Ost A, Nystrom FH, and Strafors P. Attenuation of insulin-stimulated insulin receptor substrate-1 serine 307 phosphorylation in insulin resistance of type 2 diabetes. Journal of Biological Chemistry 2005; 280(41):34389-34392.

[62] Li Y, Soos TJ, Li X, Wu J, DeGennaro M, Sun X, Littman DR, Birnbaum MJ, and Polajiewicz RD. Protein kinase C theta inhibits insulin signaling by phosphorylation IRS1 at Ser1101. Journal of Biological Chemistry 2004; 279(44):45304-45307.

[63] Gao Z, Zuberi A, Quon MJ, Dong Z, and Ye J. Aspirin inhibits serine phosphorylation of insulin receptor substrate 1 in tumor necrosis factor-treated cell through targeting multiple serine kinases. Journal of Biological Chemistry 2003; 278(27): 24944-24950.

[64] Hers I, Bell CJ, Poole AW, Jiang D, Denton RM, Schaefer E, and Tavare JM. Reciprocal feedback regulation of insulin receptor and insulin receptor substrate tyrosine phosphorylation by phosphoinositide 3-kinase in primary adipocytes. Biochemistry Journal 2002; 368(pt 3):875-884.

[65] Yu C, Chen Y, Cline GW, Zhang D, Zong H, Wang Y, Bergeron R, Kim JK, Cushman SW, Cooney GJ, Atcheson B, White MF, Kraegen EW, and Shulman G I. Mechanism by white fatty acids inhibit insulin activation of insulin receptor substrate-1 (IRS-1)-associated phosphatidylinositol 3-kinase activity in muscle. Journal of Biological Chemistry 2002; 277(52):50230-50236.

[66] Amoui M, Craddock BP, and Miller WT. Differential phosphorylation of IRS-1 by insulin and insulin-like growth factor 1 receptors in Chinese hamster ovary cells. Journal of Endocrinology 2001; 171:153-162.

[67] Gual P, Gremeaux T, Gonzalez T, Marchand-Brustel YL, and Tanti J.-F. MAP kinase and mTOR mediate insulin-induced phosphorylation of insulin receptor substrate-1 on serine residues 307, 612 and 632. Diabetologia 2003; 46:1532-1542.

[68] Werner ED, Lee J, Hansen L, Yuan M, and Shoelson SE. Insulin resistance due to phosphorylation of insulin receptor substrate-1 at serine 302. Journal of Biological Chemistry 2004; 279(34):35298-35305.

[69] Sommerfeld MR, Metzger S, Stosik M, Tennagels N, and Eckel J. In vitro phosphorylation of insulin receptor substrate 1 by protein kinase C- zeta: Function analysis and identification of novel phosphorylation sites. Biochemistry 2004; 43:5888-5901.

[70] Lehr S, Kotzka J, Herkner A, Sikmann A, Meyer HE, Krone W, and Muller-Wieland D. Identification of major tyrosine phosphorylation sites in the human insulin receptor substrate Gab-1 by insulin kinase receptor kinase in vitro. Biochemistry 2000; 39:10898-10907.

[71] Luo M, Reyna S, Wang L, Yi Z, Carroll C, Dong LQ, Langlais P, Weintraub ST, and Mandarino LJ. Identification of insulin receptor substrate 1 serine/threonine phosphorylation sites using mass spectrometry analysis: Regulatory role of serine 1223. Endocrinology 2005; 146(10):4410-4416.

[72] Yi Z, Luo M, Carroll CA, Weintraub ST, and Mandarino LJ. Identification of phosphorylation sites in insulin receptor substrate-1 by hypothesis-driven high-performance liquid chromatography-electrospray ionization tandem mass spectrometry. Analytical Chemistry 2005; 77:5693-5699.

[73] Yi Z, Luo M, Mandarino LJ, Reyna SM, Carroll CA, and Weintraub ST. Quantification of phosphorylation of insulin receptor substrate-1 by HPLC-ESI-MS/MS. Journal of the American Society for Mass Spectrometry 2006; 17:562-567.

[74] Beck A, Moeschel K, Deeg M, Haring H-U, Voelter W, Schleicher ED, and Lehmann R. Identification of an in vitro insulin receptor substrate-1 phosphorylation site by negative-ion • LC/ES-API-CID-MS hybrid scan technique. Journal of the American Society for Mass Spectrometry 2003; 14 (4):401-405.

[75] Gual P, Marchand-Brustel YL, and Tanti J-F. Positive and negative regulation of insulin signaling through IRS-1 phosphorylation. Biochimie. 2005; 87(1):99-109.

[76] Zick Y. Ser/Thr phosphorylation of IRS proteins: A molecular basis for insulin resistance. 2005; Science STKE 2005(268):pe4.

[77] Liu Y-F, Herschkovitz A, Boura-Halfon S, Ronen D, Paz K, LeRoith D, and Zick Y. Serine phosphorylation proximal to its phosphotyrosine binding domain inhibits insulin receptor substrate 1 function and promotes insulin resistance. Molecular and Cellular Biology 2004; 24(21):9668-9681.

[78] Zick Y. Insulin resistance: a phosphorylation-based uncoupling of insulin signaling. Trends in Cell Biology 2001; 11(11):437-441.

[79] Bouzakri K, Karlsson HKR, Vestergaard H, Madsbad S, Christiansen E, and Zierath JR. IRS-1 serine phosphorylation and insulin resistance in skeletal muscle from pancreas transplant recipients. Diabetes 2006; 55:785-791.

[80] Sugita H, Fujimoto M, Yasukawa T, Shimizu N, Sugita M, Yasuhara S, Martyn, JM, and Kaneki M. Inducible nitric-oxide synthase and NO donor induce insulin receptor

substrate-1 degradation in skeletal muscle cells. Journal of Biological Chemistry 2005; 280(14):14203-14211.

[81] Usui I, Imamura T, Huang J, Satoh H, Shenoy SK, Lefkowitz RJ, Hupfeld CJ, and Olefsky JM. -Arrestin-1 competitively inhibits insulin-induced ubiquitination and degradation of insulin receptor substrate 1. Molecular and Cellular Biology 2004; 24(20):8929-8937.

[82] Pederson T, Kramer DL, and Rondinone CM. Serine/Threonine phosphorylation of IRS1 triggers its degradation, possible regulation by tyrosine phosphorylation. Diabetes 2001; 50:24-31.

[83] Potashnik R, Bloch-Damti A, Bashan N, and Rudich A. IRS1 degradation and increased serine phosphorylation cannot predict the degree of metabolic insulin resistance induced by oxidative stress. Diabetologia 2003; 46:639-648.

[84] Lee AV, Gooch JL, Oesterreich S, Guler RL, and Yee D. Insulin-like growth factor I-induced degradation of insulin receptor substrate1 is mediated by the 26S proteasome and blocked by phosphatidylinositol 3′-kinase inhibition. Molecular and Cellular Biology 2000; 20(5):1489-1496.

[85] Sun XJ, Goldberg JL, Qiao L-Y, and Mitchell JJ. Insulin-induced insulin receptor substrate-1 degradation is mediated by the proteasome degradation pathway. Diabetes 1999; 48:1359-1364.

[86] Zhande R, Michell JJ, Wu J, and Sun XJ. Molecular mechanism of insulin-induced degradation of insulin receptor substrate 1. Molecular and Cellular Biology 2002; 22(4):1016-1026.

[87] White MF. IRS proteins and the common path to diabetes. American Journal of Physiology, Endocrinology and Metabolism 2002; 283:E413-E422.

[88] Thirone ACP, Huang C, and Klip A. Tissue-specific roles of IRS proteins in insulin signaling and glucose transport. Trends in Endocrinology and Metabolism 2006; 17(2):72-78.

[89] Youngren JF. Regulation of insulin receptor function. Cellular and Molecular Life Sciences 2007; 64(7-8):873-91.

[90] Lu XM, Lu M, Tompkins RG, and Fischman AJ. Site-specific detection of S-nitrosylated PKB/Akt1 from rat solues muscle using CapLC-Q-TOF^{micro} mass spectrometry. Journal of Mass Spectrometry 2005; 40 (9):1140-1148.

[91] Lu XM, Lu M, Fischman AJ, and Tompkins RG. A new approach for sequencing human IRS1 phosphotyrsine-containing peptides using CapLC-Q-TOFmicro. Journal of Mass Spectrometry 2005; 40 (5):599-607.

[92] Dong X, Park S, Lin X, Copps K, Yi X, White MF. Irs1 and Irs1 signaling is essential for hepatic glucose homeostasis and systemic growth. The Journal of Clinical Investigation 2006; 116 (1):101-114.

[93] Danielsson A, Nystrom FH, Stralfors P. Phosphorylation of IRS1 at serine 307 and serine 312 in response to insulin in human adipocytes. Biochemical and Biophysical Research Communications 2006; 342(4):1183-1187.

[94] Lowell BB, Shulman GI. Mitochondrial dysfunction and type 2 diabetes, Science 2005; 307:384-387.

[95] Manning G, Whyte DB, Martinez R, Hunter T, Sudarsanam S. The protein kinase complement of the human genome. Science 2002; 298:1912-1934.

[96] Sykiotis GP, Papavassiliou AG, Serine phosphorylation of insulin receptor substrate-1: A novel target for the reversal of insulin resistance. Molecular Endocrinology 2001; 15 (11):1864-1869.

[97] Le Marchand-Brustel Y, Gual P, Gremeaux T, Gonzalez T, Barres R, Tanti J-F. Fatty acid-induced insulin resistance: role of insulin receptor substrate 1 serine phosphorylation in the retroregulation of insulin signaling. Biochemical Society Transactions 2003; 31(pt 6):1152-1156.

[98] Sciocia M, Gumaa K, Kunjara S, Paine MA, Selvaggi LE, Rodeck CH, Rademacher TW. Insulin resistance in human preeclamptic placenta is mediated by serine phosphorylation of insulin receptor substrate-1 and -2. The Journal of Clinical Endocrinology and Metabolism 2006; 91(2):709-717.

[99] Yang J, Cron P, Thompson V, Good VM, Hess D, Hemmings BA, Barford D. Molecular mechanism for the regulation of protein kinase B/Akt by hydrophobic motif phosphorylation. Molecular Cell 2002; 9:1227-1240.

[100] Yang J, Cron P, Good VM, Thompson V, Hemmings BA, Barford D. Crystal structure of an activated Akt/protein kinase B ternary complex with GSK3-peptide and AMP-PNP. Nature Structural Biology 2002; 9(12):940-944.

[101] Huang X, Begley M, Morgenstern KA, Gu Y, Rose P, Zhao H, Zhu X. Crystal structure of an inactive Akt2 kinase domain. Structure 2003; 11:21-30.

[102] Kumar CC, Madison V. Akt crystal structure and Akt-specific inhibitors. Oncogene 2005; 24:7493-7501.

[103] Fayard E, Tintignac LA, Baudry A , Hemmings BA. Protein kinase B/Akt at a glance. Journal of Cell Science 2005; 118(pt 24):5675-5678.

[104] Brazil DP, Yang ZZ, Hemmings BA. Advances in protein kinase B signaling: AKTion on multiple fronts. Trends in Biochemical Sciences 2004; 29(5):233-242.

[105] Brazil DP, Park J, Hemmings BA. PKB binding proteins: getting in on the Akt. Cell 2002; 111:293-303.

[106] Huang BX, Kim HY. Interdomain conformational changes in Akt activation revealed by chemical cross-linking and tandem mass spectrometry. Molecular& Cellular Proteomics 2006; 5:1045-1053.

[107] Sugita H, Kaneki M, Sugita M, Yasukawa T, Yasuhara S, Martyn JA. Burn injury impairs insulin-stimulated Akt/PKB activation in skeletal muscle. American Journal of Physiology, Endocrinology and Metabolism 2005; 288:E585-E591.

[108] Carvalho-Filho MA, Ueno M, Hirabara SM, Seabra AB, Carvalheira JB, de Oliveira MG, Velloso LA, Curi R, Saad MJ. S-nitrosation of the insulin receptor, insulin receptor substrate 1, and protein kinase B/Akt: A novel mechanism of insulin resistance. Diabetes 2005; 54(4):959-967.

[109] Yasukawa T, Tokunaga E, Ota H, Sugita H, Martyn JA, Kaneki M. S-Nitrosylation-dependent inactivation of Akt/protein kinase B in insulin resistance. Journal of Biological Chemistry 2005; 280(9):7511-7518.

[110] Carter EA, Derojas-Walker T, Tamir S, Tannenbaum SR, Yu YM, Tompkins RG. Nitric oxide production is intensely and persistently increased in tissue by thermal injury. Biochemistry Journal 1994; 304(pt 1):201-204.

[111] Auguin D, Barthe P, Auge-Senegas MT, Stern MH, Noguchi M, Roumestand C. Solution structure and backbone dynamics of the Pleckstrin homology domain of the human protein kinase B (PKB/Akt). Interaction with inositol phosphates. Journal of Bimolecular NMR 2004; 28(2):137-155.

[112] Murata H, Ihara Y, Nakamura H, Yodoi J, Sumikawa K, Kondo T. Glotaredoxin exerts an antiapoptotic effect by regulating the redox state of Akt. Journal of Biological Chemistry 2003; 278(50):50226-50233.

[113] Jaffrey SR, Erdjument-Bromage H, Ferris CD, Tempst P, Snyder SH. Protein S-nitrosylation: a physiological signal for neuronal nitric oxide. Nature Cell Biology 2001; 3:193-197.

[114] Jaffrey SR, Snyder SH. The biotin switch method for detection of S-nitrosylated proteins. Science's STKE 2001; 2001(86): pl1,1-9.

[115] Greco TM, Hodara R, Parastatidis I, Heijnen HFG, Dennehy MK, Liebler DC, Ischiropoulos H. Identification of S-nitrosylation motifs by site-specific mapping of the S-nitrosocysteine proteome in human vascular smooth muscle cells. Proceedings of the National Academy of Sciences of the Unites States of America 2006; 103(19): 7420-7425.

[116] Hao G, Derakhshan B, Shi L, Campagne F, Gross SS. SNOSID, a proteomic method for identification of cysteine S-nitrosylation sites in complex protein mixtures. Proceedings of the National Academy of Sciences of the United States of America 2006; 103 (4):1012-1017.

[117] Kuncewicz T, Sheta EA, Goldknopf IL, Kone BC. Proteomic analysis of S-nitrosylated proteins in mesangial cell. Molecular & Cellular Proteomics 2003; 2:156-163.

[118] Martinez-Ruiz A, Lamas S. Detection and proteomic identification of S-nitrosylated proteins in endothelial cells. Archives of Biochemistry and Biophysics 2004; 423:192-199.

[119] Lu XM, Tompkins RG, Fishman AJ. SILAM for quantitative proteomics of liver Akt1/PKB ▪ after burn injury. International Journal of Molecular Medicine 2012; 29:461-471.

[120] Beynon RJ, Pratt JM. Metabolic labeling of proteins for proteomics. Molecular & Cellular Proteomics 2005; 4:857-872.

[121] Harsha HC, Molina H, Pandey A. Quantitative proteomics using stable isotope labeling with amino acids in cell culture. Nature Protocols 2008; 3(3):505-516.

[122] Beynon RJ. The dynamics of the proteome: strategies for measuring protein turnover on a proteome-wide scale. Brief Functional Genomics Proteomics 2005; 3(4):382-390.

[123] Moresco JJ, Dong MQ, Yates JR. Quantitative mass spectrometry as a tool for nutritional proteomics. The American Journal of Clinical Nutrition 2008; 88:597-604.

[124] Nair KS, Jaleel A, Asmann YW, Short KR, Raghavakaimal S. Proteomic research: potential opportunities for clinical and physiological investigators. American Journal of Physiology, Endocrinology and Metabolism 2004; 286:E863-E874.

[125] Krijgsveld J, Ketting RF, Mahmoudi T, Johansen J, Artal-Sanz M, Verrijzer CP, Plasterk RH, Heck AJ. Metabolic labeling of C. elegans and D. melanogaster for quantitative proteomics. Nature Biotechnology 2003; 21(8):927-931.

[126] Doherty MK, Whitehead C, McCormack H, Gaskell SJ, Beynon RJ. Proteome dynamics in complex organisms: using stable isotopes to monitor individual protein turnover rates. Proteomics 2005; 5:522-533.

[127] Hayter JR, Doherty MK, Whitehead C, McCormack H, Gaskell SJ, Beynon RJ. The subunit structure and dynamics of the 20S proteasome in chicken skeletal muscle. Molecular & Cellular Proteomics 2005; 4:1370-1381.

[128] Wu CC, Maccoss MJ, Howell KE, Matthews DE, Yates JR. Metabolic labeling of mammalian organisms with stable isotopes for quantitative proteomic analysis. Analytical Chemistry 2004; 76:4951-4959.

[129] Kruger M, Moser M, Ussar S, Thievessen I, Luber CA, Former F, Schmidt S, Zanivan S, Fassler R, Mann M. SILAC mouse for quantitative proteomics uncovers kindling-3 as an essential factor for red blood cell function. Cell 2008; 134:353-364.

[130] Gouw JW, Tops BB, Mortensen P, Heck AJ, Krijgsveld J. Optimizing identification and quantitation of ^{15}N-labeled proteins in comparative proteomics. Analytical Chemistry 2008; 80:7796-7803.

[131] Huttlin EL, Hegeman AD, Harms AC, Sussman MR. Comparison of full versus partial metabolic labeling for quantitative proteomics analysis in arabidopsis thaliana. Molecular & Cellular Proteomics 2007; 6:860-881.

[132] Mcclatchy DB, Dong MQ, Wu CC, Venable JD, Yates JR 3rd. ^{15}N Metabolic labeling of mammalian tissue with slow protein turnover. Journal of Proteome Research 2007; 6(5):2005-2010.

[133] Liao L, McClatchy DB, Park SK, Xu T, Lu B, Yates JR. Quantitative analysis of brain nuclear phosphoproteins identifies developmentally regulated phosphorylation events. Journal of Proteome Research 2008; 7:4743-4755.

[134] Bachi A, Bonaldi T. Quantitative proteomics as a new piece of the systems biology puzzle. Journal of Proteomics 2008; 71:357-367.

[135] Gan HT, Chen JDZ. Roles of nitric oxide and prostaglandins in pathogenesis of delayed colonic transit after burn injury in rats. American Journal of Physiology-Regulatory Integrative and Comparative Physiology 2005; 288:R1316-R1324.

[136] Torres SH, De Sanctis JB, de L Briceno M, Hernandez N, Finol HJ. Inflammation and nitric oxide production in skeletal muscle of type 2 diabetic patients. Journal of Endocrinology 2004; 181:419-427.

[137] Walsh CT. Modification of cysteine and methionine by oxidation-reduction. In: Post-translational modification of proteins: expanding nature's inventory. Roberts and company publishers, Colorado, USA; 2006. p95-119.

[138] Benhar M, Forrester MT, Stamler JS. Nitrosative stress in the ER: A new role for S-nitrosylation in neurodegenerative diseases. ACS Chemical Biology 2006; 1(6): 355-358.

[139] Tannenbaum SR, White FM. Regulation and specificity of S-nitrosylation and denitrosylation. ACS Chemical Biology 2006; 1(10):615-618.

[140] Hogg N. The biochemistry and physiology of S-nitrosothiols. Annual Review of Pharmacology and Toxicology 2002; 42(1):585-600.

[141] Arnelle DR, Stamler JS. NO+, NO., and NO- donation by S-nitrosothiols: implications for regulation of physiological functions by S-nitrosylation and acceleration of disulfide formation. Archives of Biochemistry and Biophysics 1995; 318: 279-285.

[142] Wu W-I, Voegtli WC, Sturgis HL, Dizon FP, Viger GPA, Brandhuber BJ. Crystal structure of human AKT1 with an allosteric inhibitor reveals a new mode of kinase inhibition 2010; PLos ONE 5(9): e12913.

[143] Carvalho-Filho MA, Ueno M, Carvalheira JB, Velloso LA, M.J. Saad. Targeted disruption of iNOS prevents LPS-induced S-nitrosation of IR/IRS-1 and Akt and insulin resistance in muscle of mice. American Journal of Physiology, Endocrinology and Metabolism 2006; 291:E476-E482.

[144] Vogt JA, Hunzinger C, Schroer K, Holzer K, Bauer A, Schrattenholz A, Cahill MA, Schillo S, Schwall G, Stegmann W, Albuszies G. Determination of fractional synthesis rates of mouse hepatic proteins via metabolic ^{13}C-labeling, MALDI-TOF MS and analysis of relative isotopologue abundances using average masses. Analytical Chemistry 2005; 77:2034-2042.

[145] Zhao Y, Lee WN, Lim S, Go VL, Xiao J, Cao R, Zhang H, Recker RR, Xiao GG. Quantitative proteomics: measuring protein synthesis using ^{15}N amino acid labeling in pancreatic cancer cells. Analytical Chemistry 2009; 81:764-771.

[146] Cho H, Thorvaldsen JL, Chu Q, Feng F, Brinbaum MJ. Akt1/PKBalpha is required for normal growth but dispensable for maintenance of glucose homeostasis in mice. Journal of Biological Chemistry 2001; 276:38349-38352.

[147] Chi H, Mu J, Kim JK, Thorvaldsen JL, Chu Q, Crenshaw EB, Kaestner KH, Bartolomer MS, Shulman GI, Birnbaum MJ. Insulin resistance and a diabetes mellitus-like syndrome in mice lacking the protein kinase Akt2 (PKB beta). Science 2001; 292:1728-1731.

[148] Wilson EM, Rotwein P. Selective control of skeletal muscle differentiation by Akt1. Journal of Biological Chemistry 2007; 282(8):5106-5110

[149] Rotwein P, Wilson EM. Distinct actions of Akt1 and Akt2 in skeletal muscle differentiation. Journal of Cellular Physiology 2009; 219(2):503-511.

[150] Braun T, Cautel M. Transcriptional mechanisms regulating skeletal muscle differentiation, growth and homeostasis. Nature Review Molecular Cell Biology 2011; 12(6): 349-361.

[151] Jespersen JG, Nedergaard A, Reitelseder S, Mikkelsen UR, Dideriksen KJ, Agergaard A, Kreiner F, Pott FC, Schjerling P, Kjaer M. Activated protein synthesis and suppressed proten breakdown signaling in skeletal muscle of critically ill patients. PLoS ONE 2011; 6(3):e18090.

[152] Xiao W, Mindrinos, Seok J, Cuschieri J, Cuenca AG Gao H, Hayden DL, Hennessy l, Moore EE, Minei JP, Bankey PE, Johnson JL, Sperry J, Nathens AB, Billiar TR, West MA, Brownstein BH, Mason PH, Baker HV, Finnerty CC, Jeschke MG, Lopez MC, Klein MB, Gamelli RL, Gibran NS, Arnoldo B, Xu W, Zhang Y, Calvno SE, McDonald-Smith GP, Schoenfeld DA,Storey JD, Cobb JP, Warren HS, Moldawer LL, Herndon DN, Lowry SF, Maier RV, Davis RW, Tompkins RG. A genomic storm in critically injured humans. Journal of Experimental Medicine 2011; 208(13):2581-90.

[153] Frost RA, Lang CH. Protein kinase B/Akt: a nexus of growth factor and cytokine signaling in determining muscle mass. Journal of Applied Physiology 2007; 103:378-87.

[154] Zhang P, Chen X, Fan M. Signaling mechanisms involved in disuse muscle atrophy. Medical Hypotheses 2007; 69:310-321.

[155] Sartorell V, Fulco M. Molecular and cellular determinants of skeletal muscle atrophy and hypertrophy. 2004; www.stke.org/cgi/content/full/sigtrans: /244/re11.

[156] Nader GA. Molecular determinants of skeletal muscle mass: getting the "AKT" together. The International Journal of Biochemistry & Cell Biology 2005; 37:1985-1996.

[157] Glass DJ. Signaling pathways perturbing muscle mass. Current Opinion in Clinical Nutrition & Metabolic Care 2010; 13:225-229.

[158] Mckinnell IW, Rudnicki MA. Molecular mechanisms of muscle atrophy. Cell 2004; 119:907-910.

[159] Kousteni S. FoxO1, the transcriptional chief of energy metabolism. Bone 2012; 50(2): 437-43.

[160] Attaix D, Bechet D. FoxO3 controls dangerous proteolytic liaisons. Cell Metabolism 2007; 6:425-427.

[161] Clavel S, Siffroi-Fernandez S, Coldefy AS, Boulukos K, Pisani DF, Derijard B. Regulation of the intracellular localization of Foxo3a by stress-activated protein kinase signaling pathways in skeletal muscle cells. Molecular and Cellular Biology 2010; 30(2): 470-480.

[162] Mammucari C, Milan G, Romanello V, Masiero E, Rudolf R, Piccolo PD, Burden SJ, Lisi RD, Sandri C, Zhao J, Goldberg AL, Schiaffino S, Sandri Marco. FoxO3 controls autophagy in skeletal muscle in vivo. Cell Metabolism 2007; 6:458-471.

[163] Senf SM, Dodd SL, Judge AR. FOXO signaling is required for disuse muscle atrophy and is directly regulated by Hsp70. American Journal of Physiology-Cell Physiology 2010; 298(1):C38-C45.

[164] Zheng B, Ohkaw S, Li H, Roberts-Wilson TK, Price SR. FOXO3a mediates signaling crosstalk that coordinates ubiquitin and atrogin-1/MaFbx expression during glucocorticoid-induced skeletal muscle atrophy. FASEB Journal 2010; 24:2660-2669.

[165] Brunet A, Sweeney LB, Sturgill JF, Chua KF, Greer PL, Lin Y, Tran H, Ross SE, Mostoslavsky R, Cohen HY, Hu LS, Cheng H-L, Jedrycowski MP, Gygi SP, Sinlair DA, Alt FW, Greenberg ME. Stress-dependent FOXO transcription factors by Sirt1 deacetylase. Science 2004; 303:2011-2015.

[166] Daitoku H, Sakamaki J-I, Fukamizu A. Regulation of FoxO transcription factors by acetylation and protein-protein interactions. Biochimica et Biophysica Acta. 2011; 1813(11):1954-60.

[167] Barhel A, Schmoll D, Unterman TG. FoxO proteins in insulin action and metabolism. Trends in Endocrinology & Metabolism 2005; 16(4):183-189.

[168] Greer EL, Oskoui P, Banko MR, Maniar JM, Gygi MP, Gygi SP. The energy sensor AMP-activated protein kinase directly regulates the mammalian FOXO transcription factor. Journal of Biological Chemistry 2007; 282(41):30107-30119.

[169] Hay N. Interplay between FOXO, TOR, and Akt. Biochimica et Biophysics Acta 2011; 1813:1965-1970.

[170] Bertaggia E, Coletto L, Sandri M. Posttranslational modifications control FoxO3 activity during denervation. American Journal Physiology-Cell Physiology 2012; 302:C587-C596.

[171] Dobson M, Ramakrishnan G, Ma S, Kaplun L, Balan V, Fridman R, Tzivion G. Bimodal regulation of FoxO3 by Akt and 14-3-3. Biochimica et Biophysica Acta. 2011; 1813:1453-1464.

[172] Aitken A. 14-3-3 proteins: A historic overview. Seminars in Cancer Biology 2006; 16:162-172.

[173] Morrison DK. The 14-3-3 proteins: integrators of diverse signaling cues that impact cell fate and cancer development. Trends in Cell Biology 2008; 19(1):16-23.

[174] Obsilova V, Silhan J, Boura E, Teisinger J, Obsil T. 14-3-3 proteins: A family of versatile molecular regulators. Physiology Research 2008; 57(Suppl 3):S11-S21.

[175] He M, Zhang J, Shao L, Huang Q, Cen J, Chen H, Chen X, Liu D, Luo Z. Upregulation of 14-3-3 isoforms in acute rat myocardial injury induced by burn and lipopolysaccharide. Clinical and Experimental Pharmacology and Physiology 2006; 33:374-380.

[176] Senf SM, Sandesara PB, Reed SA, Judge AR. p300 Acetyltransferase activity differentially regulates the localization and activity of the FOXO homologues in skeletal muscle. American Journal of Physiology-Cell Physiology 2011; 300(6):C1490-C1501.

[177] Wang F, Chan C-H, Chen K, Guan X, Lin H-K, Tong Q. Deacetylation of FOXO3 by Sirt1 or Sir2 leads to Skp2-mediated FOXO3 ubiquitination and degradation. Oncogene 2012; 31(12):1546-1557.

[178] Bell EL, Guarente L. The Sirt3 divining rod points to oxidative stress. Molecular Cell 2011; 42:561-568.

[179] Rahman S, Islam R. Mammalian Sirt1: insights on its biological functions. Cell Communication and Signaling 2011; 9:11.

[180] Guarente L. Sirtuins, aging, and medicine. The New England Journal of Medicine 2011; 364:2235-2244.

[181] Galnan DR, Brunet A. The FoxO code. Oncogene 2008; 27:2276-2288.

[182] udhary C, Mann M. (2010) Decoding signaling networks by mass spectrometry-base proteomics. Nature Reviews Molecular Cell Bioloby 11(6):427-439.

[183] Murton AJ, Constantin D, Greenhaff PL. The involvement of the ubiquitin proteasome system in human skeletal muscle remodeling and atrophy. Biochimica et Biophysica Acta 2008; 1782(12):730-743.

[184] Ciechanover A. Intracellular protein degradation: from a vague idea thru the lysosome and ubiquitin-proteasome system and onto human diseases and drug targeting. Neuro-degenerative Diseases 2012; 10(1-4):7-22.

[185] Qiang L, Banks AS, Accili D. Uncoupling of acetylation from phosphorylation regulates FoxO1 funaction independent of its subcellular localization. Journal of Biological Chemistry 2010; 285(35):27396-27401.

[186] Walsh CT, Garneau-Tsodikova S, Gatto GJ Jr. Protein posttranslational modifications: the chemistry of proteome diversifications. Angewandte Chemie International Edition 2005; 44(45):7342-72.

[187] Kraft R, Herndon DH, Al-Mousawi AM, Williams FN, Finnerty CC, Jeschke MG. Burn size and survival probability in paediatric patients in modern burn care: a prospective observational cohort study. Lancet 2012; 379(9820):1013-1021.